2002

Physiotherapy in Mental Health

Physiotherapy in Mental Health

a practical approach

Edited by

Tina Everett Grad Dip Phys, MCSP, SRP, FETC
Head of Physiotherapy Services
Oxfordshire Mental Healthcare NHS Trust
Warneford Hospital
Oxford, UK

Maureen Dennis BA, MCSP, SRP
Senior Physiotherapist
West London Healthcare Trust
London, UK

and

Eirian Ricketts MBE, FCSP, SRP Health Ed
Director of Clinical Services
Community Health Care Trust
Whitchurch Hospital
Cardiff, UK

With a Foreword by Baroness Masham of Ilton

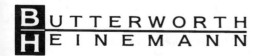

Coventry University

Butterworth-Heinemann Ltd
Linacre House, Jordan Hill, Oxford OX2 8DP

Ɽ A member of the Reed Elsevier plc group

OXFORD   LONDON   BOSTON
MUNICH   NEW DELHI   SINGAPORE   SYDNEY
TOKYO   TORONTO   WELLINGTON

First published 1995

© Butterworth-Heinemann Ltd 1995

British Library Cataloguing in Publication Data
Physiotherapy in Mental Health: A Practical Approach
  I. Everett, Tina
  616.89062
ISBN 0 7506 1700 4

Library of Congress Cataloguing in Publication Data

Physiotherapy in mental health: a practical approach/
  edited by Tina Everett, Maureen Dennis, Eirian Ricketts. – 1st ed.
  p.   cm.
  Includes bibliographical references and index.
  ISBN 0 7506 1700 4
  1. Mental illness – Physical therapy.   2. Mind and body therapies.
  3.   Mental illness – Alternative treatment.   I. Everett, Tina.
  II. Dennis, M. (Maureen)   III. Ricketts, Eirian.
  [DNLM: 1. Mental Disorders – therapy.   2. Physical Therapy.
  WM 100 P579 1995]
  RC482.P49   1995
  616.89'13—dc20
  DNLM/DLC   94-47213
  for Library of Congress   CIP

P05800

Typeset by EJS Chemical Composition, Midsomer Norton, Bath, Avon
Printed and bound by Clays Ltd, St. Ives plc

Contents

Contributors

Geoffrey Barrey CPN
Nurse Behaviour Therapist, Hafod Deg, Day Centre, High Street, Rhynney, Mid Glamorgan, UK

Diana Beaven MCSP, SRP
Physiotherapy Department, Barrow Hospital, Barrow Gurney, Bristol, UK

Peter Blythe NDT(INPP)
Director, Institute for Neuro-Physiological Psychology, Warwick House, 4 Stanley Place, Chester, UK

Kirstie Davison MCSP, SRP
Superintendent Physiotherapist, Severn NHS Trust, Wotton Lawn, Horton Road, Gloucester, UK

Maureen Dennis BA, MCSP, SRP
Senior Physiotherapist, West London Healthcare Trust, Southall, Middlesex, UK

Marie Donaghy BA(Hons), MCSP
Senior Lecturer, Department of Physiotherapy, Queen Margaret College, Leith Campus, Duke Street, Edinburgh, UK

Lynne Dunham MCSP, SRP
Head Physiotherapist, West Park Hospital, Epsom, Surrey, UK

Tina Everett Grad Dip Phys, MCSP, SRP, FETC
Head of Physiotherapy Services, Oxfordshire Mental Healthcare NHS Trust, Warneford Hospital, Oxford, UK

Jan Fletcher MCSP, SRP
Physiotherapy Department, Thanet General Hospital, St Peters Road, Margate, Kent, UK

Terri Fresko MA
Arts Therapies Department, Springfield Hospital, London, UK

Stephen T. Heptinstall MCSP, SRP
Physiotherapy Department, Whitchurch Hospital, Cardiff, UK

Elizabeth A. Holey MA, MCSP, Cert Ed, Dip Tp
Lecturer in Physiotherapy, University of East Anglia, Norwich, UK

Alexandra Hough BA, MCSP, Dip TP
Freelance Lecturer, 21 Crossfield Road, London, NW3 4NT, UK

Elaine Iljon Foreman BA(Hons), MSc, AFBPsS
Head of Adult Psychology Services, Hillington Hospital, Pield Heath Road, Uxbridge, Middlesex, UK

Christine Jones Grad Dip Phys, MSCP, SRP
Principal, The Midlands School of Reflextherapy, 5 Church Street, Warwick, UK

Lynne Kendall MCSP, SRP, Cert Couns, MBAC
Head of Physiotherapy Services, Cornwall Healthcare Trust, Physiotherapy Department, St. Lawrence's Hospital, Bodmin, Cornwall, UK

Derek Milne BSc, MSc, Dip Clin Psych, PhD
Psychology Department, St George's Hospital, Morpeth, Northumberland, UK

Valerie Pomeroy PhD, BA, Grad Dip Phys
Service Development Manager (Medicine), Salisbury Healthcare NHS Trust, Day Hospital, Salisbury District Hospital, Salisbury, Wiltshire, UK

Kathryn Poon Grad Dip Phys, MCSP, SRP
York House, Physiotherapy Department, Manchester Royal Infirmary, Oxford Road, Manchester, UK

Eirian Rickets MBE, FCSP, SRP Health Ed
Director of Clinical Services, Community Health Care Trust, Whitchurch Hospital, Cardiff, UK

Brian Roet MBBS, DA
Clinical Physiotherapist, 2 The Mews, 6 Putney Common, London, UK

Nick Rose FRCPsych
Consultant Psychiatrist, Littlemore Hospital, Oxford; Honorary Senior Lecturer and Regional Postgraduate Course Organizer, University Department of Psychiatry, Oxford, UK

Mick Skelly MCSP, SRP
Community Physiotherapy Team, 22 Clumber Street, Hull, North Humberside, UK

John Smeaton BSc, MCSP
Physiotherapy Department, St George's Hospital, Morpeth, Northumberland, UK

John Tindall MCSP, SRP
Physiotherapist and Practitioner of Chinese Medicine, The Gateway Clinic, South Western Hospital, Brixton, London, UK

Janet Ward MCSP, SRP
Physiotherapist, Mental Health Division, Priority Services NHS Trust, Lancaster, Lancashire, UK

Frank H. Willard PhD
Department of Anatomy, University of New England, College of Osteopathic Medicine, Biddeford, Maine, USA; and European School of Osteopathy, Maidstone, Kent, UK

Anne Wilson MCSP, SRP, Dip Comm Phys
Superintendent Physiotherapist, Mental Health Service, Fazakerly Hospital, Liverpool, UK

Foreword

There is sometimes puzzlement as to what physiotherapists can do for people with mental illness. This shows that the cultural split of mind and body has filtered into the consciousness of the general public, fellow professionals and the psychiatric service.

First, mental distress which has the potential for disorder, is the second most common reason for visiting the general practitioner. It is therefore a vast problem. Second, the closure of mental asylums means that people with mental distress will be found in the general hospital service and as clients in community care more than ever before. There is therefore a need for education in this area for all paramedicals. Third, there must be a greater appreciation that organic problems can exacerbate a mental state, or conversely, that mental imbalance produces vast changes in physical well-being and stability. This last fact is often ignored by the psychiatrically trained professionals, who listen rather than touch, for fear of losing that objectivity so necessary for psychological analysis.

Physiotherapy in psychiatry cannot be anything but holistic and it is perhaps in this area that the valuable skills of the so-called 'Complimentary Therapies' can be explained and introduced. They can be of help to the acutely mentally ill as well as that population of the 'worried-well' who suffer from depression, panic attacks, phobias, eating disorders or substance abuse.

This book attempts not only to define 'abnormal' mental perception from normal, in concise readable form. Some enquiry is made in the physiological basis of anxiety. It then continues to suggest that the boundaries for dealing with these mental problems must be widened. How does one handle communication with the psychiatrically disturbed especially when physical examinations have to take place? What is the role of the physiotherapist in the Community Team? How does one understand the human reaction to a major disaster as in Post-traumatic Stress Disorder? How would one handle teenagers with eating disorders who have poor physical images of themselves? How does one help physical disability in those of extreme age and confusion? What physical therapy can help substance abusers?

'High-tec' medicine has little to offer the inner turmoil of the mentally ill. However, physiotherapy at its best retains some of the essential simplicity and values necessary for healing the whole person. A listening ear and therapeutic touch plus educated insight can do much to help those who strain and drain our health resources. I recommend that this book be read by physiotherapists of all specialities.

Baroness Masham of Ilton

Introduction

In 1971 there were only 10 physiotherapists working in psychiatry in England, Scotland and Wales. Through the 1970s this small group did much pioneering work and by 1980 the Association of Chartered Physiotherapists in Psychiatry was founded. Much is owed to this early developmental work and to the members of the ACPP who have continued to extend the use of basic physiotherapy skills to help the mentally ill and promote mental health.

In 1986 members of the ACPP committee who had been writing a Foundation Course for Chartered Physiotherapists in Psychiatry achieved validation of the course by the Chartered Society of Physiotherapy. This coincided with the timely publication of Mary Hare's book *Physiotherapy in Psychiatry*, which was a source of examples and references to be used as a basis for physiotherapists needing to understand the most common mental disorders and illnesses.

Accredited courses now provide an incentive for physiotherapists to evaluate and research the work they are doing. Some have published their work and Marie Donaghy flew the flag for physiotherapists working with the mentally ill in 1990 with the presentation of her paper at the World Conference of Physical Therapists in London.

This book will be beneficial for all physiotherapists, not just those working in the specialty of mental illness. It demonstrates opportunities to show our part in improving the health of the nation, especially in the implementation of community care. It will also serve as a source of inspiration to managers and members of other professions who want to know how physiotherapy can help improve the physical, mental and social health of their patients.

Christine Dunn   BA MCSP
President of ACPP

Acknowledgements

The editors have valued the encouragement and advice all along the way from committee members of the Clinical Interest group (now renamed Chartered Physiotherapists in Mental Healthcare), some of whom have contributed chapters to this book.

Thanks are also due to all our contributors and their patients and to many friends and colleagues who have given invaluable editorial support. In particular, Marie Donaghy and Rosemary Oddy. We would also like to thank our librarians and clerical colleagues especially Paul Valentine the librarian at St Bernards Hospital, Ealing.

The front cover is designed from a sculpture by Graeme Scott. Graeme took up sculpture in the wake of a serious industrial accident. His friend Phillip Morrison was the photographer for the sculpture.

Part I

Psychiatric illnesses

Nick Rose

Introduction

One person in four will suffer from a psychiatric illness at some point in their lives, and the risk is particularly high for those who have chronic physical disability or illness. As a physiotherapist, therefore, you are very likely to be working with patients who have psychiatric illness, although since psychiatric symptoms often go undetected you may not always recognize this.

In physically ill people it is sometimes difficult to distinguish between normal emotional responses to stress, and psychiatric illness. Yet this is important, since psychiatric illnesses are generally treatable, thus making it much easier to help with the underlying physical problem. Correspondingly, failure to recognize and help a patient's psychiatric problem is likely to slow down their physical recovery, particularly where active participation in therapy is needed.

This chapter will explain what is meant by the term 'psychiatric illness', and describe the main types you are likely to encounter as a physiotherapist. It will then highlight the reasons why particular individuals become ill, and how common this is. Finally the recognition of psychiatric illnesses, the awareness of particular risk factors, the importance of personality and ways in which people can be helped are described.

What are psychiatric illnesses?

Individual psychiatric illnesses consist of particular clusters of symptoms that recur in different people at different times and places. These symptoms typically consist of a combination of abnormal thoughts and bodily sensations, usually called cognitive and somatic symptoms. For example, in the psychiatric illness of depression the cognitive symptoms include thoughts of guilt, worthlessness and hopelessness, whereas the somatic symptoms include loss of energy, sleep and appetite disturbance, and tiredness. Similarly in the illness of anxiety state the cognitive symptoms include fearful thoughts of dying, suffocating, collapsing or making a fool of oneself, while the somatic symptoms may include palpitations, breathlessness and sweating.

To recognize a psychiatric illness one must detect the cluster or pattern of symptoms. Unlike physical medicine there is rarely a laboratory test to confirm the diagnosis. This is because with most psychiatric illnesses we have yet to find any single underlying physical cause such as a virus. Thus, diagnosis of psychiatric illness is usually determined by whether sufficient key symptoms of a recognized cluster are present.

When does a symptom cluster become an illness?

In psychiatry, there is often a continuum between normality and illness. For example, after major loss or trauma it is natural to develop symptoms of sleep and appetite disturbance, features that are also found in depression. How then can one distinguish between the two?

Three things tend to point towards a diagnosis of illness. First, the presence of a full cluster of symptoms. Therefore, in someone coping with a major loss, a diagnosis of depression would need the presence of symptoms of guilt or hopelessness, together with a number of the somatic symptoms summarized in Table 1.1. Secondly, symptoms would normally be persistent, often over a period of weeks if not months. Thirdly, the intensity of symptoms is likely to impair daily living to some degree.

Thus, where an individual is experiencing psychiatric symptoms, the diagnosis of mental illness depends on whether there is a sufficient clustering of individual symptoms, and on the duration and intensity of these symptoms. If a psychiatric illness is thought to be present this is likely to have specific treatment implications.

What different types of symptom clusters are there?

Broadly speaking there are two groups of psychiatric illnesses. The first comprises those with symptoms which represent a gross exaggeration of experiences that many of us are familiar with; examples include depression, anxiety and obsessional illness. These are sometimes called *neuroses*. The second comprises those with symptoms totally different from normal experience; examples include schizophrenia and bipolar affective disorder (manic depression). These are sometimes called *psychoses*.

Less frequently, psychiatric illness can be caused by physical factors such as in drug or alcohol withdrawal, endocrine disorders or steroid use. These are usually called *organic psychiatric disorders*.

In addition to psychiatric illnesses some people suffer from abnormalities of behaviour and personality. If these abnormalities are enough to cause serious persistent disruption in relationships and in employment, then a *personality disorder* may be present. People with personality disorders are often distressed and needy, are more likely to seek medical attention, and may pose particular difficulties during treatment.

In any one individual, a psychiatric illness and personality disorder may coexist, making the treatment for the psychiatric illness less favourable. Likewise, personality disorder and physical illness or disability may coexist and result in difficulties during the rehabilitation phase of the illness.

More commonly, dominant *personality traits* may influence the clinical picture. These traits are of insufficient severity to cause the level of dysfunction associated with personality disorder, but may nevertheless present clinical management difficulties, particularly in the diagnosis and care of physical illness.

Table 1.1 Diagnosis of psychiatric illness

Diagnosis	Main symptoms	Comments
Depression	• *Depressive thinking*: sadness, thoughts of guilt and suicide • *Physical symptoms*: hopelessness worse in mornings, waking early, loss of energy, interest, appetite, weight and concentration • *In less severe forms of depression*: symptoms more variable, physical symptoms less prominent, often associated with irritability, anxiety and/or tension	• A very common disorder especially among the physically ill • Physical symptoms may predominate and be attributed to physical illness • Diagnosis often missed • Antidepressant medication generally effective • Beware suicide risk
Anxiety	• *Anxious thinking*: irrational fears of dying, falling, looking foolish • *Physical symptoms*: palpitations, sweating, breathlessness, 'pins and needles', gastrointestinal symptoms • Can be acute (weeks/months) or chronic (years) • Can be associated with avoidance of situations that trigger anxiety, e.g. crowded places (agoraphobia) or social situations (social phobia) • Often associated with coexistent depression	• Very common disorder • Physical symptoms may predominate and can be attributed initially to cardiac or gastro-intestinal disorder • Acute anxiety usually self-limiting, even without treatment • Anxiety management and relaxation techniques used in preference to minor tranquillizers (e.g. valium) which can cause dependency • Phobic avoidance behaviour may indicate need for specialized psychological treatment
Anorexia nervosa	• Characteristic over-concern about shape and weight • Active maintenance of unduly low weight by excessive dieting, exercise and less commonly self-induced vomiting • Amenorrhoea and physical effects of starvation • Associated depression, anxiety and obsessional symptoms	• Uncommon • Reluctant to seek or engage in help • Mainly affects young women aged 16–35 years • May present to physician with associated medical problems such as fainting or weight loss • Can be life-threatening
Bulimia nervosa	• Characteristic over-concern about shape and weight • Normal body weight (usually) • Frequent bulimic episodes (bingeing) involving consumption of large amounts of food in out-of-control way • Use of extreme behaviour to control shape and weight • Associated depression and anxiety, sometimes with substance abuse	• More common than anorexia • Most cases never come to medical attention • Some people have combined symptoms of anorexia and bulimia • Specialized psychological help usually needed for both anorexia and severe bulimia • Long-term outcome (years) of anorexia and bulimia: less than half remain well
Schizophrenia	*In acute form* • Bizarre false beliefs often of persecution (delusions) • Often hear frightening voices (auditory hallucinations) • Sometimes bizarre disturbed or aggressive behaviour	• Uncommon • Person may not believe they are ill, and so not seek or engage in help • Compulsory treatment sometimes necessary if person poses serious risk to themselves or others

Table 1.1 Continued

Diagnosis	Main symptoms	Comments
Schizophrenia (contd)	• May be triggered in vulnerable individuals by stress, e.g. surgery, accident, childbirth *In chronic form* • False beliefs and voices may persist • Negative features such as poor motivation and social withdrawal • Associated chronic social, occupational and personal dysfunction	• Effective help usually comprises social, psychological and pharmacological interventions • Families and carers often under stress

Hysteria	• *Disturbance of motor sensory or cognitive function in which*:
	  – There appears to be no physical cause
	  – Symptoms usually correspond to patient's level of understanding about illness, with resultant discrepancies between hysterical signs and symptoms and those of organic disease
	  – Patients may gain advantage from symptoms (secondary gain)
	  – Patients may be unconcerned by symptoms (belle indifference)
	• Dysfunction may include limb weakness/paralysis, loss of sensation, loss of memory, etc.
		• Uncommon in severe form
		• May be associated with coexistent depression
		• Beware presence of underlying organic illness which must carefully be excluded before diagnosis of hysteria made
		• Often chronic, presenting to physicians rather than psychiatrists
		• Treatment often slow and only partially effective, involving reduction of secondary gain resulting from illness

Obsessional	• *Obsessional thinking*: compulsively repetitive thoughts, images or impulses which are out of character with the person, and recognized as being nonsensical, e.g. a quiet conscientious mother has obsessional impulses to harm her child • *Obsessional behaviour*: usually associated with obsessional thoughts, e.g. thoughts of contamination may be associated with repeated cleaning. It may also be in the form of repeated senseless behaviour such as pacing in particular ways, gestures, arranging objects, etc.	• Uncommon • May be associated with coexistent depression and anxiety • Treatment may involve intensive psychological therapy sometimes combined with medication • Often of chronic duration (years)
Mania	• Grandiose thinking, over-activity, sleeplessness, irritability, disturbed behaviour • May be triggered by stress as in schizophrenia and severe depression • Usually occurs in individuals who are vulnerable to severe recurrent depression (manic depression)	• Uncommon • Reluctant to seek help because of lack of insight • Compulsory treatment may be necessary • Long-term prophylactic medication such as lithium may be needed to reduce risk of recurrent manic and depressive episodes

Table 1.1 Continued

Diagnosis	Main symptoms	Comments
Acute (organic) confusion	• Consciousness impaired with disorientation in time, place and person • Disturbed often fearful behaviour • May experience voices, persecutory beliefs, visual hallucinations • Usually acute onset	• May be caused by a variety of agents, including alcohol and drug withdrawal, toxaemia, septicaemia, etc. • May occur following surgery, childbirth, dialysis, etc.
Dementia	• Global intellectual impairment • Preservation of clear consciousness • May be progressive, depending on cause • Usually slow, insidious onset associated with uncharacteristic behaviour	• Commonest pathological cause is Alzheimer's disease • Depression with associated slowed thinking may mimic organic dementia • Some dementias are treatable, e.g.. B_{12} deficiency • Dementia may not come to medical attention until relatively late • Families and carers often under great stress

Thus, influential personality characteristics may vary across a spectrum from mild (personality trait) to severe (personality disorder). Some of the more commonly encountered personality characteristics likely to be encountered in physical medicine are described later in this chapter.

What are the characteristics of psychiatric illnesses?

Eight important characteristics of psychiatric illnesses are described below.

Common

Psychiatric illnesses are particularly common among general hospital inpatients and general practice and hospital outpatient clinic attenders. Up to a third of attenders have significant psychiatric symptoms, while up to a fifth have a specific psychiatric illness, most commonly depression or anxiety. This is 10 times what one would expect from a general population sample, and in part reflects the stressful nature of physical illness.

Those at particularly high risk of developing psychiatric disorders include people with chronic physical disability or pain, people who have life-threatening illnesses, and people who have lost a significant part of their bodily functioning, for example after a stroke, an amputation or a mastectomy. (In contrast, women undergoing hysterectomy appear to have a particularly low risk of developing psychiatric disorder after surgery.)

Recurrence

Once a person has suffered from a psychiatric illness the risk of recurrence is greater than if they had never had that illness. For example, the risk of a psychotic illness after childbirth increases from 1 in 500 to 1 in 5 if the mother has had a previous psychotic illness. Likewise, a man who has had a history of depression during his life is at particular risk of developing depression following a major health problem such as a heart attack.

Hidden

The presence of a psychiatric illness is often missed, even by experienced clinicians. At least a half of depressive illnesses are missed in hospital and GP clinics, for example. Alcohol dependence and eating disorders, particularly bulimia, are also likely to be missed.

There are reasons why certain common psychiatric disorders are so readily missed are various: Depressed patients may fail to recognize their illness, may feel unworthy of asking for help, or may attribute symptoms to physical illness; bulimic patients may be too ashamed to seek help; patients abusing alcohol may deny the problem not only to others but to themselves.

Varied presentation

Psychiatric illness can present in different ways. This is partly because individuals may attach differing importance and meaning to certain symptoms.

Psychiatric disorders presenting with physical symptoms
Both anxiety and depression may present with predominantly physical symptoms. In anxiety, for example, some patients will almost exclusively focus on physical symptoms such as palpitations, interpreting these as evidence of a failing heart. Such patients may eventually be referred to cardiac clinics, and it may be hard to reassure them that their problem is psychological. Similarly, patients suffering from depression may focus on physical symptoms such as tiredness, lack of energy or weight loss. Because they do not complain of sadness or hopelessness, physical illness may be assumed to be the cause and a treatable depression missed.

Psychiatric disorders may sometimes present as a failure of the patient to progress as expected through a physical rehabilitation care plan, particularly when the cognitive symptoms of illness are not conspicuous enough to alert carers to the possibility of psychiatric disorder.

Psychiatric disorders presenting with behaviour change
Sometimes it is not the symptoms of psychiatric disorder that present, but their behavioural consequences. For example, a depressed or anxious person may uncharacteristically shoplift or drink heavily; an anxious person may become increasingly housebound for fear of having a panic attack when not at home; a depressed person may underfunction at work or at home; or a manic depressive person during a manic phase of the illness may behave in a highly disinhibited over-active fashion, perhaps spending recklessly and getting into trouble with the law.

Stress related

Most psychiatric illness is triggered by stress. This is particularly true of the more acute illnesses. Stress usually arises from *loss* or *threatened loss, conflict* of some sort, *change*, or *relationship difficulties*. It can therefore be seen that the onset of physical illness, particularly of a chronic or disabling type, may act as a potent source of stress, especially in those vulnerable to psychiatric illness. A stroke or heart attack, for example, represents a loss of good health, and may impose substantial changes in the person's lifestyle, employment and relationships.

Distressing to patient and carers

Most psychiatric illnesses are unpleasant to experience. The degree of distress caused may be considerable, with little relief. Because much of the distress comes from the associated preoccupying thoughts, it is particularly invasive. For example, constant preoccupation with anxious thoughts of impending disaster, with obsessional thoughts of dirt and cleanliness, with distressing thoughts about bodily image (eating disorders) or persecutory thoughts (paranoid disorders) can be intensely preoccupying and exhausting. Such thoughts when combined with other symptoms may lead to ideas of suicide as the only escape route. Indeed the suicide rate in most psychiatric disorders is in excess of 10 times that of the general population.

The distress for families and carers is also great. This is particularly true of the more chronic disabling illnesses such as obsessional and agoraphobic disorders, schizophrenia and bipolar affective disorders. It is also true that stressful and over-critical home circumstances can increase the relapse rate of some of these disorders, thus creating a vicious circle of family stress contributing to illness relapse which further increases stress on the family.

Impair personal functioning

Most psychiatric illnesses have a serious effect on the sufferer's day-to-day functioning, whether at work, socially or in the family. Sometimes the impairment is found in just one area of functioning, for example a patient with bulimia may be able to perform well at work but has considerable difficulty socializing because of their eating habits. More often than not, however, the impairment is global. For example, the patient with depression or an acute anxiety state is likely to find problems in most if not all areas of functioning.

Associated with high risk

Psychiatric illnesses, as noted previously, are associated with a high suicide risk. This is particularly true of depression, but is also true of many other psychiatric conditions such as schizophrenia, eating disorders, alcohol dependence and personality disorder. Patients who self-harm, for whatever reason (usually relationship problems), also have a high risk of eventually killing themselves.

Some psychiatric disorders are associated with other forms of risk. Risk of extreme self-neglect may occur in depression and schizophrenia. Risk of harming others through assault may occur in schizophrenia and in paranoid or manic states, either as a result of the patient believing that others are against him in some way, or as a result of frightened and disorganized behaviour. More rarely, patients with very severe depression may believe that both they and their family would be better off dead and act accordingly. This is sometimes a particular risk in severely depressed mothers who have recently delivered (puerperal depression).

Why do people get psychiatric illnesses?

Although psychiatric illness is common, most people do not succumb. What then predisposes particular individuals to become ill at particular times? There is no simple answer, since usually illness results from a complex dynamic interaction between a person's vulnerability and the sources of stress in their current life situation.

Personal vulnerability

Certain people are particularly likely to develop psychiatric illness during their lives, given the right circumstances. Vulnerability comes from four main sources.

First, many psychiatric disorders appear to be *familial*. For example, the risk of developing schizophrenia or severe depression appears to be increased at least 15-fold if a first-degree relative has the disorder. Thus, while the risk of developing schizophrenia at some time during life is 1%, this increases to about 15% if a parent or sibling has the disorder. This is true even if the relatives were separated from birth, thus ruling out shared experience as the cause of the increased risk.

Secondly, there is evidence that some psychiatric disorders, particularly depression, occur more often in those who have had a *deprived or traumatized upbringing*.

Thirdly, certain enduring forms of *personality and temperament* may predispose in some cases to psychiatric disorder. For example, those with lifelong marked anxiety traits may go on to develop anxiety illnesses, whereas those with lifelong over-meticulous or melancholic temperaments may develop depressive disorder.

Fourthly, there is some evidence that psychiatric disorder, especially depression, is more likely to occur in those who are in *unfavourable social circumstances*: people who are unemployed, socially isolated or looking after young children with little support are all at particularly high risk of depression.

Sources of stress in current life situations

As mentioned previously, stress usually arises from *loss* or *threatened loss*, *conflict*, *change*, or *relationship difficulties*. Sometimes the development of psychiatric illnesses can be understood as resulting from the impact of a major life event such as bereavement, major illness or redundancy on a vulnerable individual. At other times, less conspicuous stresses may accumulate until one of them finally 'breaks the camel's back'. The relationship between personal vulnerability, stress and any resulting psychiatric illness thus depends on a number of interacting factors. For example, the greater a person's vulnerability, the more sensitive they are to stress, even minor sources of stress. The less their vulnerability, the more resilient they are likely to be.

It is probably true to say, however, that everyone has a breaking point, and massive stress may trigger psychiatric illness even in the absence of obvious personal vulnerability factors. It is also true that psychiatric illness may develop in the absence of clear stressors, particularly in very vulnerable individuals.

The relevance of an individual's personality

As already described, certain personality traits may be a risk factor for certain psychiatric illnesses. In a more general way, however, an individual's personality and temperament may be an important factor in influencing how they present and cope with physical illness, irrespective of whether a psychiatric illness is present. Four personality traits are particularly likely to be important in helping those with physical problems. These will be described separately, although in reality many individuals have features from more than one of the groups.

Somatization
The tendency to respond to life's difficulties by developing a range of physical complaints. This may result in repeated presentation of physical symptoms, with persistent requests for medical investigations in spite of repeated negative findings and reassurances that symptoms have no physical basis. If physical illnesses are present, they do not explain the nature and extent of the symptoms or the distress and preoccupation of the patient. Any attempt to discuss the possibility of psychological or social factors causing the symptoms is usually resisted. Such patients may become chronic clinic attenders (see Case Study I in the Appendix to this chapter). The term 'hypochondriacal' is usually used when patients develop a persistent preoccupation with the possibility of having one or more specific serious and progressive physical disorders.

This tendency to express emotional stress through physical complaints may be acutely exaggerated by superimposed depressive or anxiety illnesses. When this is the case, the depression or anxiety should be treated and this may relieve the somatization symptoms.

In its severe form, persistent somatizing behaviour can be regarded as an illness in itself, the two main forms being somatization disorder characterized by multiple bodily symptoms, and hypochondriacal disorder characterized by preoccupation with a specific disease. Specialized psychological treatment for these disorders can be of benefit in some cases.

Anxiety
The tendency for the individual to experience persistent and pervasive feelings of tension and apprehension, often associated with poor confidence, sensitivity to rejection, and restricted lifestyle. Individuals may be especially at risk of developing fears and physical symptoms of anxiety when medically ill. Reassurance, careful provision of relevant information, and relaxation techniques are likely to help.

Over-dependency
The tendency to allow others to take over, often at the expense of their own needs. This includes powerful feelings of helplessness when alone or abandoned because of the patients' exaggerated fears of being unable to care for themselves. Individuals may find everyday decisions difficult without an excessive amount of advice and reassurance from others, and they may also regress to an immature level of functioning when faced with what to them may feel overwhelming difficulty. Often tolerance to loss, particularly of a partner, is poor, and the sick role may be particularly rewarding (see also some aspects of Case Study II in the Appendix).

Antisocial
The tendency to antisocial behaviour, with poor ability to keep friendships, impulsivity, and low tolerance to frustration. Also the tendency to be demanding, blame others and not feel guilty themselves. Individuals may present with fictitious illnesses and other attention-seeking behaviours. Firm boundaries as to what behaviours are acceptable and what are not, together with social and personal support may help.

How to recognize that someone has psychiatric illness?

Given the tendency for psychiatric illness to remain hidden, is it worth trying to detect it and if so how should this be done?

Most psychiatric illnesses are treatable, and since they are associated with suffering, with reduced ability to engage in physical rehabilitation, and in the case of depression with risk of deliberate self-harm, then detection is clearly worth while. How should you go about this? Three things are important:

First, you should develop a *low threshold of suspicion*. This is particularly important if you see people who are at a special risk of psychiatric illness, for example young mothers, those with chronic physical illness or those coping with very stressful circumstances. It is important always to consider the possibility of a psychiatric disorder even when the individual may not be complaining of psychiatric symptoms specifically. In some circumstances it may be worth while using a screening questionnaire in order to detect the most commonly ocurring illnesses. The self-report Beck depression inventory, which takes about 5 minutes to complete, can be used in this way. Patients who score highly could then be assessed in more detail for possible depressive illness. Similarly, the Spielberger anxiety questionnaire can be used to screen for anxiety. It may be particularly useful to do this before and after surgery, since high anxiety levels are associated with increased postoperative complications such as chest infection.

Secondly, you need to have a *working knowledge of the rånge of symptoms and features that occur in the more common psychiatric disorders*. You are then more likely to recognize the symptom patterns involved, understand their significance, and mobilize relevant help or advice. A brief description of the psychiatric illnesses you are likely to encounter is given in Table 1.1, together with a commentary on key points to note.

Thirdly, you need to develop the necessary *listening and interview skills* which enable your patients to disclose their feelings and problems. For example GPs

Table 1.2 Example of structured interview

Recent events and symptoms

A 57-year-old man, physically well, working and living alone until having a mild stroke 2 months ago

Slow progress in physical rehabilitation, when he was noted to be increasingly irritable and socially withdrawn. He denied problems, and subsequently took a massive overdose one weekend from which he only just survived

Closer enquiry revealed increasingly low mood over a period of 6 weeks, mood was particularly low in the early part of the day. There was also early-morning waking, together with general loss of energy and interest

Relevant past history, focusing on vulnerability factors

Lifelong dependency on capable spouse who died a year ago. Has few close friends to turn to for support. Previous depression treated by GP after patient's mother died 8 years ago

Father died of a stroke in his early 60s, and patient fears same outcome for himself

Current behaviour and state of mind

Able to 'put on a brave face' but cannot sustain this, with his underlying sad expression emerging. Poor self-care, 'letting himself go'

On persistent enquiry, reveals he is preoccupied with joining his dead wife, believing he has lost his health, his job and his only friend, and now has nothing to live for. Also feels guilty and worthless, believing he is beyond hope. Regrets surviving the overdose. Unable to see that he is ill and in need of help

Opinion

A man with a number of vulnerability factors who succumbed to a severe depression following a stroke. The depression remained hidden because of his reluctance to disclose his true feelings, and the way his symptoms were attributed to the physical consequences of his stroke. This resulted in him taking a near fatal overdose

Lessons to be learnt

- Awareness that depression is common in the physically ill, but may remain hidden; thus vigilance is important
- Early detection and intervention with depression may reduce risk of serious self-harm
- People who have increased vulnerability to developing mental illness should be particularly carefully observed

who give their patients little opportunity to talk about difficulties in their own way are particularly likely to miss treatable underlying psychiatric disorders such as depression.

Listening skills involve the capacity to show interest and sympathy towards the other person, encouraging them to talk in confidence about things that are bothering them, and providing sufficient quiet and confidential 'space' for this to be possible.

Interview skills refer more to the capacity to elicit particular areas of relevant information through a process of careful probing and questioning. Important information to establish would include the nature of any stress or personal vulnerability factors, and the presence of specific psychiatric symptoms. In this way, the likelihood of psychiatric illness and the possible causal factors, together with any associated risk factors such as suicidal thoughts, can be ascertained. An example of a structured interview covering a patient's recent circumstances, past history, and current behaviour and state of mind is given in Table 1.2. A more detailed version of this framework would be used by a psychiatrist when doing a formal psychiatric assessment.

What help is available for those with psychiatric illness?

The treatment of psychiatric illness usually involves a combination of psychological, physical and social approaches:

Psychological help

Psychological help is most often in the form of support, together with problem-focused counselling which aims to understand and tackle any difficulties which may have triggered the illness in the first place. Explanation about the nature and effects of the psychiatric symptoms may also be important, particularly where physical symptoms of anxiety and depression are prominent. The teaching of relaxation techniques in anxiety and distraction techniques where preoccupying thoughts and worries are present may also be useful. These forms of help can be given by a variety of health professionals.

More specialized psychological treatment may be needed in certain conditions. For example, cognitive behavioural psychotherapy for those with eating disorders; exposure therapy for those with phobic avoidance disorders such as agoraphobia; and psychodynamic counselling for those with certain types of persistent difficulties in relationships.

Psychological help is usually given on a one-to-one basis, but can also be given to groups (e.g. learning anxiety management or exploring relationship difficulties), and to families or couples. A family or couple approach is especially valuable if domestic problems have contributed to the illness.

Physical help

Physical help is usually in the form of medication, although in very serious intractable or life-threatening depression electroconvulsive therapy (ECT) may be given under a brief general anaesthetic. Medication for the treatment of psychiatric illnesses can be divided into antidepressants, including mood stabilizers; antipsychotics; and minor tranquillizers.

Antidepressants

These will help about 70% of those who have a depressive illness. However, they do take 1–3 weeks to be effective, some have unpleasant side effects, and care must be taken when prescribing for people who have physical illnesses, especially those of the heart, liver and kidneys. Although tricyclic antidepressants such as amitriptyline are effective and have been available for over 30 years, the newer serotonin specific reuptake inhibitors (SSRI) antidepressants such as paroxetine and fluoxetine are gaining popularity because they are safer in overdose, have fewer side effects, and can be used with fewer problems in many physical illnesses, particularly cardiac ones.

Where a person appears resistant to a trial of antidepressants, alternative medication strategies are available which are usually, although not always, successful. Antidepressant-resistant depression is a common reason for referral to a psychiatrist.

Antidepressants have two purposes. First to shift depression and secondly to prevent depression returning. It is for the latter reason that antidepressants are continued for at least 6 months after the illness has resolved, since to discontinue them sooner increases the risk of relapse. Some people, however, need to continue taking prophylactic antidepressant medication for many years. In addition to antidepressants, mood stabilizers such as lithium and carbamazepine can be used for the treatment and long-term prophylaxis of manic depressive disorder.

Antipsychotics

These are used to treat the acute symptoms and associated behavioural disturbance of psychotic illnesses, particularly schizophrenia amd mania. They may also be used in severe agitated depression. The older antipsychotics such as chlorpromazine and haloperidol cause sedation and may also cause unpleasant muscular side effects. Where sedation of disturbed or agitated behaviour is not needed, newer antipsychotics such as respiridone and sulperide may be used since they produce fewer side effects. Whatever medication is used, the antipsychotic action will take at least 1–4 weeks before being effective in resolving the underlying symptoms of illness such as delusional ideas or the hearing of voices.

Like antidepressants, antipsychotics have two purposes: initial treatment of the acute illness and prevention of relapse. During the prevention phase, antipsychotics can be given in intramuscular depot form, usually on a fortnightly basis.

Minor tranquillizers

These are used less and less because of the ease with which people can become physically dependent on them. They are sometimes valuable, however, for brief interventions of up to 3 weeks in severe acute anxiety, after severe trauma or loss, and in combination with antipsychotics in the management of acute psychotic illness.

One of the most common reasons for the failure of any medication treatment is that some patients do not take their tablets. Compliance is better if the purpose of medication is continually reinforced, and side effects can be kept to a minimum either by careful dosage control or, where appropriate, choosing medication with the fewest side effects.

Electroconvulsive treatment is used in life-threatening depression (either because of very serious suicide risk or failure to take fluids and food), and may also be used when medication treatments have failed. A brief electric shock is given while the patient is lightly anaesthetized. The underlying antidepressant mechanism is almost certainly the same as for antidepressant medication, but the effectiveness may be slightly greater, particularly in the most severe depression, and the speed of action faster. Side effects include a short-lived headache and temporary memory problems for a week or so. There is no evidence of any lasting side effects or damage, and the temporary side effects that do occur are usually more acceptable to patients than those of high doses of medication.

Social help

Just as social stress factors can predispose to or trigger psychiatric illness, help with social difficulties may aid recovery and reduce the risk of relapse. Help with housing, physical problems, finance, social supports, links with self-help groups, and the building up of structured day activities may all have a part to play. Support to families and carers is also very important and may greatly reduce the risk of the patients' illness relapsing.

How to deliver help to those with psychiatric illness

Often help may be provided by a number of different people. A GP or psychiatrist may prescribe and give support; a counsellor, health visitor, physiotherapist, psychologist or nurse may give psychological help; and a friend, family member, social worker, pastor or employer may help with social interventions of one sort or another.

Two things are particularly important. First, it is important for all those professionally involved to establish a *trusting therapeutic relationship* with the patient. Without this, your helping potential will be greatly undermined. Indeed a poor relationship may actually make things worse, particularly if it is rejecting in anyway.

Secondly, especially if a number of people are involved in helping, it is important to have a *clear care plan* so that they do not conflict with one another. The care plan should be agreed jointly between the patient, carers or relatives where appropriate and the relevant professionals. A *keyworker* is usually responsible for ensuring that the care plan is carried out and that it is reviewed from time to time.

Appendix

Case Study I

The chronic somatizer	Commentary
A 55-year-old with a 10-year history of severe low back pain. Retired on medical grounds 5 years ago from a stressful job. Increasing dependency on family, use of walking aids, hospital transport, analgesia, etc. No objective evidence of deterioration on physical examination and investigations. Regular physiotherapy meets with no progress	• No objective evidence of severe physical dysfunction • Secondary gain of sick role includes retirement on medical grounds, attention of family, no responsibilities • Gain of continued sick role sabotages motivation to improve through progress with physiotherapy and other medical interventions • Recovery must be based on advantages of health outweighing those of sickness

Case Study II

Overdependent self-harmer	*Commentary*

A 25-year-old woman who jumped 10 ft (3 m) and sustained bilateral fractured ankles in an intentional self-harm attempt. Long history of failed relationships, impulsivity, overdoses, and poor ability to live independently or take full responsibility for herself. Resistant to physiotherapy and attempts to help her mobilize, yet frequently demanding of attention and constantly managing to get nurses to do things for her that she in fact could do for herself. Very slow physical progress towards eventual discharge from hospital to returning to live alone in her isolated bedsit	• Self-harm not clearly suicidal, and may have been in part at least a cry for help in order to ensure subsequent medical care and attention
	• Isolated impulsive individual who relates to others in a childlike fashion, and has high dependency needs
	• Gain of sick role includes constant professional attention, and the shifting of her responsibilities onto others. Thus poor motivation to become well, and poor capacity to become truly independent
	• Management must:
	  – Emphasize advantages of progress to full mobility (e..g. by helping with more supported accommodation, befriending schemes, day activities, etc.)
	  – Not collude with dependency by never doing for her the things that she can reasonably do for herself, thus increasing her sense of control and self-esteem
	  – Consider contract approach (e.g. appropriate behaviour could be reinforced by regular talking sessions with a member of staff)

Further reading

Rose, N. (ed.) (1994) *Essential Psychiatry*, Blackwell Scientific, Oxford (an introductory text with a wide-ranging coverage including psychiatry in general medical settings, eating disorders, terminal illness, bereavement, reactions to trauma, psychiatric ethics, psychological treatments, etc.)

2

Models of mental disorder

Marie Donaghy

Introduction

Models are defined, for the purpose of this chapter, as representations of a particular body of knowledge, that are put forward as an explanation and interpretation of events. They are intended to give the reader insight into the way a theoretical approach may be applied in a clinical setting. Models may be broad based or narrow based, each trying to explain a broad or narrow range of phenomena. The function of models is to predict and to generate forms of therapeutic intervention.

A review of the history of psychiatry over the past 100 years suggests that there is an optimism about its future development. There is no doubt that the role of psychiatry within medicine has become more prestigious, in both the undertaking of successful research (Weller and Eysenck, 1992) and in the application of increased therapeutic efficacy (Dryden and Rentoul, 1991). Since the turn of the century several different models have been proposed, in an attempt to organize knowledge and test theories within psychiatry in an orderly manner. Therapeutic models have been developed by different schools of psychology to provide a basis for clinical treatment; for example, psychoanalysis, behavioural therapy, cognitive therapy, family therapy and client-centred therapy.

The delivery of health care to the mentally ill within the specialized branch of medicine known as psychiatry has greatly influenced the subsequent scientific models such as neurophysiology, human genetics and neuropharmacology. However, models have also been developed to challenge and reject the established views of mental illness (Szasz, 1961; Laing, 1967; Kovel, 1982). Like diseases, models are abstractions (Siegler and Osmond, 1974) and are not necessarily true or false. As described here, models are similar to theories in that they are not static constructs but dynamic, being influenced by new knowledge and events occurring with the passage of time.

Goldberg and Huxley (1992) suggest that mental disorders can be studied from two major standpoints: how the brain works or from knowledge about how man interacts within the environment as a social animal. The first approach is from the medical perspective and considers the scientific disciplines of neuropsychology, neurophysiology, immunochemistry and the genetics of psychiatric syndromes. The other approach is from the social sciences and considers methods of enquiry derived from epidemiology, sociology and psychology. Within physiotherapy the current climate of thinking is to place greater emphasis on the integration of knowledge from both perspectives.

Physiotherapists are unlikely to focus on cerebral dysfunction as the only explanation of mental illness. To be eclectic in approaches to treatment, an understanding of abnormal behaviour in psychological and social terms will also be required. Clearly knowledge of models from both the medical perspective and the social sciences will enable physiotherapists, psychiatrists and other medical personnel to take the most appropriate intervention for the management of mental ill health.

In this chapter, several different models are introduced, focusing on the way the model is conceptualized and the application or influence of the model on approaches to treatment. There is no attempt to include all the models that have been proposed over time. Models have been selected that describe the most widely practised treatment approaches in the Western world today. It is hoped that these will be of value to physiotherapists in informing their own practice. The models reviewed in this chapter include the following: biomedical; neurophysiological and genetics; social control; family therapy; humanistic; psychoanalytical; behavioural; and cognitive.

Biomedical model

The medical model of abnormality has been existent since the fourth century BC. It was at this time that the Greek physician Hippocrates attempted to explain behaviour disorders such as depression and epilepsy as physical diseases (Bernstein *et al.*, 1994). Hippocrates' views were later developed by the Greek and Roman physicians into what became known as mental illness or psychopathology. This model is dominant in psychiatry today, with the remedicalization of psychiatry being a current slogan at national and international meetings (Weller and Eysenck, 1992). The model is based on the belief that mental disorder is an illness which can usually be diagnosed and categorized into distinct conditions with recognizable symptomology. Classification is made under the International Classification of Disease ICD-10 or the Diagnostic and Statistical Manual of Mental Disorders (DSM-IIIR) framework, first developed in 1980 and revised in 1987 by the American Psychiatric Association. Within psychiatry it is recognized that these conditions may or may not respond to medical intervention; for example, the use of antidepressant drugs to treat unipolar depression. Success in treatment is therefore not seen to be imperative to sustaining the model. In medicine it is generally accepted that there are major diseases which defy explanation in terms of aetiology, favourable prognosis and successful outcome. If we consider illness to be the presence of disease, do we then assume that the absence of disease is wellness? The concept of health and wellness has been well documented elsewhere (French, 1992) and further discussion is beyond the scope of this chapter. However, in relation to this topic it is important to identify what it is we mean by mental illness.

The way in which people become defined as mentally ill and reach mental illness services has been illustrated in a five-level framework by Goldberg and Huxley (1980). This framework suggests that a large number of the population will suffer minor bouts of mental illness lasting less than 2 weeks. This has been identified as levels 1 and 2 within the framework and medical intervention is not always required. The majority of distressed people will consult their doctor, but often they will do so for associated physical symptoms. At level 3, mental disorders are identified and treated by primary care physicians, with only a small minority of the population, those at levels 4 and 5 in the framework, being seen by mental health professionals. The latter levels contain the more severe illnesses such as schizophrenia and bipolar affective disorders, with unipolar depression and anxiety disorders being more prevalent at levels 1, 2 and 3. Definitions of mental illness that are based entirely on symptoms may be entirely appropriate for severe illnesses such as psychotic depression and schizophrenia (Goldberg and Huxley, 1992), but may be less appropriate for short-term bouts of anxiety or depression. For these illnesses, Williams (1986) offers a triaxial model consisting of symptoms, personality and social functioning, as a more appropriate definition. In assessing whether someone has a mental disorder, the person will have experienced a discernible number of symptoms from an identified constellation of symptoms and these within a known time frame.

The biomedical model is criticized by Eisenberg (1986) who argues that the causal relationship between bodily malfunction and problems in living is a complex one. He elaborates this by suggesting that medical personnel have to identify the presenting symptoms and find agreement from patients about their significance. For instance, it has to be established to what extent bodily malfunction is related to problems in living and how far the symptoms are the somatic embodiment of problems in living. The physician then has to indicate which treatments are available. He puts forward the suggestion that working within the biomedical model alone is not sufficient for this process and that doctors' dialogue with patients has to be informed by the social sciences.

Many scientific theories have been postulated in support of the biomedical model. These theories claim biochemical, genetic and organic abnormalities to be the underlying causation of mental illness. The classification of all psychiatric disorders, including personality disorder, alcoholism, depression, anxiety and schizophrenia have been associated with genetic or organic factors. The neurophysiological model and genetic links with psychiatry will briefly be examined in an attempt to gain a better understanding of the rationale underpinning this model.

Neurophysiological model

Attempting to relate psychiatric systems to the underlying physiological disturbance is extremely difficult (Craggs and Carr, 1992). Technological advances have enabled rapid expansion of several non-invasive brain imaging techniques. Two such techniques are nuclear magnetic resonance (NMR) imaging, and positron-emission tomography (PET). These techniques enable psychiatric disorders to be investigated at a cellular level in greater detail (Andreasen, 1989). One area of research where this technology is seen to offer potential, when linked with electroencephalography (EEG), is in the investigation of neural substrates and neurophysiological mechanisms that underlie the psychoses of temporal lobe epilepsy (Craggs and Carr, 1992). Some progress has already been made in studying epilepsy using telemetry, EEG and video, allowing electrical changes to be monitored alongside behaviour (Binnie, 1987). Most of the early work in this area has been with animals and the use of the technology is at an early stage. However, it offers the potential of enhancing our knowledge of understanding brain functions and the treatment of psychiatric illness.

In the most common severe mental illness, schizophrenia, there is ongoing debate with regard to the causal links of the disease with visible brain damage. Schiebel and Kovelman (1981) have observed disorientation of hippocampal pyramidal cells and their processes in a small number of patients. They have also put forward evidence to suggest left hemispheric dysfunction and deficits in information processing between the two hemispheres (Kovelman and Schiebel, 1986). There have also been reports of enlargement in the corpus callosum, cerebral atrophy accompanied by enlarged ventricles, and reduced blood flow in the frontal lobes (Weinberger *et al.*, 1986; Silverton *et al.*, 1988; Bruton *et al.*, 1990). However, the evidence to support these abnormal changes is still limited. It had been hoped that the findings from NMR and PET would have enabled the prediction of the type of impairment likely to accompany any observed damage, but to date this has not been the case. Future developments may lead to a better understanding of the neurochemical mechanisms, allowing the development of rational treatment for some of the mental illnesses.

Altered pathologies have been found in psychiatric conditions of an organic nature such as Alzheimer's disease, multi-infarct dementia and Korsakoff's syndrome. These conditions are known as the organic mental disorders. The identifiable biological cause of these diseases has ensured that the biomedical model remains influential, even though it has yet to explain fully most behaviour disorders.

Failure to identify specific abnormalities in the brain for the majority of psychiatric illnesses has resulted in extensive examination of neurotransmitters as the possible root of psychological illness (de Fonseca, 1989). Synaptic conductive agents such as noradrenaline, 5-HT, dopamine and acetylcholine have been singled out for attention. Causal relationships between schizophrenia and malfunctions in dopamine, noradrenaline, serotonin, and abnormalities in spinal fluid circulation and various viruses, have all been proposed (Meltzer, 1987). In depression and anxiety also, the cerebral monoamines have been linked with the aetiology of the illness. Goldberg and Huxley (1992) propose that general psychological processes such as reward, punishment, attention and memory are related specifically to these chemicals. For example, dopamine is related to reward systems, noradrenaline is associated with attention and memory and may transmit information with regard to the magnitude of reinforcement. In recent research, postsynaptic receptors have been investigated as a causal link with depression (McNeal and Climbolic, 1986). The results of these studies should be regarded with caution. Although they demonstrate an unarguable association of biochemical changes with psychological illnesses such as depression and schizophrenia (Claridge, 1990), a causal relationship has yet to be established.

This research suggests that advances in psychiatric medicine from the bio-medical perspective is dependent on a breakthrough in biochemical research that will inform the pharmaceutical industry of future progression in treatments.

Genetics and psychiatry

The fear of madness being inherited and infiltrating throughout communities has led to forced sterilization of supposedly mad people throughout the nineteenth and twentieth centuries (Ussher, 1991). The premise that all psychiatric illnesses are linked to genetic factors was formed and nurtured in the 1930s by the eugenics movement (Ussher, 1991). The attempt of the Nazi campaigns to eliminate mental illness, by using genetic theories to justify mass murder (Pilgrim, 1990), resulted in genetic research in psychiatry being neglected for many years. More recently, ethical concerns have arisen in relation to issues surrounding developments in molecular genetics. An example of this is the controversy surrounding the genetic testing for Huntington's disease.

It has been suggested that recent developments in the understanding of the pathogenesis of psychiatric disorders and molecular genetics enables prediction of common psychiatric disorders, such as depression and schizophrenia (Goldin *et al.*, 1986; Hayden *et al.*, 1988; Sherrington *et al.*, 1988; Crauford, 1989). However, the ethical issues surrounding genetic links with common psychiatric disorders are complex. The potential risks and benefits to individuals and society as a whole have been highlighted in recent reviews of these issues (Pelosi and David, 1989; Gill, 1991).

Links between genetic factors and psychiatric illness have been reported in the literature and a few have been selected to introduce the reader to the debate. McGuffin and Murray (1991) highlight recent research developments in molecular genetics covering a wide spectrum of psychiatric disorders. The research emphasizes the links with specific disorders and how they interact with environmental influences. With regard to studies of families of depressed patients, McGuffin *et al.* (1988) concluded that the complexity of the association between life events and depression is greater than that previously reported by sociologists. People react differently to life events and whether there is a pre-disposition to react that is determined by intrafamilial culture or whether there is a genetic predisposition is unclear and awaits further investigation.

Studies involving monozygotic (MZ) twins have been used extensively in an attempt to separate genetic from environmental factors. Since MZ twins share the same genes, any phenotypic differences can be attributed to environmental factors (Rosenthal, 1970). Studies involving other family members thought to possess high genetic risk are also frequently used (Dorman *et al.*, 1988). Much of the research related to familial links and alcoholism has used this approach. Adoption studies have provided evidence of genetic influence, with a similar increased risk found in the sons of alcoholics adopted by non-alcoholic parents (Anthenelli and Schuckit, 1990). However, studies to investigate genetic links with alcoholism have to date failed to identify a genetic marker. The work of Blum *et al.* (1990) suggests that there may be a genetic susceptibility to alcoholism located in chromosome 11, but the findings of this work have yet to be confirmed by further research. Indications from the research (Adava, 1989) suggest that while family influence contributes to the development of alcohol problems in later life, a significant fraction of the association is genetically, rather than environmentally, determined.

Familial links with schizophrenia have also been extensively researched in this way. In general, the genetic studies of schizophrenia have shown that the more closely related an individual is to a person with this diagnosis, the greater the risk of developing the disorder. It has also been found that children of schizo-phrenics who are adopted by normal parents have a higher incidence of schizo-phrenia than the normal population (Kety *et al.*, 1975). This has been challenged by Abrahams and Taylor (1983) who failed to find familial links. However, their study was quasi-experimental, they had no controls and their diagnostic criteria have been criticized for being too narrow (Kety, 1983). Studies have failed to find a single causal gene defect that could account for schizophrenia. The disorder is considered to be the interaction of both genetic and environmental factors (McGue and Gottesman, 1989).

The only disease gene that can be located in psychiatry at the present time is Huntington's disease. The growing body of evidence for a genetic link with other disorders is complicated due to the apparent multifactorial nature of these illnesses.

Influence on treatment

The effect of both research in neurophysiology and genetics has been to look for a biologically identifiable problem that resides within the individual. This possibility of biological or genetic factors causing mental illness has inevitably led to physical treatments being seen as the most appropriate. Past treatments have included lobectomy, insulin therapy and electroconvulsive therapy (ECT). The former two treatments ceased in the 1950s. ECT is still used as a treatment for depression. The treatment of choice today is invariably pharmacological. Psychiatrists will often use psychological therapies, but these are invariably seen alongside other treatments such as physiotherapy and occupational therapy, as adjuncts to pharmacological intervention. However, the influence of psychology and the success of associated therapies in treatment is gaining increasing recognition (Dryden and Rentoul, 1991).

Physiotherapy assessment and treatment have been and will continue to be influenced by the biomedical model, particularly where there is a known organic pathology. The pattern and progression of a disease such as Alzheimer's will be considered in the assessment and treatment plan for patients suffering from these disorders. The degree of neurotransmitter depletion and altered brain pathology associated with Alzheimer's disease is assessed by the extent of cognitive impairment. There is a tendency for medical personnel to categorize these patients depending on their cognitive function as 'mild, moderate or severe'. While physiotherapy treatment will tend to concentrate on maintaining function in terms of general mobility and activities of daily living, this is often modified in the light of cognitive ability. There is a risk in this approach that the 'stage of illness' determined on initial examination may direct the assessment and treatment plan and ultimate overall management of the patient. It is essential that physiotherapists and other medical personnel see each patient as being unique and that the medical, cognitive and functional problems are viewed alongside the needs of carers and the availability of social support.

Typically, physiotherapists have worked in psychiatry alongside psychiatrists and their role has therefore been shaped by this relationship. In particular, physiotherapists see their role as supportive. Exercise regimens used within psychiatry have been and will continue to be justifiable on biomedical grounds. However, recent research, for example in exercise psychology (Steptoe *et al.*, 1988; Martinsen *et al.*, 1989; Martinson, 1990; Biddle and Mutrie, 1991; Plante, 1993), suggests that exercise may in the future be considered an important psychological treatment, in its own right, for the management of anxiety and depression.

Despite its widespread influence, the biomedical model has been criticized for its failure to take into account cultural and other sociological and psychological perspectives. The narrow cultural premise on which this model is based can be evidenced with regard to the choice of treatments for different groups of people. In the lower socioeconomic classes there is an increased likelihood of receiving medication, as opposed to therapy (Mollica and Mills, 1986), with ECT being chosen twice as often as a treatment for depression for women than men (Showalter, 1987). This is indicative of certain assumptions about gender and class. The major attack on the established views in psychiatry came in the 1960s and 1970s from a group of people who became known as the anti-psychiatrists. Critiques of the model have continued, with much of the criticism coming from psychologists and sociologists.

Models of social control

The biomedical model was rejected by critics such as Laing (1960) and Szasz (1961) on the grounds that their views of mental illness and insanity were morally judgemental, based on value-laden conceptualizations of health and illness. Szasz (1961) proposed that mental illness was a myth; he based this on his view that a clear distinction between organic illness and mental illness could be made, arguing that the latter was in reality a problem in living. His theory postulated that physical and mental illness can clearly be separated, a view supported by Goffman (1968). Diagnosis of the former is based on underlying physical pathology that can be scrutinized by rigorous scientific enquiry, whereas the latter is based on a social construction of normality. He proposes that the mind is not an organ and for this reason cannot be diseased in the same sense as the body (Szasz, 1971). This shift from the medicalization of mental illness towards what Szasz sees as the real problem, that of society, was an extremely radical view. At the time it attracted a great deal of attention from the media, health professionals, and from people who themselves had been diagnosed as being mentally ill. Professionals were seen to be 'labelling' people as mentally ill to fit with their own philosophical views of 'illness' (Ussher, 1991).

Scheff (1966), who was one of several labelling theorists at that time, argued that madness is dependent on social and cultural values not scientific objectivity. This theoretical construct suggests that mental illness may be interpreted by society in ways that allow psychiatry to be used as an agent of social control. Behaviour may be seen to be deviant or normal depending on the context within which it ocurs, and whether the person is in a social category vulnerable for labelling (Sedgewick, 1981). Working class people living in cities are more often given a diagnosis of schizophrenia (Levontin *et al.*, 1984) than people in a higher socioeconomic class. Ethnic minorities also have an increased likelihood of being labelled mentally ill (Collins *et al.*, 1980).

The views of Szasz have been criticized for essentially ignoring the evidence for biological and psychological factors that may contribute to disorders of behaviour. However, his views prompted increasing recognition of the value of non-medical concepts of abnormal behaviour (Bernstein *et al.*, 1994).

Laing (1960) took a different view of mental illness, conceptualizing madness as a state of hyper-wellness, where the individual sees reality as something beyond the socially constructed reality. He argued that madness, and specifically schizophrenia, should be considered as a 'special strategy that a person invents to enable them to live in an unlivable situation'. Laing points out that there is an expectation within traditional psychiatry that the patient will abandon their subjective perspective for the psychiatrist's 'objective' reality. This is seen by Laing as detrimental to the patient. Ingleby (1982) has criticized psychiatry and its assumption that it takes an 'objective' value-free scientific approach, arguing that much of the diagnosis is based on subjective opinion with regard to a constellation of symptoms and behaviour. This criticism challenges the very basis of diagnosis and the validity and reliability of classification of psychiatric disorders. However, the view of mental illness that assumes that objective diagnosis can then be categorized within a known set of syndromes such as depression, has a certain political power. It serves to glorify the role of the 'expert' (Ussher, 1991).

The dissension raised by these critics caused public debate surrounding power and authority, the role of experts, the relationship between biological and social phenomena and perhaps more fundamentally it challenged value judgements about mental illness.

Their criticism with regard to the subjective, value-laden, political nature of diagnosis, challenged the ethos of applying physical medicine to mental ill health problems. However, this presumes that physical medicine is a purely objective science that is not socially constructed. This is a view that is not shared by several authors; for example, Sedgewick (1982) argues that all medicine, including psychiatry, contains an element of subjectivity, politics and value judgements. For instance, a disease acknowledged in one culture may be accepted as health in another (Sanders, 1985).

The views projected by the anti-psychiatry movement can briefly be summarized as seeing madness as something that is experienced by individuals and that causes these individuals distress. However, the suffering is seen to be a response to societal pressures. These are exacerbated by inequalities and conflicts within society. Laing (1967) saw problems lying predominantly within the family, whereas Szasz (1971) saw symptoms resulting from conflicts inherent in the tensions between individual needs and the collective needs of society. The concept of mental disorder can thus be seen as reflecting the political views of society in relation to power structures, oppression within certain groups, and discontentment with socioeconomic inequalities.

While the models based on the concept of social control have not of themselves prompted the development of treatment approaches ('treatment' being anathema to their conviction), they have been influential in the conception of a number of psychosocial models, for example the family therapy model.

Psychological models

Family therapy model

Laing and Esterson (1964) were among the first British writers to express the view that individuals with mental illness were the victims of a pathological family process. Fundamental to their theory, which has its roots in psychoanalysis, is the notion that those aspects of the human psyche denied legitimate expression in the value system of a family will manifest themselves in other ways (Skynner, 1976). This concept of the family being at the root of the individual's problem was further developed by several writers over the next two decades. Selvini-Palazolli *et al.* (1978) put forward an influential systems theory suggesting that it is not individuals who are mentally ill but the family system in which they live. Dysfunctions within a system are seen to be manifested by the individual. This model is characterized by the individual manifesting problems inherent within the family. The individual is reflecting conflicts, communication problems and other difficulties in the family as a whole (Minuchin *et al.*, 1978; Goldenberg and Goldenberg, 1980). An example of this is described by Minuchin (1974) who proposes that family structure is hierarchical, consisting of subsystems, parental and sibling being an obvious one, with the parental subsystem assumed to be in the position of leadership. Problems of mental illness are seen to be present within the family when this difference between the subsystems, for example, is absent, allowing family members to be enmeshed together or, alternatively, perhaps entirely fragmented within individual subsystems. Therefore, treatment based on the individual in isolation from the family will be inappropriate. Family therapy usually begins by an approach which encourages all members of the family to work together in resolving the conflict.

Family therapy is designed to identify and change relationships where necessary. The therapist pays attention to family interactions, especially to alignments and discord and the engagement and disengagement of the different group members. The aim of treatment is often to engineer changes in communication (Minuchin and Fishman, 1981). For example, parents may be taught to engage in conversation without interruption. Whatever the strategy employed, the treatment approach is based on modifying the present situation, not on exploring or interpreting the past. The overall goal of family therapy is not just to resolve an existing problem, but to assist families in gaining a better understanding of interactions within the family and the problems they create (Gurman *et al.*, 1986). The success of this approach is dependent on the full co-operation of key family members, and any sustained resistance to the efforts of the therapist is likely to result in failure of this approach. The other barrier to success is where a key family member has a psychological disturbance, such as a paranoid personality, that prevents them from gaining insight into their own situation or that of another family member. Physiotherapists involved in the treatment of patients with anorexia nervosa and bulimia may find it useful to be informed of family therapy sessions to gain an understanding of the family dynamics. The treatment approach adopted by the phsyiotherapist may include other family members.

Model of humanistic psychology

The humanistic model sees behavioural problems arising as a signal that an individual is failing to reach their potential and that psychological growth has stopped (Bernstein *et al.*, 1994). The theory of 'self-actualization' (Maslow, 1971) suggests that everyone has the potential to reach peak experiences as long as certain necessary conditions are met. The philosophy of client-centred therapy was developed from the work of Carl Rogers and was based on caring and equal respect for others. It was felt that if mental illness was recognized within a therapeutic setting, and the distress was acknowledged and understood, the person would progress in recovery. It was felt that by empathizing with the person, demonstrating warmth and genuineness and treating them with unconditional positive regard, they would be facilitated in their personal development.

This model has been influential in forming the foundation of counselling (Rogers, 1980) and as such has been a useful model for dealing with 'problems in living'. It aims at increasing people's autonomy to enable them to take greater control over their lives. The approach requires the therapist, who is acting as a counsellor, to be able to listen intently to what is being said and to help the individual recognize and clarify the feelings being experienced. The counsellor, in a non-directive manner, offers a safe environment where the individual can talk freely and explore these feelings, while still maintaining a sense of control.

This model would seem less appropriate for dealing with more serious problems of mental illness such as severe depression, obsessive compulsive disorders and schizophrenia. Rogers (1967), however, has provided some limited evidence to dispute this. In a study of client-centred therapy with hospital inpatient schizophrenics who were extremely withdrawn, he reported that they responded positively to this form of treatment. The humanistic model focuses on the individual and the interpretation of situations. Group therapy sessions using this approach are often run with the focus on shared distress and shared support. Critics of the approach argue that therapists, although portraying a non-directive approach, may in fact lead their clients more than they think by reflecting selectively on the things that the therapist deems to be important (Gray, 1991).

This model is one that many physiotherapists working in psychiatry have found to be pertinent to their everyday communication with people suffering from mental illness and in the application of specific counselling techniques. It requires a relationship between the physiotherapist and the individual that is based on trust and the sharing of information. The knowledge possessed by the physiotherapist is shared with the individual, thus establishing a partnership in the therapeutic relationship.

Psychoanalytical model

The psychoanalytical model depicts the problems of mental disorder as residing within the individual. However, treatment differs quite radically from a bio-medical approach; talking with the therapist is seen as the key to therapeutic intervention. Freud (1856–1939), undoubtedly the most influential of all the psychoanalysts, developed his theory of psychoanalysis in response to his clinical work with neurotic patients. He acknowledged the influence of the unconscious mind on behaviour, and related adult distress to childhood experience. The main tenet of his theory related the importance of infantile sexuality, and various defence mechanisms, to the formation of identit ̄ motiva-tion and behaviour. Neurotic anxiety was seen to be caused by inner (the battle for dominance between aspects of the unconscious mi to realize sexual desires or to express anger, for example, may be somatically as anxiety or depression.

The therapeutic relationship established between therapist and p the resolving of conflicts at the root of distress through facing a repressed feelings in the security of the analytic setting. Behaviour is interpreted symbolically and it is the therapist's role to interpret and explore the meaning with the patient. Freud's theories have been influential in the development of psychology, and their influence can be seen in Western culture and in present-day views on mental disorder. Perhaps the most important of all his contributions was the conceptualization of defence mechanisms, which include denial, repression, resistance, transference and counter-transference. These mechanisms, as described by Anna Freud (1968), are devices that come into play when the person's 'ego' is threatened. The 'ego' is the part of the personality that mediates between the instincts and biological drives of the 'id' that desire immediate gratification, and the demands of the outside world. The 'ego' is the part of the personality that learns through experience how far it can accommodate the needs of the 'id' and under what conditions. It is a process that allows the avoidance of conflict.

The post-Freudians, such as Anna Freud, Melanie Klein and Donald Winnicott, further developed clearly delineated schools of therapy for the treatment of psychological problems. Psychotherapy is being used to treat mental disorders by an array of people trained in specific techniques; it is no longer just the tool of the medical practitioner. Psychotherapy refers to any systematic treatment that is theory based and utilizes psychological rather than physiological means for the treatment of mental disorders. During this century, it is estimated that over 400 different 'psychotherapies' have appeared, each with a different name (Karasu, 1986).

Psychotherapy has been influential with regard to physiotherapy practice. One example of this has been in the development of psychomotor therapy (Bunkan and Thornquist, 1990), a specialist branch of physiotherapy which has its roots in psychotherapy, merging psychotherapy with knowledge about patterns of breathing and movement. It is being used by physiotherapists, who have trained in psychomotor therapy, as a treatment approach for a wide range of problems, but with a particular application in psychiatry. More generally, the influence of this model can be seen in everyday practice of physiotherapy. The defence mechanism of denial is one that physiotherapists may see in patients who have had recent news of terminal illness. This coping mechanism allows the person to deal with feelings that cannot be dealt with in any other way, and is a means of protecting one's self-concept. It is important that the physiotherapist does not disrupt this defence by reiterating factual information with regard to the prognosis to the patient. Neither should information be withheld, but should be given to the patient when requested.

Within psychiatry the defence mechanism of resistance may prevent the person with anxiety from facing fears that perpetuate their underlying distress. For example, the person with extreme anxiety symptoms may be continually failing in all attempts at relaxation. This may be seen by the physiotherapist as an unwillingness by the person to co-operate with treatment, and as continual attempts to divert the therapeutic process. An awareness of how resistance may interfere with the patient's attempts to change behaviour will enable the physiotherapist to understand the situation. Transference is a process within the therapeutic relationship that can influence the progress of therapy. Feelings, such as anger, hatred or love are transferred from the person undergoing treatment to the therapist. For example, the anger the person feels towards someone else but 's unable to direct towards them is directed at the physiotherapist. The physiotherapist may be subject to an aggressive outburst and continued hostility. Again an understanding of this mechanism can enable the physiotherapist to cope more effectively with the situation. The physiotherapist with knowledge of this process will not view the anger as a personal insult, but rather the response will be interpreted in a way that will support the therapeutic relationship. However, the behaviour surrounding anger may be complex, and should not always be assumed to be pathological.

In Britain, as in many other countries, psychoanalysis is not the dominant therapy, unlike in Southern Europe where psychoanalysis is still more prevalent than other models of therapy. The theories of psychology that have been empirically based and which are seen to be within the 'objective' science have proved to be more popular in treating mental illness. These include a behaviourist model and a cognitive model.

Model of behavioural therapy

This model suggests that mental disorder occurs as the result of maladaptive learning or problems in the environment. The unconscious mind is not considered; it is observable behaviour that is the focus of this theory. The theory has developed from the initial work of Pavlov on classical conditioning, and the subsequent work of Watson (1924) and Skinner (1953) on operant conditioning.

This model has been applied extensively with regard to the treatment of phobias, anxiety and depression. The treatment of phobias and anxieties has been based on classical conditioning. Learned associations between a feared situation and an unpleasant stimulus are seen to be at the root of the phobia or anxiety with the person learning to avoid the situation. However, this only serves to reinforce the initial fear when the situation is met again. The treatment of phobias and other anxieties by desensitization and related techniques has been particularly successful (Bernstein *et al.*, 1994). Treatment consists of gradual exposure to the feared situation or object for increasing lengths of time (relaxation is used during the exposure) until the anxiety is no longer experienced. This is called systematic desensitization (Wolpe, 1958). The approach utilizes the theory of counter-conditioning which is based on the premise that if the individual is practising relaxation when exposed to an anxiety provoking situation the anxiety will subside. The introduction of a range of 'exposure' oriented therapies (Marks, 1987), which includes flooding, where the person is exposed to a fearful situation and remains there until the fear subsides, has overtaken systematic desensitization as the treatment of choice for anxiety reduction (Hawton *et al.*, 1989). However, the contribution to the treatment of anxiety made by Wolpe is enormous due to his rigorous methodology and explicit descriptions of treatment.

Operant conditioning, which is also based on principles of learning, relates to the reinforcement of desired behaviour, and the ignoring or punishment of less desirable behaviours. Societal values based on a monetary system that rewards us financially for work is an example of positive reinforcement. Behaviour can be shaped using operant conditioning. This occurs when part of the behaviour or behaviour closely related to that desired is observed and rewarded. Token economies have been used in the past two decades in institutions with residents who have learning disabilities or mental illness. The tokens, which can be later exchanged for commodities not readily available elsewhere, are given out to reward desired behaviours. The key concept is that this will encourage performance of the behaviour on which, by association, the availability of these commodities is contingent. There is debate as to the usefulness of this practice. It has been suggested that token systems have helped prepare people with severely disturbed behaviour to live outside of institutional care (Paul and Lentz, 1977). Antisocial behaviour in children has also been said to respond to this treatment approach (Kirigen *et al.*, 1982). However, it has been criticized as being potentially coercive.

Another approach used to change behaviour is a procedure known as 'time out'. The individual is removed from a situation which is providing a positive reinforcement until the undesirable behaviour has ceased. An example of this technique as applied by physiotherapists when working with brain-injured patients has been described by Wood (1987). During aggressive outbursts, the physiotherapist disengages eye contact, turns her head away and discontinues with any interaction for a short period of time, in this way attempting to avoid reinforcing the behaviour by reacting to it. The patient may be placed in a non-stimulating room, which has been set aside for this purpose, for a brief pre-determined period of time, or until the aggressive behaviour has subsided.

The practice of 'time out' has recently come under criticism when used as a form of punishment. An example of this was the practice of 'pin down' in British children's homes highlighted by the media in 1991 (Ussher, 1991).

Modelling, where it is suggested that we learn from observing others to behave in a particular way, is another form of behaviour therapy. Social skills can be learned by observing others in real-life situations or using the media of video. Learning to become more assertive, developing interpersonal skills and dealing with anger are frequently practised through role play. People with mental illness often display a lack of assertiveness and find decision-making extremely difficult. This is perhaps not surprising, as the skills required for decision-making relate to thought and behaviour (Nelson-Jones, 1983) and it is likely that these skills will have been disturbed during the illness.

Physiotherapists have intuitively applied behavioural techniques in practice. The use of praise is commonly a positive reinforcement, when a patient succeeds in reaching a desired goal or often when they partly succeed. Setting appropriate aims of treatment and appropriate goal steps can be seen as shaping behaviour, if they are successfully completed and reinforced. The logging of a diary, noting progression, is another useful technique for reinforcement often used by physiotherapists. Physiotherapists have also successfully applied specific behavioural therapy techniques in a variety of clinical settings (Cauldrey and Seeger, 1981; Hill, 1985; Williams, 1989; Hughes and Alltree, 1990).

Physiotherapists have an important role to play in helping people who are recovering from mental illness to regain their ability to take decisions and be more autonomous. Many physiotherapists in psychiatry plan programmes of intervention jointly with patients, encouraging them to consider the implications and consequences of treatment, the alternatives and setting performance indicators to assess outcome. The patient is given the task of monitoring their own progress and setting new goals. The physiotherapist, and other professionals, may be viewed as role models by their patients. An understanding of the different models of mental disorder, and an awareness of their own beliefs, prejudices and health-related behaviours, is thus imperative to the provision of an appropriate role model.

Although the model of behaviour therapy is seen to have a wide applicability and its usefulness as a treatment approach is generally accepted (Rachman and Wilson, 1980), it fails to provide a satisfactory explanation for the complexities of mental illness. The utility of the model in the treatment of anxiety disorders is undisputed, but in many other 'neurotic' disorders cognitions appear to play a clear functional role. Issues such as patient compliance are not accounted for and there are numerous psychiatric problems that do not lend themselves to observable behaviour (for example, obsessional ruminations). The theory can thus be criticized for being reductionist and simplistic. The cognitive model and the cognitive–behavioural approach in particular attempts to bridge the gap, utilizing the clinical success of the behavioural approach into a more problem-solving approach which has wider application.

Model of cognitive therapy

The cognitive model starts from the assumption that people become mentally ill through disturbance in their own thoughts. The focus is on conscious mental experience, with the role of thoughts, beliefs, attitudes and memories being seen as determining factors of behaviour. Maladaptive thoughts are seen as the cause of anxiety and depression (Beck, 1976) and schizophrenia (Frith, 1979). Beck proposed that negative thoughts are stored in memory in the form of schemata based on prior experience. These schemata are activated when similar events occur, resulting in automatic negative thoughts and corresponding emotional responses. Ellis (1962) developed the approach which he called rational-emotive therapy (RET). Ellis viewed mental illness as the result of people's irrational interpretation of their experience, creating negative emotions that were not based on the objective experience itself. Treatment is based on training the individual to identify and challenge these beliefs that give rise to emotional, cognitive and behavioural consequences. Strategies used include self-monitoring with feedback, direct challenging of beliefs by the therapist, and the rehearsal of more rational statements by the individual. The cognitive therapy (CT) approach of Beck (1976) to the treatment of problems associated with anxiety and depression was developed independently of RET, although the assumptions made with regard to how the individuals problems develop and how they are maintained are similar. Wessler (1986) suggests the following as the critical difference between the two approaches. RET will focus on the irrational nature of the individual's appraisal of the event and what the likely outcome will be. The therapist is looking for the person to provide evidence that if the event occurred it would be catastrophic. CT by contrast focuses on the distorted nature of the content of the thought, with the therapist exploring with the individual the evidence to support the irrational belief. Beck also argues that negative thinking is a central part of emotional distress, and his approach is less confrontational than Ellis's.

The third most influential approach in cognitive psychology is self-instructional training (Meichenbaum, 1977). Similar to Beck and Ellis, Meichenbaum attempts to help individuals to identify irrational beliefs and negative thoughts. However, the approach differs in that he is more concerned with the internal dialogue (what people say to themselves before entering stressful situations) that serves to maintain behaviour. This treatment approach involves the identification and modification of negative self-statements and may involve some training in coping and problem-solving skills. The role of the therapist is to assist in this training process by providing the necessary guidance and reinforcement. These three treatment approaches remain influential in guiding therapeutic interventions alongside the numerous other less well-known variations (Newell and Dryden, 1991).

The aim of the cognitive therapist is to help the individual recognize and change errors in thinking patterns; for example, over-generalization; selective abstraction; minimalization; catastrophizing – any of which may be self-defeating. The changing of thinking patterns that are well established may appear threatening to the person, as they may be deeply rooted in childhood experience and cultural beliefs. The therapist has to be skilled in this therapeutic approach to assist the person to gain insight into this particular mode of thinking and to enable them to challenge irrational beliefs and to replace them with more realistic thoughts. Within this framework the individual is seen as being responsible for identifying the problem and being able to select, implement and evaluate the chosen intervention. The individual is encouraged to take responsibility for identifying where reinforcement of a particular behaviour is desirable and to ensure that this is self-administered. This differs from the traditional behavioural approach where the therapist remains in control of the reinforcer.

This approach has been used by clinical psychologists in the treatment of anxiety and depression, in stress management programmes, and with other clinical problems. Physiotherapists with knowledge and experience of this approach may find it useful in helping patients to identify and challenge maladaptive thinking patterns that are detrimental to their progressive recovery. Some physiotherapists have been using this approach in conjunction with clinical psychologists in the management of stress and the treatment of anxiety. It requires an understanding of the theory and training in the application of the technique. It is recommended that it is undertaken with the knowledge and guidance of a clinical psychologist.

The cognitive–behavioural approach has developed empirically from both the behavioural and cognitive therapies. It is more concerned with the factors maintaining a disorder than the factors that initiated the problem. The approach encompasses a wide range of models of human disorder and a diversity of approaches to treatment. These include problem-solving, coping skills acquisition, cognitive restructuring and combinations of some or all of these. An example of this is in the application of the model to relaxation training. Skills to enhance the patient's judgement with regard to self-efficacy in anxiety-provoking situations are included along with instruction in relaxation. The aim is to teach patients how to identify, evaluate, control and modify negative anxiety-provoking thoughts, anxiety-provoking cues and associated behaviours (Hawton *et al.*, 1989).

Cognitive–behavioural strategies can be applied within psychiatry to enable individuals with eating disorders, obsessional disorders, sexual problems, alcohol and drug addictions to maintain their changed behaviour following a programme of intervention (Marlatt and Gordon, 1985). The reader is directed to Dryden and Rentoul (1991) for a further account of this approach to a wide range of adult clinical problems.

Conclusion

The explanations offered to account for mental disorder are multitudinous, resulting in a diverse range of models that influence and direct the current approaches in the treatment and management of the mentally ill. The medical profession are still holding on to the position of power, with the biomedical model still dominant, in the diagnosis and care of the mentally ill. However, this position is increasingly being challenged by other professional groups such as psychologists, psychotherapists, nurses, occupational therapists, physiotherapists and social workers (Ussher, 1991), all of whom are increasing their expertise and proficiency in the care of people with mental ill health. Within physiotherapy, for example, the past decade has witnessed the inception of a special interest group in psychiatry, development of post-registration education, and an increased number of physiotherapists specializing in this area. In concluding this chapter, the following questions require to be addressed: which model is best, and are all models effective?

The debate with regard to the effectiveness of therapy has been going on for 40 years. The efficacy of the different models of psychotherapy have been established through controlled research studies (see Lambert *et al.*, 1986, for a review of this literature). In a large meta-analysis study undertaken by Smith *et al.* (1980) it would appear that therapy seems to be effective in alleviating symptoms of distress for the majority of people, with one therapy seeming to be as effective as another. The placebo effect and the influence of the therapeutic relationship have not been controlled for in the majority of studies that have looked at the efficacy of therapy. Future research should attempt to address this issue. It may be that the benefits of therapy are due to contact time and the enthusiasm of the therapist. It would seem therefore that the most appropriate way forward is to use the model that fits best with the identified needs of the person requiring treatment and in keeping with the skills of the professional. Consideration should be given to the patient's views with regards to treatment and in deciding whether to work with the individual, with the group or with the family.

Physiotherapists have historically worked within the biomedical model. However, increasingly other models are being applied in approaches to treatment; for example, the client-centred approach as a way of communicating with people and specifically as applied to counselling. Intuitively physiotherapists may find they are applying a behavioural approach in treatment with the use of positive reinforcement. This can be further developed in psychiatry for more specific application, for example in the treatment of anxiety management, in social skills training and in working with people with chronic psychiatric problems. The cognitive and cognitive–behavioural models will be appropriate for the treatment of anxiety, stress management programmes and depression. As previously stated, this approach will require the physiotherapist to work alongside the clinical psychologist to integrate the approach within the therapeutic framework. The role of the physiotherapist and the psychologist may overlap, but there are boundaries of delineation and each profession has a different knowledge base and clinical skills. Eclecticism encourages a diversity of therapeutic process; however, the goals should be clearly identified for each individual and for all professionals involved in the management plan.

For the future, physiotherapists will continue to influence existing theoretical models by evaluating practice, undertaking research, and by debating the issues pertinent to the health care provision for people with mental health problems.

References

Abrahams, R. and Taylor, M.A. (1983) The genetics of schizophrenia: a reassessment using modern criteria. *American Journal of Psychiatry*, **140**, 171–175

Adava, S. (1989) Problem drinking and alcohol problems. *Recent Developments in Alcoholism*, **8**, 173–201

Andreasen, N.C. (1989) *Brain Imaging: Applications in Psychiatry*, American Psychiatric Press, New York

Anthenelli, R.A. and Schuckit, M.A. (1990) Genetic studies of alcoholism. *International Journal of the Addictions*, **25**(1), 81–94

Beck, A.T. (1976) *Cognitive Therapy and the Emotional Disorders*, International Universities Press, New York

Bernstein, D., Roy, E., Srull, T. and Wickens, C. (1994) *Psychology*, 3rd edn, Houghton Mifflin, Boston

Biddle, S. and Mutrie, N. (1991) *The Psychology of Physical Activity and Exercise: A Health Related Perspective*, Springer-Verlag, London

Binnie, C.D. (1987) Ambulatory diagnostic monitoring of seizures in adults. In *Advances in Neurology*, Vol. 46, *Intensive Neurodiagnostic Monitoring* (ed. Gummit, R.J.), Raven Press, New York

Blum, K., Noble, E.P., Sheridan, P.J. *et al.* (1990) Allelic association of human dopamine D2 receptor gene in alcoholism. *Journal of the American Medical Association*, **263**(15), 2055–2060

Bruton, C., Crow, T., Frith, C., Johnstone, E., Owens, D. and Roberts, G. (1990) Schizophrenia and the brain: a prospective cliniconeuropathological study. *Psychological Medicine*, **20**, 285–304

Bunkan, B.H. and Thornquist, E. (1990) Psychomotor therapy: an approach to the evaluation and treatment of psychosomatic disorders. In *Psychological and Psychosomatic Problems* (eds Hena, T. and Sveram, M.), Churchill Livingstone, Edinburgh

Cauldrey, D.J. and Seeger, E.R. (1981) Biofeedback devices as an adjunct to physiotherapy. *Physiotherapy*, **67**(12), 371–376

Claridge, G. (1990) Can a disease model of schizophrenia survive? In *Reconstructing Schizophrenia* (ed. Bentall, R.P.), Routledge, London

Collins, J.L., Rickman, L.E. and Mathura, C.B. (1980) Frequency of schizophrenia and depression in a black inpatient population. *Journal of the National Medical Association*, **72**(9), 851–856

Craggs, M.D. and Carr, A.C. (1992) Neurophysiological aspects of psychiatry. In *The Scientific Basis of Psychiatry* (eds Weller, M. and Eysenck, M.), W.B. Saunders, London

Crauford, D. (1989) Progress and problems in Huntington's disease. *International Review Psychiatry*, **1**, 249–258

de Fonseca, A.F. (1989) Psychiatry in the 1990's. In *Human Psychopharmacy: Measures and Methods*, Vol. 2 (eds Hindmarsh, I. and Stoner, P.), New York, Wiley

Dorman, J.S., Trucco, M., LaPorte, R. and Kuller, L.H. (1988) Family studies the key to understanding genetic and environmental etiology of chronic disease? *Genetic Epidemiology*, **5**, 305–310

Dryden, W. and Rentoul, R. (eds) (1991) *Adult Clinical Problems: A Cognitive–Behavioural Approach*, Routledge, London

Eisenberg, L. (1986) Mindlessness and brainlessness in psychiatry. *British Journal of Psychiatry*, **148**, 497–508

Ellis, A. (1962) *Reason and Emotion in Psychotherapy*, Springer-Verlag, New York

French, S. (ed.) (1992) *Physiotherapy: A Psychosocial Approach*, Butterworth–Heinemann, London

Freud, A. (1968) *The Ego and Mechanisms of Defence*, Hogarth Press, London

Frith, C.D. (1979) Conscious information processing and schizophrenia. *British Journal of psychiatry*, **134**, 225–235

Gill, M. (1991) Ethics, molecular genetics and psychiatric disorders. In *Ethical Issues of Molecular Genetics in Psychiatry* (eds Sram, R.J., Bulyzhenkov, V., Prilipko, L. and Christen, Y.), Springer Verlag, London

Goffman, E. (1968) *Stigma: Notes on the Management of Spoiled Identity*, Penguin, Harmondsworth, UK

Goldberg, D. and Huxley, P. (1980) *Mental Illness in the Community: The Pathway to Psychiatric Care*, Tavistock, London

Goldberg, D. and Huxley, P. (1992) *Common Mental Disorders: A Bio-social Model*, Tavistock, London

Goldenberg, I. and Goldenberg, H. (1980) *Family Therapy: An Overview*, Brooks Cole, Monterey, CA

Goldin, L.R., Nurnberger, J.I. and Gershon, E.S. (1986) Clinical methods in psychiatric genetics II: The high risk approach. *Acta Psychiatrica Scandinavica*, **74**, 119–128

Gray, P. (1991) *Psychology*, Worth, New York

Gurman, A.S., Kniskern, D.P. and Pinsof, W.M. (1986) Research on marital and family therapies. In *Handbook of Psychotherapy and Behavioural Change*, 3rd edn (eds Garfield, S.L. and Bergin, A.E.), Wiley, New York

Hawton, K., Salkovskis, P.M., Kirk, J. and Clark, D.M. (1989) *Cognitive Behavioral Therapy for Psychiatric Problems: A Practical Guide*, Oxford University Press, Oxford

Hayden, M.R., Robbins, C., Allard, D. *et al.* (1988) Improved predictive testing for Huntington disease by using 3 linked DNA markers. *American Journal of Human Genetics*, **43**(5), 689–694

Hill, L.D. (1985) Contributions of behaviour modification to cerebral palsy habilitation. *Physical Therapy*, **65**(3), 341–344

Hughes, S. and Alltree, J. (1990) A behavioural approach to the management of functional disorders. *Physiotherapy*, **76**(4), 255–258

Ingelby, D. (ed.) (1982) *Critical Psychiatry: The Politics of Mental Health*, Penguin, Harmondsworth, UK

Karasu, T.B. (1986) The specificity versus nonspecificity dilemma: toward identifying therapeutic change agents. *American Journal of Psychiatry*, **143**, 687–695

Kety, S.S. (1983) Response to Abrams and Taylor. *American Journal of Psychiatry*, **140**, 1111–1112

Kety, S.S., Rosenthal, D., Wender, P., Schulsinger, F. and Jacobson, B. (1975) Mental illness in the biological and adoptive families of adopted individuals who have become schizophrenic: a preliminary report based on psychiatric interviews. In *Genetic Research in Psychiatry* (eds Fieve, R.R., Rosenthal, D. and Brill, H.), Johns Hopkins University Press, Baltimore

Kirigen, K.A., Braukmann, C.J., Atwater, J.D. *et al.* (1982) An evaluation of teaching family (Achievement Place) group homes for juvenile offenders. *Journal of Applied Behaviour Analysis*, **15**, 1–16

Kovel, J. (1982) The American mental health industry. In *Critical Psychology: The Politics of Mental Health* (ed. Ingelby, D.), Penguin, Harmondsworth, UK

Kovelman, J. and Schiebel, A. (1986) Biological substrates of schizophrenia. *Acta Neurologica Scandinavica*, **73**(1), 1–32

Laing, R.D. (1960) *The Divided Self: A Study of Sanity and Madness*, Tavistock, London

Laing, R.D. (1967) *The Politics of Experience*, Penguin, Harmondsworth, UK

Laing, R.D. and Esterson, A. (1964) *Sanity, Madness and the Family*, Tavistock, London

Lambert, M., Shapiro, D. and Bergin, A. (1986) The effectiveness of psychotherapy. In *Handbook of Psychotherapy and Behavior Change* (eds Garfield, S. and Bergin, A.), Wiley, London

Levontin, R.C., Rose, S. and Kamin, L.J. (1984) Not in our genes. *Biology, Ideology and Human Nature*, Pantheon Books, New York

McGue, M. and Gottesman, I.I. (1989) Genetic linkage in schizophrenia. *Schizophrenia Bulletin*, **15**, 453–464

McGuffin, P., Katz, R. and Bebbington, P. (1988) The Camberwell Collaborative Depression Study

III: depression and adversity in the relatives of depressed probands. *British Journal of Psychiatry*, **152**, 775–782

McGuffin, P. and Murray, R.M. (1991) *The New Genetics of Mental Illness*, Butterworth–Heinemann, Oxford

McNeal, E.T. and Climbolic, P. (1986) Anti-depressant and biological theories of depression. *Psychological Bulletin*, **99**, 361–394

Marks, I.M. (1987) *Fears, Phobias and Rituals: Panic Anxiety and their Disorders*, Oxford University Press, Oxford

Marlatt, G.A. and Gordon, J.R. (1985) *Relapse Prevention: Maintenance Strategies in the Treatment of Addictive Behaviours*, Guilford, New York

Martinsen, E.W. (1990) Benefits of exercise for the treatment of depression. *Sports Medicine*, **9**(6), 380–390

Martinsen, E.W., Strand, J., Paulsson, G. and Kaggestad, J. (1989) Physical fitness level in patients with anxiety and depressive disorders. *International Journal of Sports Medicine*, **10**, 58–61

Maslow, A.H. (1971) *Motivation and Personality*, 2nd edn, Harper and Row, New York

Meichenbaum, D. (1977) *Cognitive Behaviour Modification*, Plenum Press, New York

Meltzer, H. (1987) Biological studies in schizophrenia. *Schizophrenia Bulletin*, **13**(1), 77–111

Minuchin, S. (1974) *Families and Family Therapy*, Tavistock, London

Minuchin, S. and Fishman, C. (1981) *Family Therapy Techniques*, Harvard University Press, Cambridge, MA

Minuchin, S., Rosman, B.L. and Baker, L. (1978) *Psychosomatic Families: Anorexia Nervosa in Context*, Harvard University Press, Cambridge, MA

Mollica, R.F. and Mills, M. (1986) Social class and psychiatric practice: a revision of the Hollingshead and Redlich model. *American Journal of Psychiatry*, **143**(1), 12–17

Nelson-Jones, R. (1983) *Practical Counselling Skills*, Holt, Rinehart and Winston, London

Newell, R. and Dryden, W. (1991) An introduction to the cognitive–behavioural approach. In *Adult Clinical Problems: A Cognitive–Behavioural Approach* (eds Dryden, W. and Rentoul, R.), Routledge, London

Paul, G.L. and Lentz, R.J. (1977) *Psychosocial Treatment of Chronic Mental Patients: Mileu versus Social Learning Programs*, Harvard University Press, Cambridge, MA

Pelosi, A.J. and David, A.S. (1989) Ethical implications of the new genetics for psychiatry. *International Review in Psychiatry*, **1**, 315–320

Pilgrim, D. (1990) Competing theories of madness. In *Reconstructing Schizophrenia* (ed. R. Bentall), Routledge, London

Plante, T.G. (1993) *Aerobic exercise in prevention and treatment of psychopathology in exercise psychology. The influence of physical exercise on psychological processes* (ed. P. Seraganian), John Wiley, New York, 358–379

Rachman, S.J. and Wilson, G.T. (1980) *The Effects of Psychological Therapy*, 2nd edn, Pergamon, Oxford

Rogers, C.R. (1967) *The Therapeutic Relationship and Its Impact: A Study of Psychotherapy with Schizophrenics*, University of Winconsin Press, Madison

Rogers, C.R. (1980) *A Way of Being*, Houghton Mifflin, Boston

Rosenthal, D. (1970) *Genetic Theory and Abnormal Behaviour*, McGraw-Hill, New York

Sanders, D. (1985) *The Struggle for Health*, McMillan, London

Scheibel, A. and Kovelman, J. (1981) Disorientation of the hippocampal pyramidal cell and its processes in the schizophrenic patient. *Biological Psychiatry*, **16**, 101–112

Scheff, T.J. (1966) *Being Mentally Ill*, Weidenfield, London

Sedgewick, P. (1982) *Psychopolitics: The Politics of Health*, Pluto, London

Seigler, M. and Osmond, H. (1974) *Models of Madness, Models of Medicine*, Macmillan, New York

Selvini Palazolli, M., Cecchin, G., Boscolo, L. and Prata, G. (1978) *Paradox and Counterparadox*, Jason Aranson, New York

Sherrington, R., Brynjolfsson, F., Petursson, H. *et al.* (1988) Localisations of a susceptibility locus for schizophrenia in chromosome 5. *Nature*, **336**, 164–167

Showalter, E. (1987) *The Female Malady*, Virago, London

Silverton, L., Mednick, S., Schulsinge, F., Parnas, J. and Harrington, M. (1988) Genetic risk for schizophrenia, birthweight and cerebral ventricular enlargement. *Journal of Abnormal Psychology*, **97**, 496–498

Skinner, B.F. (1953) *Science and Human Behavior*, New York, Macmillan

Skynner, R. (1976) *One Flesh: Separate Persons*, Trowbridge and Esher, London

Smith, M.L., Glass, G.V. and Miller, T.I. (1980) *The Benefits of Psychotherapy*, Johns Hopkins Press, Baltimore

Steptoe, A., Moses, J., Edwards, S. and Mathews, A. (1988) Effects of aerobic conditioning on mental wellbeing and reactivity to stress. In *Sport, Health, Psychology and Exercise Symposium Proceedings*, London, The Sports Council/Health Education Authority, London

Szasz, T. (1961) *The Myth of Mental Illness: Foundations of a Theory of Personal Conduct*, London, Secker

Szasz, T. (1971) *The Manufacture of Madness: A Comparative Study of the Inquisition and the Mental Health Movement*, Routledge, London

Ussher, J. (1991) *Women's Madness: Misogyny or Mental Illness?* Harvester Wheatsheaf, London

Watson, J.B. (1924) *Behaviourism*, W.W. Norton, New York

Weinberger, D.R., Berman, K.F. and Zec, R.F. (1986) Physiologic dysfunction of dorsolateral prefrontal cortex in schizophrenia, 1. Regional blood flow evidence. *Archives of General Psychiatry*, **43**(2), 114–124

Weller, M. and Eysenck, M. (1992) *The Scientific Basis of Psychiatry*, 2nd edn, W.B. Saunders, Philadelphia

Wessler, R.L. (1986) Conceptualising cognitions in the cognitive–behavioral therapies. In *Cognitive–Behavioral Approaches to Psychotherapy* (eds Dryden, W. and Golden, W.L.), Harper and Row, London

Williams, J. (1989) Illness behaviour to wellness behaviour. *Physiotherapy*, **75**(1), 2–7

Williams, P., Tarnopolsky, A., Hand, D. and Shepherd, M. (1986) Minor psychiatric morbidity and general practice consultations: The West London Survey. *Psychological Medicine Monograph Supplements, 9*

Wolpe, J. (1958) *Psychotherapy by Reciprocal Inhibition*, Stanford University Press, Stanford, CA

Wood, R.J. (1987) *Brain Injury Rehabilitation: a Neurobehavioural Approach*, Croom Helm, London

3

Communication in the clinical mental health setting

Maureen Dennis

Introduction

Most of the time we communicate our anxieties to one another. However, at some time in our lives we may decide there is a need to seek the help of doctors – we adopt the 'sickness role', which assumes that we have some problem which is detrimental to our health and that if we lay the problem in their hands, we will receive advice and relief.

This chapter will discuss the interaction between doctor and patient, therapist and patient. Outpatients in the clinical mental health area have nearly always been through a clinical interview with a physician before they seek the advice of a physiotherapist. We should be aware of the problems which may arise in communication which happen partly because doctors are under pressure of time to 'increase productivity', as are many other professions.

Mentally ill patients who are having acute phases of their particular illness may be experiencing confusions and distortions of reality. It is important that we understand some of these, so that when communication does break down we have the insight and skills to re-establish mutual co-operation. The second half of the chapter will discuss some of these confusions, and approaches which might reduce them.

The clinical interview: doctor and patient communication

Both categories of patient have to go through some kind of selection process within the medical interview. Decisions and recommendations are made on their behalf which may involve other medical professionals such as the psychologist, community nurse or physiotherapist.

There are elements in the doctor–patient interview which can be examined by other professionals to their benefit. First, if the encounter is satisfactory for the patient, their anxiety will be reduced and they are likely to be more co-operative in any sequential interviews with health professionals. If it has not been carried out with skill or empathy, other professionals can allow space for patients to express their anxieties and can do a great deal to repair the damage of an insensitive encounter. It is also necessary for physiotherapists to make their own judgements as a result of history-taking and examination. The greater length of time physiotherapists are with patients means they can reach a deeper understanding of particular predicaments. The quality of that contact may have a profound effect on the patient's insight, anxiety and levels of motivation. However, paramedical professionals must not assume that they are automatically good communicators.

Good communication skills in day-to-day interaction are based on

- listening to each other
- eye contact which permits 'meshing' or the taking of turns to speak
- physical or auditory acknowledgement of the information given
- attentive body posture and suitable body language
- reciprocal questioning to obtain more information
- pauses which also indicate opportunity for the other person to speak
- empathy which implies emotional warmth during the act of communication

There are, in addition, a number of more subtle assumptions which influence our attitude to the person to whom we are speaking regarding age, gender or cultural group. Also, it is important to maintain our own identity or role in the interaction and our sense of the other person's identity in relation to that role.

Doctor–patient interaction

Pendelton and Hasler (1983) have analysed the doctor–patient interaction in order to understand better what actually happens in a cultural context of the clinical interview.

'Locus of control': What caused my problem?; Who controls my problem?
First, a patient does not live in a cultural limbo, but brings to the interview beliefs about their own health. They may have remained indifferent to these beliefs until symptoms occur, when a sense of their own 'locus of control', i.e. an idea of how much they are able to control or influence their sick role, comes to the fore. This in turn is influenced by a wider set of cultural beliefs drawn from their upbringing, environment and social setting. Patients may believe that the cause of their malaise is external or internal; equally they may rationalize that the control of their illness is largely external or internal. One external factor is a sense of fatalism, as if one was predestined for such an experience. People will examine their family medical history to justify such an outlook, but they can either underplay or accept realistically the preventative factors which could have been taken.

This can have a profound effect on outcome, especially if one is dealing with problems with a high stress/anxiety/depression induced factor. For example, Freeling and Harris (1984) analysed the depressive response of individuals to new experiences, and cited four classes of events which constitute threats:

1. The failure of events to develop in the way one has come to expect from past experience, e.g. redundancy versus employment, so that habitual reaction is no longer appropriate.
2. The effects of prolonged stress, often appearing after its removal, e.g. the death of a relative for whom one was caring.
3. The chronic frustration of some social situations, when the expression of anger is inhibited, e.g. when a skilled employee feels undervalued and ignored.

4. The chronic boredom and tedium of some situations and jobs which is reflected in the low skill, part-time work especially of women.

Added to these can be the problems of adjustment to physical disablement due to dramatic or gradual events.

The above factors are all distressing, but one might ask why do some people show great resilience when faced with such events and others do not? It may be that some people's 'locus of control', i.e. their concept of causality, may be heavily distorted by their reasoning. They may see themselves as the victim of circumstances when they are not actually so. Not only will these people as patients react negatively, but they will have negative expectations of the future, and the more firmly these are believed, the more difficult it will be for health professionals to obtain their co-operation for a positive adaptation and outcome.

Ironically also, as an external factor, if the patient believes the doctor (or the physiotherapist) has a high measure of 'control' over their problem, they are more likely to listen to their advice. However, as Pendleton and Hasler (1983) indicate, there may be a mismatch between the cultural expectations of the doctor and the patient. The patient may want a 'quick-fix' prescription, whereas the doctor may omit prescription but recommend life style changes, which would require persistence, practice and patience.

Communication: breakdown or breakthrough?

A consultation can be roughly divided into four sections:

- the introduction and explanation of symptoms (reason for visit)
- the medical examination which may require undressing on the part of the patient, and some physical contact with the patient by the doctor
- a diagnosis, or suggestion of one, requiring further investigation
- prescription, reassurance or advice

Patients of any age may suffer sensory loss and be unable to hear clearly what the doctor is saying, especially if the language is mixed with medical jargon. Also, if either doctor or patient speaks with a heavy local or foreign dialect, misunderstandings may arise. Therefore, if there is a mixture of anxiety, sensory loss, strange colloquialisms and jargon, there is a potential for enormous misunderstandings. Some doctors are aware that the use of certain words, such as 'serious', 'operation' and 'cancer', can trigger such alarm that the patient does not hear any more, but may sit in a state of stunned shock.

The doctors themselves may unknowingly discourage the patient to question because of their authoritative presence, which may be very inhibiting. A clinic itself communicates something of the aura that doctors wish to project. A white coat and/or formal dress can enhance an image of authority and separateness. Before a word is spoken, patient and doctor will have made some assumptions about each other, which may or may not be modified by further questioning. These can be based on prejudices towards class, gender, age or ethnic type.

An example of communication barriers
For example, Root (1986), in Oklahoma, studied the 'communication barriers' of doctors and older women patients to identify the prejudices which exist on both sides. She comments that the aging process is not standard in any individual,

but stereotypes may exist in both the doctor and the patient herself. Therefore, symptoms may be dismissed as part of the aging process when in fact they may be the 'atypical or vague presentation of symptoms' and part of an insidious disease process. The body manifests 'disease processes' less dramatically and definitively 'when it is older'. Women may be reluctant to provide information which they think is trivial or embarrassing or may actually be ashamed of their symptoms. They may be shy to admit to growing confusion or depression which may well have an organic and treatable basis. So both doctor and patient fall into the stereotypes of the 'deity-like doctor' and the 'crabby old woman' who does not expect good health in her mature years.

Touch and examination
Touch gestures are socially useful ways of reinforcing attention during speech, especially with the older patient, but professionals may be too inhibited and resting on their authority to use this humane way of reinforcing communication.

Doctors may ask the patient to indicate the site of symptoms, unlike physiotherapists who palpate for the source of symptoms. But patients usually have a poor idea of where the main organs are situated in the body. For example the 'stomach' may be indicated in any area below the ribs and above the pubis, and patients have little idea of the size of the lungs in the chest cavity or the position of the kidneys at the back.

Medical examinations by a doctor differ from that of a physiotherapist, because for a physician there is usually a clearly demarcated space for interviewing and for examining. In the examination area, privacy is given for undressing and often the patient is asked to wear a clinical robe which in a sense objectifies the patient's body from himself. This permits examination of the more personal areas of the patient's body in a detached manner. Both the doctor's white coat and the patient's clinical gown mask the characteristics of gender identity which are emphasized by personal dress (Young, 1989).A physiotherapist has no such ritual and therefore can perhaps observe more closely the subtle postures and body tissue changes which reveal so much of a person's psyche and state of health.

Questioning

Interviewing can involve two types of questions: open questions and closed questions. Closed questions stick to a strictly biodynamic level of enquiry as to the degree of severity, duration and physical complexity of the presenting symptoms. Patients may comply with this limitation and describe only the immediate and localized symptoms when there is a more general malaise being experienced. The complaint is often a 'somatic cry' in a wilderness of personal despair which can be helped by skilled counselling. Open questions ask more of the psychosocial circumstances of the patient and may therefore have to cope with more complex or initimate replies.

The second type, closed questions, give the patient an opportunity to describe anxieties and social problems, but only if phased in at the right time of the interview. If asked too early in the consultation they can be seen as judgemental and perhaps threatening. This calls for a counselling role on the part of doctors, which can be continued by therapists but can be time consuming. But if doctors are trying to find a pattern of social breakdown which is indicative of mental breakdown, they may have to ask more 'intrusive' questions than 'How well do you sleep?' and 'Why do you want to continue to be absent from work?'. The interview has to build up gently to asking the more personal questions concerning alcohol consumption or quality of personal relationships, including sexual behaviour.

Some patients 'don't wish to bother the doctor' and do need help, whereas others fill the interview with tales of their woes. Pendelton and Hasler note that middle class patients tend to ask more questions than working class patients, and doctors are more willing to offer explanations to those whom they see as social equals. Others, including older people of all social classes, may accept without question prescriptions or advice which they may or may not adhere to, since they may lack the personal confidence to be seen to be challenging the doctor in any way.

Note taking, prescription writing or form filling for further tests can all provide the doctor with opportunities for avoidance of eye contact with the patient. By this means they can avoid or ignore the emotional anxiety or curiosity which may be expressed on the patient's face. In fact, often due to pressures of time, some doctors may show little empathy for the patient and maintain a barrier of professional detachment.

First encounters with the physiotherapist

The majority of patients therefore have been through a selection process before the appointment with the physiotherapist. The patient will bring with them their problem, now influenced by their degree of satisfaction with the doctor's clinical interview. Thornquist (1990) studied first encounters between physiotherapists and patients to discover the 'complexity and social organization of the interaction'. The professional's contribution can influence strongly 'the patient's attitude towards his own body and health problems and his motivation for treatment'.

There is, by nature of the profession, a great deal more touch between therapist and patient than there is between doctor and patient. However, Thornquist questions whether physiotherapists disembody the patient and refer to 'it' – the body – as a thing apart, something which is a 'sheath or a container' for the inner self. Or do they regard the human frame as integral to the person themselves, with experiences, emotions, needs and energies?

Her researches identified a therapist who focused her attention on 'local conditions and joint mobility' and who explained the symptoms only as a local problem. The therapist explained to the patient 'what she found important and relevant' and prescribed treatment accordingly. This undemocratic narrow approach by the physiotherapist was reinforced by talking to the half-dressed patient who lay on the treatment couch, i.e. in a position of vulnerability. The treatment and exercise recommendations were presented didactically by the physiotherapist, with no consultative process with the patient as to her social and emotional well-being.

A second interview presented a physiotherapist who was much more concerned with the total physical and emotional health of her patient. She did not present herself as the expert, but involved her patient in the 'consultative process'. She did not ask the patient to undress before questioning her, and maintained the communication as between equals. The dialogue was 'semi-structured', with both open and closed questions and with opportunities for two-way communication.

Thornquist is concerned that the first interview reinforces the mind/body dichotomy which besets Western medical thinking, and though verbally the physiotherapist showed 'acknowledgement, acceptance and interest', her examination showed 'distance and neglect' of the whole person.

This surely is 'safe' treatment by a physiotherapist: to attend to a series of symptoms rather than the person who is experiencing those symptoms; to present oneself as the expert, with a series of treatments which can be applied as a set formulae over a set period of time. This reinforces a stereotypical form of professional behaviour, at the expense of establishing real communication with the patient. It ensures the therapist relates to patients as 'objects' rather than complex personalities whose bodies are inextricably part and expression of who they are.

How much more crucial is it, in the psychiatric field, that physiotherapists consult democratically with the patient? Face-to-face discussion is important because it enables the patient to feel secure and accepted when they may have many fears about even being sent into the mental health area. Public stigma still exists against those who seek help for mental disorder. It is very important that an opportunity is given for patients not only to express their anxieties concerning their physical symptoms, but of the moods and emotions that are part of their malaise. Often, outpatients in phases of acute mental anxiety or inpatients with more evident mental illness feel disorientation and despair within their bodies and in their relationships to the world around them. To 'objectify' symptoms, indeed their whole body, is to reinforce this sense of dichotomy.

In a further paper, Thornquist analysed the interviewing procedures of physiotherapists to discover how much the therapist, in their questioning of the patient, acknowledges or ignores points raised by the patient, i.e. how much the questioning is confined within the therapist's own narrow range of reference, thereby implicitly defining what is relevant. Patients may only be difficult because their relationship with their therapist is defined within such a narrow context. If they feel excluded from the consultative process, objectified and perhaps even dictated to, enthusiastic co-operation cannot be expected.

Non-compliance

Having received recommendations from the doctor and advice from the physiotherapist, why do patients not comply?

As previously mentioned, patients have their own beliefs regarding the quality and maintenance of their own health and ideally will draw upon them when considering life-style habits, preventative measures against illness, and acceptance of risk factors given with medical advice. Calnan (1987) advises that there is a fallibility in the theory because people only consider it when they are ill, rather than using it as a premise to keep them well.

Patients do not comply because they sometimes do not understand instructions or forget them. Others consciously ignore what they are requested to do because of mistrust of prescribed medication, scepticism or resistance or inability to change. Also, if the advice given is unrealistic within the patient's social culture, there will be very little compliance.

Compliance, therefore, is based on negotiation with the patient to avoid a mismatch between their needs and the therapist's expectations. The counselling skills of physiotherapists are just as important as their ability to help physical disorder. Saunders and Maxwell (1988) emphasize the importance of 'effective personal relationships' with patients. The physiotherapist spends 'longer in a one-to-one relationship with patients than any other member of hospital staff'. This results in patients invariably revealing 'their innermost feelings and emotions ranging from fear, anxiety and inadequacy on the one hand to hope, progress and achievement on the other'.

The physiotherapist 'listens, observes, interviews, instructs, persuades, and recommends'. Returning to the point that a doctor's questions can be 'closed or open', the same principle applies to the questioning of the physiotherapist. 'Where does it hurt?' is more closed than "Tell me about your problem'. Saunders and Maxwell emphasize the need for 'reflecting', i.e. statements of facts or feelings representing the essence of the patient's message which are fed back for 'verification, clarification and extension'.

It is important that the physiotherapist has time for the patient and is not attempting to attend to two patients in alternating cubicles. The physical set-up of the clinic is also important, to ensure privacy. Also, there should not be too much distracting noise in the area, and the patient and therapist should be able to sit face to face with equal status. This allows each to read the other's body language and to establish eye contact. Although it is professionally important to keep medical records, this should not be at the expense of giving full concentration to the patient.

Saunders and Maxwell emphasize that the physiotherapist does not echo the patient's words, but must select the essential from the inessential, without distortion or interpretation. This is not psychoanalysis, but getting to the core of what that human being is feeling in that particular circumstance. They warn, however, that it is important not to raise the subject of feelings and then to leave the patient 'in mid-air' without a natural supportive conclusion to the encounter. Patients particularly value such support and interest from therapists.

A supportive conclusion is also important, to identify what effort the patient has to make to help himself, to re-emphasize instructions which may have been given, and to organize follow-up. It is helpful to have some exercise class into which a patient can be placed when they have progressed from individual treatment. This allows supervision to continue without undue demands on the physiotherapist's time.

Communication with the mentally ill

Communication with the very mentally sick is a challenge: first, the patient's perception of themselves in relation to the world may have become very distorted; secondly, they may lack or have abandoned the social skills needed for normal social interaction; thirdly, by hospitalization, the patient has adopted the sick role and renounced their autonomy as an individual. This latter point is a mixed blessing because although their personal risks are reduced, it encourages passivity, and they are removed from their normal social context.

Physiotherapists may encounter these patients because they have need of the physiotherapist's skills for an additional acute or chronic physical disability or are participants in a recreational exercise group which involves social interaction and co-operation. In groups, character traits of the respective illnesses are exaggerated and a therapist must not accept patients if it is obvious they will be disruptive or threatening to others.

The role of the 'other'

Argyle (1969) cites, as the basis of most inappropriate behaviours, the inability to identify with the other, i.e. the skill to imagine oneself in the role of the listener and observer to one's own interactions. Mentally ill people may fail to do this. Whether the cause is genetic, familial or organic can never be known. However, it is important to give clear instructions, responses and support to such patients, and also to keep the interactions focused on practical situations in the immediate time span.

For brevity's sake, the examination will confine itself to the social interaction problems of two categories of mental illness – but such categorization should be treated with caution – those of schizophrenia and depression.

Schizophrenia

Schizophrenia is the most common form of psychosis whose cause has yet to be discovered. The symptoms of schizophrenic behaviour manifest themselves as 'withdrawal from social relationships, disturbance of thought and speech, failure of persistent goal-directed behaviour, and flattening of emotions' (Argyle, 1969). Their voices will lose emotional colour and they fail to 'emesh' or to interact within conversational pauses satisfactorily. They will either maintain an inordinately long silence or interrupt. This can be because they do not use eye contact to read the interpersonal signals of the person with whom they are communicating. They will stare rather blankly or avoid eye contact. Their physical spacing can either be too close or beyond communication range. They are not happy when asked to socialize and become isolates in general society. They often neglect personal grooming and their dress becomes scruffy, which is also a detraction. Schizophrenics may appear detached and unresponsive to the friendliness of the staff because of their insensitivity to other people's emotional stimuli. This is called a 'lack of affiliative motivation'.

Falloon *et al.* (1984) give advice to assist the family of schizophrenics who often suffer to the point of breakdown from the lack of affiliation of their afflicted member. It is very important that schizophrenics have the 'long-term continuity of a supportive relationship'. This means that if, for example, a physiotherapist is running a recreational group in the community, consistency of staffing is important. Equal to recreational benefit is the need to enhance the social training and to encourage functional (as opposed to dysfunctional) methods of communication. They list the following skills as the 'minimum sufficient repertoire':

1. Communication of positive feelings for specific positive behaviour.
2. Communication of negative feelings for specific negative behaviour.

3. Making positive requests for change of specific behaviours.
4. Attentive listening behaviour when discussing problems.

The physiotherapists must be aware of these social skills and try to reinforce their implementation in the immediate social situation in which they encounter this group of patients. It is important to:

- establish face-to-face communication
- deal with the immediate practical situation
- use specific direct rudimentary instructions without imagery (which in a patient in a delusional state can be misinterpreted)
- state how you would feel if the patient co-operated with your request
- give reinforcing praise for compliance and co-operation – even the smallest improvement must be given recognition.

Schizophrenics are sensitive to criticism and also will become upset if there is any disturbance among other members of the group. If they are manifesting anti-social behaviour, however, it is necessary to communicate your disapproval clearly in words. They are unable to read emotion from body language alone (Argyle, 1978).

Sometimes, delusions and hallucinations are imposing themselves in the patient's mind and a host of other powers, voices and persons, deified or demonic, are persuading, cajoling or confusing the mind of the patient. Empathic contact helps to dispel the acute paranoid experience, but the patient's body language may well be in tune with this internal conflict rather than with that of the people around him. Do not collude with the delusions when the patient tells you about them. Acknowledge that you have heard what the patient is saying, but focus them back on the activity or task in hand.

Arieti (1974) states that in the acute phase patients experience 'an increased acuity of perception. Noises seem louder, colours are more pronounced'. Added to this may be a failure of cognitive processes to understand perception. This perception has regressed often to an 'inability to see wholes'. People, objects and the background environment are not perceived in scale to each other. A patient's psyche is dominated by one part at one time of a person, object or background. This is a regression to the early stages of postnatal development: babies can only focus on 'parts' such as the mother's face or breast and not on her as a whole person.

If the physiotherapist therefore brings the patient who has been hospitalized in an acute state into an environment with too much auditory and visual stimuli, she will be inadvertently creating more confusion and a tendency to regress, instead of co-operation and communication.

It must also be remembered that any patient suffering from states of paranoia may interpret extraneous sound, movements and interruptions, for example people walking past the window, as a threat. Therefore, physiotherapists should bring such individuals into pleasant, secure and reasonably private environments.

Depression

Depression is a 'disturbance of mood' (Arieti, 1974) which can vary in severity. A description of depression, especially as it afflicts the elderly, is included in other chapters and discussion will be given to the necessity to obtain the co-operation of the depressed patient. Their illness can be complicated by physical illness or disability which may be primary or secondary to the depression. In either, this will greatly affect the patient's ability to comply or co-operate with the programme of rehabilitation.

The physiotherapist will not be greeted with any enthusiasm. The whole aura of the person will pervade a sense of flatness, fatigue, sullen silence and un-willingness. They may express little confidence in any measures designed to help them and become passive, dependent patients. Fatalism and low self-esteem will colour their thoughts and actions. They will often withdraw from activity groups because the social interaction skills required prove too much for them.

Manic states are the very opposite in their behaviour and a physiotherapist will find the person loquacious, self-opinionated and dominating to the point of disruption. They will not withdraw from a group but will be insensitive to the other members within the group. Bipolar depressives can go from one state to another, but this is uncommon.

Alongside the medical treatment of depression and the organic cause is the need for the establishment of therapeutic relationships between therapist and patient. It will be non-productive to tell the patient their anxieties are groundless, or to become too subjectively caught up in the necessity to establish a relation-ship with a depressed person. It is, however, important to set realistic routines for their patterns of daily living while they are hospitalized and gently and firmly to insist on the maintenance of the routines. Within this framework, the patient is encouraged to deal with immediate practical events. At a deeper level is the need to adjust or come to terms with causative social factors. This takes time, thera-peutic support and a certain amount of self-analysis for cognitive retraining.

Establishing communication with the depressed patient
In order to establish communication with the patient suffering from depression, consideration must be given to the following:

1. There is obviously a greater need for the counselling role in dealing with depression; therefore it is important to know the full social history of the patient and to not confine one's knowledge solely to the physical symptoms.
2. To be prepared to spend time with the patient before any physiotherapy practices can be carried out. This may be necessary in order to establish rapport and to enable the patient to relax.
3. To be empathic but objective in order to maintain a firm construct to the therapeutic process. In deep depression, patients need their symptoms and often fail to respond to the most well-intentioned treatments. Be realistic about compliance.
4. To make initial contact on a one-to-one basis before asking them to join a group. Patients often do not have the confidence to cope socially during the acute stage of their illness. Request the company of a ward nurse for reassurance initially.
5. To maintain good contact with the rest of the therapeutic team in order to present a consistency of effort and programme.
6. To also use this contact to support oneself. The treatment can drain one's energy!
7. To approve and reinforce any initiatives or participation by the patient, particularly with the use of supportive gestures and smiles.

8. Pendleton and Hasler (1983) advise that patients may provide information which is not verifiable, but which may be responses in order to obtain what they want; for example, 'I am no longer in pain', 'I want to go and lie on my bed' or, more likely, 'I don't know', 'I don't want to today', which may be an attempt to be left alone and not interfered with. This is characteristic of their introverted mood. If co-operation cannot be achieved on one particular day, it is important to negotiate that some kind of participation will take place on another agreed day.

9. If there is continued refusal, it may be because there is distortion and confusion in the mind of the patient and this should be checked by finding out the inferences and assumptions which may be in their minds.

10. It must never be forgotten that the patient's needs are more important than the therapist's perception of those needs. As an 'expert', the therapist may assume they know what is best for the patient without listening to and negotiating with the person involved.

Heron (1986) describes six basic categories of authoritative and facilitatory interventions, which are divided into:

Authoritatively and facilitatory interventions

1. Prescriptive advice, which attempts to guide the behaviour of the patient to making their own decisions (rather than giving advice directly which may be ignored.)
2. Giving information which again enables the patient to take more responsibility for their own decisions.
3. Confronting in a positive manner the negative communication signals of the patient. It is important that the physiotherapist does not take on the parental role, nor imply criticism of the patient as a person rather than just the behaviour of the patient at that time.
4. Cathartic – that is, permitting the patient to express grief or anger or other strong emotions safely. This may involve re-experiencing the trauma which caused disability.
5. Catalytic – that is, to encourage the patient to change by reflecting not only on their immediate circumstances but on the greater possibilities.
6. Supportive – that is, to encourage and praise efforts made by the patient.

Patients within the community

Community care emphasizes the psychosocial approach to care rather than the medical methods of intervention. It is more accessible, therefore providing intervention at an earlier stage, and combines the skills of a multidisciplinary team and contacts with the resources in the community at a voluntary and social services level (Sheppard, 1991).

The role of the physiotherapist within this team is discussed in Chapter 5. It is obvious that a negotiated and agreed programme of effort must be organized realistically within the patient's lifestyle rather than superimposed dictates. Communication with the closest and most caring family member is important. Three case examples illustrate the psychosocial approach to care:

A man suffering from schizophrenia broke both ankles in a suicide attempt. A visit to his home enabled his mother, with whom he still lived, to express her concern regarding his ability to get to the first-floor bedroom. It was realistically put to her that her son must remain mobile instead of being waited on by an already stressed mother.

A bachelor in his fifties suffered a left hemiplegia. He was admitted several months later for depression, where his mobility was maintained but always with one person's support. A visit to the nursing home where he resided proved he was being treated as a dependent elderly like the rest of the inhabitants. It was not possible to move him from the nursing home, but instructions and demonstrations were given to the staff. Also it was arranged for him to visit the local Stroke Club and he was befriended by somebody from the local MIND organization who took him out for weekly visits.

A 58-year-old woman was hospitalized for depression, associated with the development of Parkinson's disease which was still in its early stages. Her 26-year-old daughter gave up her job to be with her mother. A home visit was arranged to encourage more independence in the mother. It was apparent that considerable strain was being put on the daughter by the invalid role the mother was adopting. There was a certain inconsistency between the activity she demonstrated for the physiotherapist and that she found unable to do at home. The daughter was able to discuss openly the increasing restriction on her life created by her mother's apparent unwillingness to help herself. The mother, on the other hand, spoke of her fear of being left alone. Both were able to express their anxieties, which considerably eased the atmosphere. The physiotherapist visited the mother when she was on her own to establish confidence in mobility and also brought the matter to the attention of the social services team. The daughter, who had professional qualifications, was able to look for part-time employment.

On these occasions, the physiotherapist is, in fact, interviewing and assessing the domestic situation. The initial part of the interview will be establishing relationships and only when a certain amount of trust has been developed will the therapist become aware of the truth of the quality of the relationship between the individuals concerned. Communication thus needs to

- interview – that is, to ask questions which discover the quality of lifestyle of the patient and their carers
- discover the quality of the emotional relationship between the patient and the carer; a stressed carer will not be able to reinforce any activity suggested by the physiotherapist
- establish confidence that the present activities and more can be accomplished safely
- informing – only a percentage of information given is remembered, so the most important information should be stressed first, while the rest should be rationed
- encourage exercises – as they do not form part of the average person's culture, teaching exercises is in most cases unrealistic; however, recreation can be encouraged if it is associated with a pleasurable environment and provided that whatever is requested is negotiated with and not imposed upon the patient
- setting goals (again, negotiated and not imposed); the goals to be achieved in a mental health setting may be aimed at a subjective reduction in symptoms, more varied social functioning or more positive cognitive reasoning – these are less tangible but just as important as the pragmatic aims set by general physiotherapy practice

- follow-up – this should be promised and carried out, either by phone or in person, and should reflect the growth in rapport and trust between therapist and patient, even if there has not been too much tangible progress: the patient needs praise if only just to keep trying.

Conclusion

It is not intrusive or medicalizing a patient's life unduly to make the effort to discover a true picture of (a) the patient's needs, (b) the patient's anxieties and expectations, and (c) the wider social circumstances.

A proper 'contract of care' emphasizes the need for the 'expert' to be modest in their approach. The patient has more insight and understanding of their problem than is realized, but often is too inhibited to give the share of the information needed. Health professionals must give time to listen and must encourage participation rather than passivity. It is vitally important, therefore, that therapists listen with an open mind, and 'negotiate with' rather than 'talk at' someone who seeks help. Even the most disturbed patients will sense intuitively those who approach them with respect and calmness. It is a skill which must not be taken for granted but which must be studied like any other skill. Remember the Scottish proverb: Hear twice before you speak once!

References

Argyle, M. (1969) *Social Interaction*, Tavistock

Arieti, S. (1974) *Interpretation of Schizophrenia*, Crosby, Lockwood Staples

Calnan, M. (1987) *Health and Illness: The Lay Perspective*, Tavistock

Falloon, T., Boyd, J. and McGill, C. (1984) *The Family Care of Schizophrenia*, Guilford Press,

Freeling, P. and Harris, C.M. (1984) *The Doctor Patient Relationship*, Churchill Livingstone

Heron, G. Quoted in Lyttle (1986) *Mental Disorder*, Balliere Tindall, P. 116

Pendleton, D. and Hasler, J. (1983) *Doctor–Patient Communication*, Academic Press,

Root, M. (1986) *Women and their Health Care Principles: A Matter of Communication*. Health Reports

Sheppard, M. (1991) *Mental Health Work in the Community*, Falmer Press

Thornquist, E. (1990) What happens during the first encounter between patient and physiotherapist. *Scandinavian Journal of Primary Health Care*, **8**, 133–138

Young, K. (1989) The phenomenology of the body in medical examinations. *Semiotica*, **73**, 1–2

4

The multidisciplinary team approach to group practice

Tina Everett

Introduction

Group work in physiotherapy during the past 30 years has developed to give less formal instruction and more time for the expression of anxieties and the sharing of symptoms. This chapter discusses the powerful feelings and emotions raised by bringing people together in a therapeutic group. A psychotherapist is not always available, but it is hypothesized here that co-leaders from different disciplines and different experiences of group work can together effect more change, sufficient to justify joint leadership both therapeutically and financially. This, of course, must be demonstrated by careful evaluation of each group using standard rating scales and questionnaires. Help for this may be obtained from the clinical psychology department (see Chapter 6).

Recognition of the unconscious processes which develop in any therapeutic group are best learnt, first, through a look at the individual counselling process and, secondly, in studying the development of group psychotherapy. A physiotherapist running a therapeutic group would be wise to share the leadership with another member of the multidisciplinary team and clients will benefit from the joint experiences of both leaders. They in turn can support each other and preferably be supported by an external supervisor.

Development of group work in physiotherapy

Why groups? When the author trained as a physiotherapist in the late 1960s, much of our work was in groups. There were classes on the wards every morning during which students had to untuck the end of the beds so patients could wiggle their toes, and so on. Most outpatients were selected for a particular exercise group following a brief assessment. These had names such as 'Back extension', 'Shoulder raising' or 'Strong men's leg group'. The taught advantages were that people responded better to exercise when there was an element of competition and a mutual sharing of symptoms. Group work in physiotherapy has moved a long way since then, but the effects of sharing a common problem are still recognized as being of profound benefit and substantiated by the research of group psychotherapists. We now have the development of 'Cardiac rehabilitation' and 'Stress management' groups, 'Back schools' and 'Antenatal classes'. Although these groups are primarily educational, most physiotherapists recognize the necessity of listening to individual needs and fears and to allow time for the sharing of anxieties.

In the area of mental health, physiotherapists are often involved in groups for 'Anxiety management', 'Hyperventilation' or 'Chronic fatigue'. Where possible these groups should be run in conjunction with another member of the multi-disciplinary team (such as a social worker, a nurse trained in cognitive therapy, or an occupational therapist); the importance of co-leadership is expanded upon later. In leading such a group it is important to understand the relationships which will develop in the group and the feelings and emotions which are bound to surface if clients are allowed time to express themselves.

The individual counselling process

To appreciate the emergence of feelings and emotions it is first necessary to look at the individual counselling process which is done here through a fictitious character (based on real ones) and then to follow this person through to a phys-iotherapy group. We shall look at Sarah, a lady in her late thirties who reports to her GP with panic attacks, lethargy and lost ability to concentrate at work. The GP refers her to the practice nurse, Kate, a trained counsellor who after an initial one-hour interview agrees to see her for a programme of counselling for 10 consecutive weeks and then review the progress.

At the first session, Kate welcomes Sarah and introduces herself. She explains that she will keep strictly to the one-hour time and that the purpose is for Sarah to talk about her problems and any other issues which she finds important. Kate will not give advice but she may ask occasional questions. It will be up to Sarah only to disclose what she wants and in her own time. Kate assures her of complete confidentiality, but informs her that she (Kate) will attend her own supervision group where she might offload some of Sarah's problems without mentioning names or give-away details.

Kate has arranged the room where she can see the clock easily and positioned herself at near right angles to her client. There is no telephone in the room and interruptions are not allowed. Sarah is asked if she would like to outline her problem but to take her time. She is obviously nervous and is silent for a while, avoiding any eye contact. After a few minutes she says she feels really embarrassed and a complete failure at needing to take up the counsellor's time when there are far more needy people about. It is because of the difficulties at work that Sarah has decided she must get help. After a few more minutes' silence, Kate asks if it would help to explain what she finds difficult at work. .Tears flow as Sarah talks about the panic attacks that started a few months ago and how she is avoiding responsibility at work where possible, for fear of further attacks. She describes chest pain and headaches that are increasing as she tries to carry on with work and cope with two young teenagers. She says it would be easier to accept if it was just a physical problem, but she has seen the cardiologist and has been reassured there is nothing wrong with her heart or lungs. She knows the doctor is right and that it is induced by anxiety, but it makes her feel so very inadequate.

Sarah spends the rest of the session exploring her current situation. She describes how her husband's small business is struggling for survival in the recession, which puts an added burden of responsibility on her to be the main breadwinner. She tells how she tries to hide difficulties from her husband as he has enough problems of his own and is seldom around to give her any attention. The children seem to have become more argumentative of late, but she realizes that this may be related to her diminishing patience/tolerance. The older one is also tending to stay out late, causing her worry and making her husband very angry with him.

Kate listens intently, realizing that this is the first time Sarah has had so much time just to focus on her own despair. By accepting Sarah as she honestly presents herself, she is enabling her to begin to accept herself.

Near the end of the session Kate reflects back to Sarah that she must feel life is very difficult just at the moment, but she has been very courageous to admit to it. Next week she may want to explore her feelings of anxiety and where they are coming from.

There are many clients who attend for physiotherapy treatment and who for years are unable to make connections of their physical symptoms with their present anxiety or their past emotional trauma. Sarah has already begun to make links which will help enormously in the healing process. As Kate writes notes on the session, she realizes that she identifies closely with Sarah. She also has two difficult teenage children and must be careful to remain empathic without over-identification. She resolves to bring this up at her supervision group so that her own feelings do not intrude into the next counselling session.

At the next two sessions Sarah describes events from her past which relate to her present anxieties. Her mother was also 'the anxious type' and was very restrictive. Sarah felt she hardly had time to grow up and become independent before she started her own family. Her mother died just when her youngest was starting school and Sarah decided the best diversion from both events was to go back to work, which proved a wise decision at the time.

At the fifth session Sarah arrived five minutes late and sat down and sighed heavily before she began. She said she had had a panic attack just as she was getting ready and was sure that the counselling was not helping her. She said it was her own fault and thought it best not to come any more. It was difficult to spare the time and Kate would be better helping someone else. Kate felt angry and guessed Sarah was projecting angry feelings onto her, even though her words disguised this.

Discussion

This case history is now examined in more detail. Freud was one of the first analysts to consider the stages of development of a young baby and named them the oral, anal and genital stages. Jacobs (1985) calls these 'the oral, dependency, trust stage, the anal authority, autonomy stage and the genital, oedipal, rivalry, social stage'. Problems in developing and or parenting at any of these stages can lead to neuroses and other psychological problems in adult life. Psychodynamic counselling is a way of looking back at these stages and helping to put right what has gone wrong. It is not a quick or easy process, as people build up defences to protect themselves from deeper levels of pain and often these can only be looked at over a long period of time. Sarah's anxiety about dependency on her counsellor and feeling she is wasting her time is related to her mother's over-protectiveness, and is known as experiencing transference in the client/counsellor relationship.

Melanie Klein, who was a student of Freud but later went her separate way, looked more closely at the infantile development of the mother/child relationship. She describes the first 4 months of a baby's life as a time when it can only be attached to objects which are part of the whole mother and are divided into good and bad (e.g. the good breast and the bad breast). She calls this the paranoid–schizoid position, where the child has both an idealized and a terrifying picture of the mother, and is only later able to recognize these as parts of the same person.

Just as the child is terrified of destroying the mother by attacking the bad object, so the adult patient may fear destroying the counsellor or her relationship with her. The counsellor's task is then to remain available and non-judgemental, allowing expression of bad feelings, e.g. anger and envy. Klein suggests the baby separates good and bad feelings into separate compartments by 'splitting', believing the good experiences come from a good mother and the bad from a bad mother; in this way the bad cannot damage the good. This is seen in the adult in the concept of good and bad political ideals, or in the religious belief of God and the Devil.

In Sarah's case splitting may occur if she idealizes her counsellor as the perfect person and sees only bad in herself. Kate's task is first to recognize this and then to point out to Sarah that in idealizing her she is denying her own value and strength.

Occasionally this idealization in the counsellor/client relationship becomes so extreme that she is almost worshipped and the dependency becomes nearly impossible to cope with. This is called eroticized transference and is another situation that needs detailed and regular discussion with a skilled supervisor and very careful handling.

The group process

From Sarah's experience of individual counselling we can go on to suppose she is invited to attend a 'Hyperventilation' group run by a physiotherapist. The aims of this group are to educate the members about the causes and effects of hyperventilation and to look for practical ways to make changes which will relieve symptoms. Groups like this should allow time for some mutual sharing of symptoms and for some rapport to build up with the leader and the co-members. Opportunity must be given for asking questions, homework may be set and progress discussed from week to week. Much work has been done on group therapy and a physiotherapist should never aim to run her group as in-depth psychotherapy. However, it is helpful to look at the development of group psychotherapy and to be aware of the unconscious processes which develop within any group which meets for a set purpose. In studying this, the physiotherapist may consider the advantages of sharing the leadership with another member of the multidisciplinary team (MDT) who is trained in counselling techniques and preferably has some experience in running groups. As co-leaders they will allow time for the expression of feelings within the group and to look at life events in order to relate the past with present symptoms. From this type of group some clients may recognize their need to explore this further and for the first time find it acceptable to consider individual counselling. Others may find that sufficient connections can be made through the short 8–10-week group to make significant life changes.

The 1940s has been called the 'group decade', largely due to the work of Wilfred Bion in developing group techniques for the 'war effort' and then afterwards in pioneering therapeutic communities to help the 'war wounded'. He studied medicine and psychiatry and Melanie Klein was his psychoanalyst. The study of group behaviour began much earlier, at the latter part of the nineteenth century, and was initially based on observations of crowd behaviour. Le Bon, in 1895, observed that when individuals are transformed into a group they are 'put in possession of a sort of collective mind which makes them feel, think and act in a manner quite different from which each individual would feel, think and act if he were in a state of isolation'. In other words, Le Bon saw group behaviour as a type of hypnosis, whereas Freud saw the group merely as a vehicle in which the individual could be freed from the repressions of his unconscious impulses. Trigant Burrow was one of the early psychoanalysts to see the possibility of analysis in a group setting and is known for the view that 'an individual discord is but the symptom of a social discord'. About the same time, Moreno was working with groups in Vienna and was more concerned with social interaction. He later developed methods of psychodrama and sociodrama which focused treatment on providing reality-testing situations.

Bion (1955) describes the two levels of group functioning: first, where the group sets about its task for which it was set up; and secondly, the emotional functioning which may work in opposition to the conscious work and take over the energies of the group. He describes three ways in which this may happen: (a) the group may be dependent on the leader to provide the answers and do the work for them; (b) they may set up two members to find a solution; or (c) they may 'take flight' and claim the task is too difficult or they have not enough information, etc. These are all described as defences and in the therapeutic group are the individual's way of avoiding rejection. Bion and Ezriel saw the task of the leader as non-directive and passive, offering an interpretation of what is going on and demonstrating that despite any of the defensive behaviour the individuals are accepted, not thrown out, and allowed to express their true feelings. In learning to do this in the therapeutic group they can transfer this skill to other relationships and abandon more neurotic behaviour.

Foulkes (1975) initiates a method which he termed 'group analytic psychotherapy' in which he believes that the group members could give more meaningful interpretations to individuals than the leader. In fact, he uses the terms 'conductor', 'guardian' and 'guide' rather than 'leader'.

A common phenomenon in all group work is the recognition of 'scapegoating'. Foulkes feels it important that in selecting members for a group there should be no major differences between one person and the rest in age, class, colour, sect, etc. However carefully the group is selected (and this may not always be possible or advisable), there will be times when one member is scapegoated and all the bad feelings are projected onto that person. Some people unconsciously set themselves up to be the scapegoat. The leader will need to recognize and interpret this and sometimes protect the 'scapegoat' from the aggressive feelings of other members.

One of the main reasons for a careful selection interview is to assess whether the client will be able to function in a group setting. The author's personal experiences of clients unsuitable for our particular groups include those with very fixed beliefs/values related to religion or the position of women in society; or the expression, in a powerfully disruptive way, of psychotic ideas. Although Whitely and Gordon (1979) have found that patients suffering from schizophrenia and acute psychosis can benefit from group therapy, it is unlikely that they would be helped by a physiotherapy stress management or hyperventilation group and could be very disturbing to other patients.

The initial interview also enables the client to meet the group leaders, ask questions about the group, and establish whether they are prepared to make a commitment of 8–10 weeks. The referring agent (GP or psychiatrist) may be of help where there is uncertainty, but the final decision must rest with the group leaders and the client themselves. In some instances the client may have been coerced into attending the group (e.g. by their doctor) via the mechanism of withholding further treatment until after completion of the group. This in itself is not a reason for exclusion, but should be recognized and worked through.

In the ongoing group, transference relationships predominate. The group leader and the other group members take on images of key figures from the individual's past and present life situation. How far this can be explored within the group will depend on the level of trust which has built up, but it is important to recognize that angry, jealous and suspicious feelings from the past begin to surface in the group and need careful handling. Counter-transference is also likely to occur where the group leader experiences similar negative feelings towards one or more group members. This is where supervision for the group leaders becomes essential. In fact, sometimes the supervisor may be the first to recognize the unconscious transference and counter-transference processes going on and can interpret these to the leaders.

Yalom (1975) believes that co-leaders should be of equal status and experience, but Whitely and Gordon (1979) feel that this may be a disadvantage and that the less experienced leader can add fresh insight as well as being supported in difficult situations. The present author suggests that in a hyperventilation group co-leaders of different disciplines will have complementary skills and can benefit from each other's experience. The physiotherapist who is not used to this type of group work will benefit from the insights of a community psychiatric nurse, social worker or occupational therapist, while bringing her own skills in teaching relaxation or explaining the relationship between physical symptoms, incorrect breathing patterns and the build up of stress and anxiety. Joint planning of the programme and supportive evaluation of each group will lead to a more effective outcome. Debriefing at the end of each session will prevent too much unwanted 'baggage' interfering with the next patient contact or being taken home at the end of the day.

Boundaries

In psychotherapy and psychodynamic counselling the counsellor or conductor do not talk about themselves or give information about their own personal circumstances. Physiotherapists may be accustomed to talking about their family or social life in making conversation with patients, though hopefully do not offload their own problems onto them. Teachers of antenatal classes will find mothers are always interested in the physiotherapist's own birth experiences, though the more mature teachers will minimize the details.

It is important for the group leaders to discuss boundaries before starting any therapeutic group, and issues of self-disclosure and sharing of experiences is a major boundary. Direct personal questions can be deflected with 'I'm wondering if its important to you to know that' or, more bluntly, 'I don't think it's helpful to talk about my own situation here'. Often other group members will back the leader on this and ease any difficult tension. Group members will be very sensitive to any feelings of embarrassment, anxiety or annoyance on the part of the leaders. Sometimes it helps to say 'I'm picking up feelings of anxiety (or anger) and wonder if anyone knows what that's about', so that the feelings are brought into the open and given back to the group.

Another important boundary is confidentiality, and this must be discussed at the first session. In a hospital setting, members may be anxious about what reports will be written and the information that will be fed back to other professionals. It might be wise to offer to show any written report to the individual concerned. If the group is being used for any form of research, permission must be obtained and individual identities disguised by more than just names. It is always helpful to explain the reason for the leader's own supervision and the confidentiality maintained within that. Group members are then invited to share only what they feel comfortable with and to maintain confidentiality about their peers.

One of the selection criteria for a group might be an assessment of the client's ability to maintain an acceptable level of discretion, but in any event it will take time to build up trust with one another.

Touch is another sensitive issue, and psychotherapists tend to avoid any physical contact with their clients. Physiotherapists are used to touching their patients in the course of physical treatments and may feel it is appropriate and sometimes even essential to touch someone when teaching relaxation or diaphragmatic breathing exercises in the group situation. Sensitivity is required, and permission must be sought first and reticence accepted. Massage may be introduced as a form of relaxation, along with a discussion on the benefits of other complementary therapies. In one of the author's groups, participants asked for a demonstration of foot massage, with one member volunteering as model. They did not feel comfortable about massaging each other's feet, but some felt they could try it out at home with members of their own family. An interesting discussion on feelings about touch occurred as a result of this. In another group, at a residential regional secure unit, the clients enjoyed learning to massage each other's hands and feet in a safe non-threatening situation.

Curative factors

Yalom (1970) discusses at length the curative factors in group therapy. We will look at these as experienced by our imaginary client Sarah in the physiotherapy 'Hyperventilation' group. First, the 'imparting of information' which can be divided into two areas.

The group programme will include information on the physiological responses to stress, normal and abnormal breathing patterns, anatomy of the heart and lungs, respiration, etc. Sarah did not realize that her lungs reached from her shoulders nearly to the bottom of her rib cage. She was never quite sure exactly where her heart was (people always said it was on the left side). She had never realized that she only breathed in the upper part of her chest. All these facts were relevant and interesting, but the most important learning was that she could now have some control over her panic attacks. Even if the breathing did not help every time, it was something to work at. The second obvious area of imparting of information would happen more subtly over the whole course of the group. That is, Sarah began to understand how talking through her problems, past and present, could bring about change. Yalom feels that the group gives patients a major opportunity to gain insight into their own behavioural patterns. This then leads to an awareness of and control over emotional disturbance.

The next curative factor is the 'installation of hope', and now that Sarah understood what actually happened in her body when she was over-anxious she had hope that she could gain control of the frightening symptoms. The author usually starts a group by asking the clients to talk through their symptoms in pairs and then we list them all together on a flip chart. There are seldom many symptoms that are not shared by others.

Yalom's third factor is 'universality', and Sarah was heartened to find two other women and one young man who also suffered panic attacks. Yet another woman, Marie, was extremely distressed by her teenage children and, in sharing this problem, Sarah was also able to benefit from the fourth factor 'altruism'. She found she was able to support this woman through a shared experience and to tell her how helpful it was to have individual counselling. Marie had always thought counselling was for the mentally ill and would be a very scary process. She was most interested in Sarah's enthusiasm for it.

Another curative factor which Yalom describes is 'corrective recapitulation of the family group'. He feels that patients entered group therapy with a history of bad family experiences, and the developing transference relationships allowed early relationships to be re-explored. Sarah was able to tell the group how her mother's own fears and anxieties had restricted her freedom for as long as she could remember. She was aware from her individual counselling experience that there were still some areas here that would need working through either individually or in a longer term therapy group.

Two further factors are the 'development of socializing techniques' and 'imitative behaviour'. Sarah enjoyed the sharing of experiences with other adults and felt she had missed out on socializing. She noticed how other equally busy women were able to give themselves some time and space and was determined to join an evening class for her own relaxation, possibly a yoga or pottery class.

Yalom puts great importance on 'interpersonal learning' and sees it as a broad and complex therapeutic factor. In order to understand it, one must first recognize the importance of interpersonal relationships and the social microcosm. The dying, the imprisoned and even the very wealthy often fear loneliness and isolation more than anything else. He states that those who leave a therapeutic group may depart for a variety of reasons but never because of boredom or indifference. Every group member is deeply involved in the group and if this is not openly acknowledged it will be expressed in other ways, e.g. dreams, increased anxiety before or after the group, or acting-out behaviour.

Yalom conducted some research into the 'corrective emotional experience'. He looked at whether the emotional experience in itself was sufficient to affect change or what other ingredient was necessary. Much of the 1970s expressed the importance of experience – the 'primal scream', bioenergetics, and other techniques of the encounter group. The necessary ingredient for effecting change was found to be cognitive, i.e. acquiring information and personal insight (as seen above). He also found that whatever school of counselling was followed, either individually or in groups, a good client/counsellor relationship was essential. However, he quotes a team of researchers who asked clients to evaluate the source of help they had received from a short-term crisis group in a 12-month follow-up: 'Forty-two per cent felt that the group members and not the therapist had been helpful, and twenty-eight per cent responded that both had been of aid. Only five per cent stated that the therapist alone was a major contributor to change.' This outcome is backed up by numerous other studies.

Douglas (1976) draws up a list of the basic assumptions upon which group-work practice is founded. These are:

1. That group experience is universal and an essential part of human existence.
2. That groups can be used to effect changes in the attitudes and behaviour of individuals.
3. That groups provide experiences that can be monitored or selected in some way for beneficial ends. Life outside the group is in no way neglected, it tends to be put out of focus in favour of considering the 'here and now' situation within the group.
4. That groups offer experience shared with others so that all can come to have something in common with the sense of belonging and of growing together.
5. That groups produce change which is more permanent than can be achieved by other methods and change which is obtained more quickly also.
6. That groups assist in the removal or diminution of difficulties created by previous exposure to the process of learning.
7. That groups as instruments of helping others may be economical in the use of scarce resources, e.g. skilled workers, time, etc.
8. That a group can examine its own behaviour and in so doing learn about the general patterns of group behaviour (process).

Conclusion

The powerful feelings and emotions raised by bringing people together in a therapeutic group have been discussed. A psychotherapist is not always available, but it is the hypothesis here that co-leaders from different disciplines and different experiences of group work can together effect more change, sufficient to justify joint leadership both therapeutically and financially.

Possible research projects have been considered to attempt to prove this hypothesis, but they would be swamped by many other variables. However, in a stress management group run jointly by the author and a social worker in a care-fully evaluated project, it was noted from verbal evaluation and from a symptom checklist that significant changes had taken place.

Adams (1991) describes her research into running a 'Body orientated therapy (BOT)' group to reduce depression and improve self-esteem. She writes: 'Personal clinical experience from leading the group suggests that emotional maturity is required to deal professionally with the feelings expressed by the group. For BOT to be effective, access to psychotherapy should be available to help patients accept realised feelings and return to emotional health.'

The group leaders, together with their supervisor will be aware of those clients who, because of the complexity of their past lives, are in need of long-term psychotherapy. They may then be able to steer these people in the direction of further skilled help. If the client is not acknowledging this need for themselves, the leaders can only discuss available options and leave the client to access further help if and when he or she feels it appropriate.

References

Adams, H. (1991) *Free to Move: Free to be Me*, ACCP Foundation Course
Douglas, T. (1976) *Groupwork Practice*, Tavistock
Foulkes, S.H. (1975) *Group-analytic Psychotherapy, Method and Principles*, Gordon and Breach
Jacobs, M. (1985) *The Presenting Past*, Open University Press
Whiteley, J.S. and Gordon, J. (1979) *Group Approaches in Psychiatry*, Routledge and Kegan Paul
Yalom, I.D. (1975) *The Theory and Practice of Group Psychotherapy*, Basic Books

5

Community care and working with carers

Mick Skelly

Introduction

This chapter is not a prescriptive guide for physiotherapists working in the community mental health psychiatry setting. The author intends to provide his own particular perspective based upon the collective practice of the multidisciplinary team of which he is a member. To understand the team's developing approach, a broad knowledge is required of the different models of mental disorder and an awareness of the effectiveness of cognitive–behavioural approaches as detailed by Paul *et al.* (1977). It will also be assumed that any readership composed of health care professionals are conversant with both *The Black Report*, the update on it – *The Health Divide* (Whithead, 1987) – and the work of Totman (1987) on the social causes of ill health.

The actuality of community care has been profoundly influenced by political, ideological and financial considerations. This may continue to be the case in the future. Despite this, there remain health care professionals who wish to distance themselves from the sociopolitical context in which community care is taking place.

The Community Care Act also made commitments for both Health and Social Services. In effect, this amounts to meeting as many of the clients' needs as resources allow so that they can remain in their own homes as long as possible. Where residential provision is required, it is as likely to pass into the private sector as to the public sector or to partnerships between the two. The government has promised 'adequate' resources. This is intended to provide a 'needs' rather than a 'service' led system which will provide overall a higher quality of care at a lower cost.

A service led system is also a 'results led' system, i.e. it selects out those clients who best fit the system and with whom the system can get the fastest results. In terms of health care, the focus is upon technical skills. The working mode is 'condition centred', symptomatic, and addresses physical needs as narrowly as possible. It tends to be authoritarian and treatment centred, with an individual therapist approach or via a 'fragmented' multidisciplinary team (MDT). The author would support this kind of approach as being viable with some clients and ensuring a rapid throughput.

A needs led system is also a 'process led' system, i.e. it attempts to provide a service which fits the individual client and their needs. High interpersonal skills may be primary in such a system; however, high technical skills are also required. A process led system is person centred – it is global, attempting to meet all the client's needs in a package of care arising from the formulation of a care programme.

This latter approach requires a unified MDT which is authoritative yet works collectively with the client, their carers, or client advocate. If anything, its orientation is educational rather than being limited to the provision of treatments.

Within the community mental health team the physiotherapist is considered to be a specialist providing a particular perspective and approach to intervention. Their primary function is to provide a specialist assessment of the client's needs and the possible physiotherapeutic interventions which might meet these needs and to identify who might best provide these interventions. Certain interventions might be specialist, i.e. they can only be provided by the physiotherapist, whereas many interventions can be provided by properly educated carers and/or care staff. Therefore, if the primary role of the physiotherapist is assessment, the secondary role is an educational one in a 'needs' or 'process' led system.

Figures 5.1–5.4 illustrate various models and services in the community mental health/psychiatry setting.

Historical perspective

As Illich *et al.* (1982) argue, the twentieth century has seen an increasing 'medicalization' of many aspects of human experience and this has been

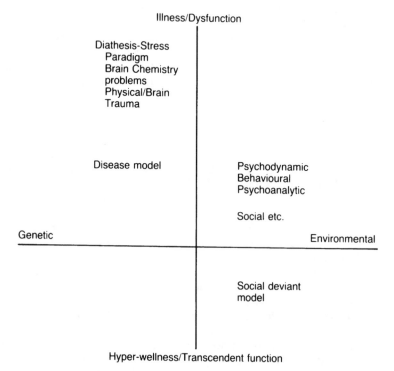

Figure 5.1 Diametrically opposed models influencing community care in mental health/psychiatry

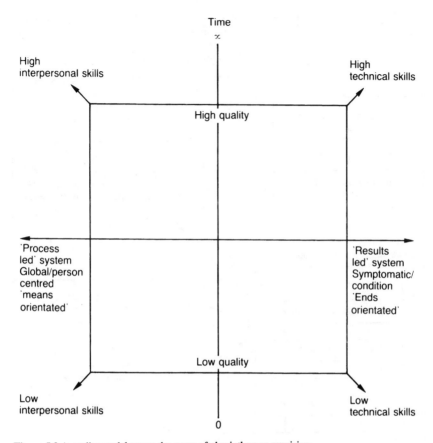

Figure 5.2 A quality model across the range of physiotherapy provision

Quality = Skill(s) + Commitment + Time + Resources

where   Time   = $\dfrac{\text{Clients per day} \times \text{Skills}}{\text{Client type, i.e. 'Results' or 'Process'} + \text{No. of clients}}$

Commitment   = $\dfrac{\text{Morale} + \text{Dedication/Interest in job} + \text{Perceived ability}}{\text{Distress}}$

Skill   = $\dfrac{\text{(Training)}\ \text{Interpersonal ability} + \text{Technical ability} + \text{Eustress}}{\text{Negative perceptions}}$

especially so with regard to psychological distress. There have been powerful critiques of this, the most recent being Breggin (1993), and many other perspectives have evolved; see Kovell (1978). These perspectives have generated, in general, language-based approaches to working with people suffering this kind of distress and the recognition that physical suffering is also likely to generate psychological suffering (and vice versa). It was in this critical environment where, if Paul's research was correct, and to paraphrase Laing

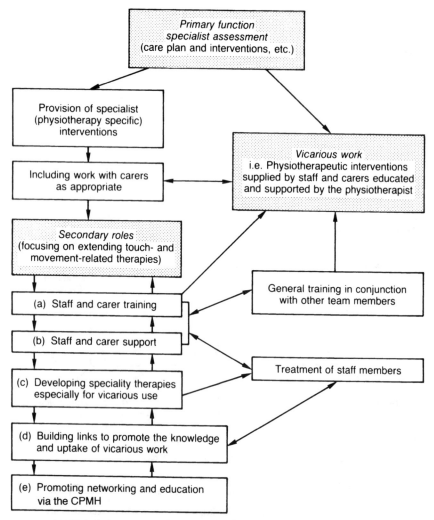

Figure 5.3 Physiotherapy services in the community – evolving functions showing flow of work/care provision (CPMH, Chartered Physiotherapists in Mental Healthcare)

(1967), the people operating an exclusively disease model approach were characterized as the single greatest danger to psychiatric clients and charities as client advocate/pressure groups were formed.

Goffman (1961) was not alone is identifying the potential for abuse in the 'total institutions' which the misnamed asylums afforded. The many scandals and the arguments of both the pressure groups and many concerned practitioners were to provide a reasonable justification for community care. In practice, community care was elevated to Community Care and then hamstrung by several factors:

- erroneous or biased baseline data
- lack of coherence of structure

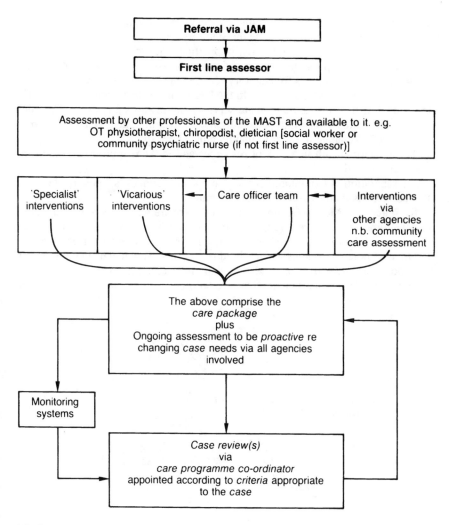

NB. *The case* = Named clients + Carer(s) + Identified relevant 'others' with support or educational needs around the quality of *client care*

Monitoring systems include all types of outcome and quality assurance measures being used plus the carious types of audit

Figure 5.4 Multi-agency support team – provision of services (JAM,Joint Allocation Meeting; MAST, Multi Agency Support Team; OT)

- lack of resources
- competing models of care.

The concept of 'community' has never been clearly defined. The closest to a working definition has perhaps been held within the government's term, 'a mixed economy of care', i.e. where responsibility is shared, presumably equally, between family, neighbours, voluntary services, private provision, and the disparate agencies which comprise the statutory services.

There is no clear single authority, in practice, with the overall responsibility to co-ordinate all possible avenues of care provision from whatever source. Furthermore, the agencies for statutory services provision are being consistently squeezed within a cost led system. In the NHS this has been complicated by the traditional drift of resources to acute services and towards areas of work which health care professionals find personally most rewarding; also generally there is a resistance to change in order to maintain the status quo.

These factors result in a lack of resources and in the inappropriate use of the resources available.

The separation of Community Trusts from acute services is a positive factor in this context, as thereby resources are separate.

Resources for Mental Health Community Care are based upon the number of clients currently being referred to the mental illness services. According to the figures of Goldberg and Huxley (1992), this represents less than one-tenth of the total of potential clients as identified by doctors. This means that there is an enormous disparity between the potential need and the available resources. Indeed it can be argued that services are tailored to fit resources rather than to

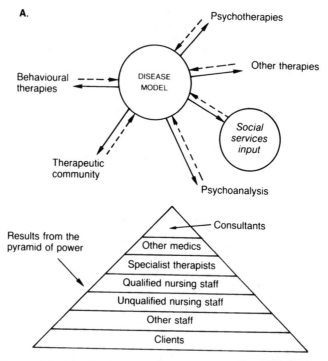

Figure 5.5 Three models of psychiatric care. A, The 'traditional' medical model (the actual provision of care is dominated by the disease model, medication, etc., and doctors). B, The 'eclectic' model (Tyrer and Steinberg, 1984, claim this is the actuality of the 'medical' model). C, The 'psychosocial' model – a functional model in which the most effective approaches are central, with other techniques being fed by specialist staff (see Paul *et al.*, 1977)

meet real needs, this being the gist of the argument of Graham (1984) concerning community care, i.e. it is a 'results' led system masquerading as a 'process' led system.

There are further complicating factors:

1. A purchaser–provider split, where the purchaser is not the consumer.
2. Statistical monitoring systems which focus on face-to-face contacts with named clients rather than the needs around the whole 'case' inclusive of carer support, educational and liaison work, etc.
3. Demographic and other factors, the most important being wealth, which increase disparities in health care provision.
4. The legacy of traditional, institutionally-based practice and competing models of care both within the psychiatric establishment and between it and other agencies which provide care (Figure 5.5).

Another complicating factor is that despite the assertions of Tyrer and Steinberg (1987) that psychiatrists are eclectic in their practice (if this were true, then no more than one in five clients would be on medication) in the present author's experience the dominant model is the disease model. If the dire warnings of Breggin (1993) are accurate, this is likely to remain so. To a large extent the unified and more collective approach of the service the writer works within avoids this kind of problem, as will be outlined later.

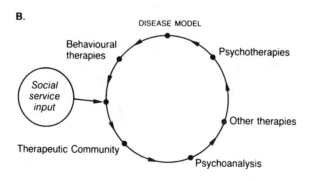

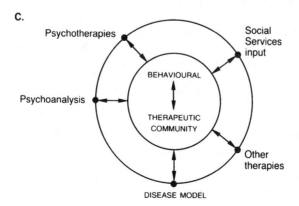

The physiotherapeutic role

The research quoted by Ader is eloquent testimony to the unity of the 'body-mind'. The underlying premise of the physiotherapeutic role in psychiatry is that body and mind are one, like the two ends of a piece of string – one 'gestalten' or pattern existing within four dimensions.

Cognition: what you know or think you know, your thoughts.

Affect: what you feel, your emotional state.

Physiology: your physical state and your chemical state.

Behaviour: what you do, how you do it and how your actions influence your life through their effect upon others.

This four-dimensional pattern does not stand alone, but can be characterized as a subsystem of larger systems such as the family, the neighbourhood, etc. This point was made by Laing in the 1960s.

People do not *have* bodies, they *are* bodies. As Merleau-Ponty (1962) argues, states of mind are validly to be seen as psychophysical states. The 'whole person' is worked with when you work with the body. Conversely, when interpersonal skills are used to work with the client's 'mind', you are also working with the body. Aproaches such as the 'Body-Psychotherapy' of Gerda Boyeson, the Alexander Technique (Maisel, 1969), Shiatsu, and modern Cognitive–Behaviourism come to mind – Yoga, T'ai Chi, etc. Upon careful observation it is apparent that many psychiatric clients are as locked into patterns of body use as they are into patterns of cognition, affect and social behaviour. These can exacerbate stress, become a causal factor in physical conditions through imbalanced muscular use, or affect interpersonal interactions via a posture perceived by others as aggressive for example. Furthermore, self-esteem is largely bound up with how we feel about ourself as a body moving in social space, whether we feel clumsy, ugly, ungainly, unapproachable, etc.; whether we feel fit and physically capable, at home being a body or whether we feel that we 'have' a body which is somehow not 'us', which is both alien and a kind of a trap. In the author's experience many, if not most, psychiatric clients also have a problem with the quality of touch in their lives.

Physiotherapists, like other manual therapists, have a powerful non-linguistic dimension for communication literally at their fingertips. Touch-related therapies, from the various types of massage to mobilizations and manipulations, provide ways of 'listening to', diagnosing and empathizing with the client.

Analysis of posture and movement dynamic can also be used in this way. The author uses a conceptual framework derived from Mclarg-Anderson (via Leslie Crosier), the Alexander Technique, Laban, and T'ai Chi Ch'uan. Other people use different bases, such as Feldenkrais, Dance Movement Therapy, Bobath, etc. Whatever the framework, it provides a way of working and being with the client, a way of mutual discovery and communication, a way of enabling change. It is the physiotherapist's ability to use their skills, whether interpersonal or technical, to enable change in a positive way, from pain relief to radical changes in body use, which affect the client and others around them, focusing upon the bodily aspect of the 'gestalten'.

The above is what makes physiotherapists different from the other practitioners in the Community Mental Health Team (CMHT).

Especially, but not exclusively, with the elderly there is often a problem of increasing disability exacerbated by disabling seating and handling which is so poor that it borders on abuse. It is the elderly who provide the greatest challenge regarding the provision of creative programmes of intervention for the physiotherapist.

It is precisely those clients who do not fit the paradigm of being easily able to be talked with, or counselled, that physiotherapists can work with and provide proactive programmes for. The background of movement/exercise training, massage, handling and mobilizing skills common to all physiotherapists provide a ready facility to further develop knowledge and skills in touch- and movement-related therapies and also provide a perspective that no other member of the CMHT will have. The client will best benefit from the close rapport that a physiotherapist within the CMHT will have with the other members of the team.

The realm of touch- and movement-related therapeutic approaches is just beginning to be explored. They are proving popular with the 'worried well' and individuals in the private market. Within the public system, physiotherapists are required to develop these areas and to complement what the system already offers. It is the physiotherapist who, because of their initial training, is best able to develop and research working practices from this perspective and to establish a working rapport with a client which is beyond, although it includes, the linguistic dimension.

The function of the care programme approach

In the evolving system in Hull, the flexible use of the care programme approach has bridged the chasm of social- and disease-based models of care by the simple expedient of discarding rigid theoretical ideological stances or working practices in favour of addressing the client's needs in a global way.

The team, via the Client Centred Care Programme Approach identify collectively with the 'case' (client/carers/related others in need) – the client's real needs as they experience them. The specialized members of the team each provide a perspective on these needs and subsequently identify all the possible interventions which might help to meet these needs. The Care Programme Approach is a public document in the sense that it goes to the client/carer and the GP, and can be used to identify unmet needs and the shortfall of resources to meet these needs.

In providing coherence of care in the global provision of services for the individual client, the general lack of coherence in the system is sidestepped. This is because it is more concrete and, therefore, easier to consider care provision in the context of the real needs of a person than in the context of a principle of care provision.

In practice, the physiotherapist has to juggle with a number of factors:

- their own scarcity as a resource
- which physiotherapeutically-based interventions can be safely given by others or done by the client themselves (NB client enabling)
- prioritization of clients
- physiotherapist only/specialist interventions
- the inability to ensure the consistency of many other carers as intervention providers

These factors are ever present and are dealt with, in part, by the physiotherapist referring back to their core abilities.

It is the core abilities related to physiotherapeutic practice which make the physiotherapist different from the other members of the MDT. These are briefly considered from the author's perspective below.

The core of physiotherapeutic assessment should be the ability to assess the client across the breadth of their physical needs, including posture, movement dynamic and the influence of environmental stimulation on their overall physical condition.

The core of physiotherapeutic interventions should be touch and movement approaches/therapies plus the use of electrical modalities, among others, where needed.

Counselling, should already be provided by other professionals and cannot

---

Needs

1. Postural re-education

2. Reduction of overall muscular tension, possibly both reflecting and influencing her state of mind

3. Maintenance of mobility; improvement if possible

4. Maintenance/improvement of joint ranges

5. Reduction of pain

6. Increased interaction with others

Strengths

1. Mobile with minimum of assistance

2. Alert and chatty

3. Reasonably compliant

Risk factors
- Increased pain with negative effects on mobility and state of mind.
- Increased stiffness and loss of mobility.
- Posturally-related problems are likely to increase without intervention.
- Increasing likelihood of falls. NB: 'Sudden' movement dynamic.

Possible Interventions
Needs addressed   Intervention

1, 3, ?5, ?2   a Prone lying, before rising and immediately on going to
                      bed, beginning with 5 min and progressing to 15 min.
                      Daily. Care staff

Figure 5.6 A specimen care programme

3, 6, ?5	b	Regular mobilizing, i.e. walking no less than 15 steps hourly (at least). Care staff
2, 6, 5, ?3 ?4	c	Massage. Daily. Physiotherapist and care staff
3, 6, ?4 ?5	d	Patella mobilization. Daily. Physiotherapist and care staff
5, 3, ?4 ?2 ?6	e	Pain relief via electrotherapy. Two to three times weekly. Physiotherapist
1, 2, 4, 6	f	Postural work from an Alexander base. Twice weekly. Physiotherapist. ?Care staff
4, 2, 3, 6, ?5	g	Passive/active-assisted movements plus PNF. Daily. Physiotherapist and care staff
2, 5, 6	h	Relaxation using language-based techniques. NB: Covert rehearsal. Three to four times weekly. Physiotherapist. ?Care staff
3, 4, 5, ?5 ?2	i	Participation in an exercise group and OT. As frequently as possible. Physiotherapist, care staff and OT

The physiotherapy assessment would be included at this point.

Note that this represents only the physiotherapy input of the total care programme. The complete care programme would contain input from other members of the team and would fully consider such issues as the client's social needs, etc.

An outcome measures system which evaluates the success of intervention in a way which makes sense to the client, carer or client advocate is a necessity, especially in the context of the three-way split between purchaser, provider and consumer in the organization of the health market.

Outcome measures – A short note
'What gets measured gets done' (Peters, 1982)

Quality = Skill + Commitment + Time + Resources

where resources are expressed both in terms of 'hardware' – equipment, buildings, staff numbers and profile (human resources), etc.; or 'software' – the accessibility of 'rolling training' and updating/development for staff.

A 'results' led system can use quantitative outcome measures plus qualitative 'snapshots' via Customer Satisfaction Questionnaires and corporate standards.

A 'process' led system, which the Client Centred Care Programme represents, requires a qualitative outcome measures system which is equally as client centred as its primary system.

The Le Roux system, TELER, which is based upon single-case study research methodology dovetails neatly into the philosophy of the Care Programme Approach.

It uses three indicators of effect. Indicators of effect are goals which are functional, simple, and relevant to the client/carer(s)/client advocate and which measure progress in the case.

Each indicator has to be broken down into five steps from the baseline, i.e. where the baseline is 0 the indicator goal is 5. (NB: The position of the baseline can be varied on the scale when the aim of intervention is maintenance or the retardation of decline.)

Each indicator step must be considered as a clinically useful measure by peers and, especially, as a useful measure by the client, etc.

be claimed as a primary role by the physiotherapist, even where they have been trained as counsellors (though counselling skills are useful for the physiotherapist). Language-based relaxation systems, such as guided fantasies, etc., can also be provided just as well by other members of the team, depending on their individual skills.

Due to the relationship a particular practitioner builds with a client, it may be appropriate for the practitioner to do trans-disciplinary work which in theory ought to be the role of another professional. No profession should be over-protective regarding its territory if this is to the detriment of the client.

Much of the physiotherapist's work is likely to be from a consultancy model as they focus away from passive treatment and concentrate instead upon what the client can learn to do for themselves or that their carers can do with them. The Care Programme Approach regards the whole 'case' in a sophisticated way and will therefore support and involve relatives and/or other carers in order to provide the interventions to meet the client's needs.

In future, a large proportion of the hands-on work will go to skilled semi-professionals. These workers, e.g. the Social Services based Care Officers, are already been employed and are certainly being considered within the Health Service. In this sense, the die is cast. Physiotherapists must ensure the quality of care which reaches our clients via these semi-professionals.

An 'enabling' approach to case management plus the rise of a new type of worker means that physiotherapists will have to move from the narrowest medical paradigm to an educational paradigm which encompasses the disease model at the heart of the medical paradigm. The physiotherapist must also sustain and develop their particular high standard and breadth of 'hands-on' treatment skills. Within such a paradigm, the client and/or carers are primarily conceptualized as active and equal participants rather than passive recipients. The Care Programme Approach, with its 'process' orientation, is a means of enabling this paradigm shift with the appropriate clients, arguably all the clients who present in mental health/psychiatry.

Figure 5.6 shows a specimen Care Programme, to provide an illustration of the physiotherapy input for an imaginary female client.

It is within the context of a complex sociopolitical environment that the physiotherapist in community mental health/psychiatry is having to 'sell' the worth of what they do. The author believes that we should create our 'marketing strategy' around the role we play, based upon the core skills and abilities, as noted above, that make us different in the CMHT. We should be seen as team players not as an isolated or 'stand-alone' service with a narrow protectionist stance.

Despite the resurgence and extension of biopsychiatry described by Breggin (1993), French (1992) is correct to assert the drift towards more truly psychological, psychosocial, humanistic and holistic approaches to the provision of interventions with this client group. The physiotherapist can feel secure in operating from a developing core base of touch- and movement-related interventions and therapeutic approaches which are growing ever more marketable.

The community is the future for the provision of services for this mental health psychiatry client group. Physiotherapists have a powerful extending role and a crucial part to play in ensuring quality of care for the whole person. This will be enhanced as we develop our awareness of ever more sophisticated biopsychosocial models of those influcences upon the self which result in individuals being referred to the mental health/psychiatric system.

Indicator steps have to be observable, objective, behavioural, simply under-standable and therefore measurable by anyone. When three indicators of effect are used, the chances of any change being spontaneous and not the result of the interventions given is statistically less than one.

The system produces a simple numerical record of the level of outcome at any given time during the course of intervention. This can allow for large-scale research while tailoring goals/indicators to the individual.

Combined with less sophisticated quantitative measures and CSQs, this should provide a clear picture of the volume and quality of the service provided.

The TELER system appears to combine adaptability across the range of professions while remaining client centred, providing not merely a monitoring tool but also an engine for quality enhancing the Care Programme Approach.

A case weighting system would be useful if it could predict, even roughly, the overall likely resource demand of a particular case over time. This would help clients to avoid the trap of practitioners being pressured to withdraw because they have reached the limit of treatments that this condition is supposed to need, i.e. 'results' led thinking dominating the needs of 'process' clients.

Conclusion

The conclusions of research demonstrate that equity in health is impossible without equity in wealth. The first principle of *Health For All 2000* is, therefore, unachievable without enormous social change.

In real terms, those within the 'caring professions' have no logically and behaviourally consistent commitment to the health of the nation. For those who are most at risk within the community, a 'needs' led client centred system of care/intervention has to be in place to attempt to create equity of service provision. The physiotherapy profession appears to be firmly committed to a policy of equity of service provision in the NHS. Physiotherapists should approach this in a sophisticated way, clearly differentiating between those clients who fit a 'results' led system and those clients who require a process led system which meets their individual needs.

In the community setting this should be facilitated by the Care Programme Approach which, in effect, does commit us to a 'needs' led and therefore 'process' oriented system. The right outcome measures system will help us to meet client needs in the most effective way.

Observational and research evidence, plus historical/retrospective analysis, has demonstrated that, in the main, institutional care is not particularly helpful to the majority of mental health/psychiatric clients. Indeed the bulk of the evidence, from Goffman to Breggin, seems to suggest that it is detrimental. Even so, it is also true that some people will always need 'asylum' from a hostile environ-ment and some people will need continuing care, neither of which needs to be provided from a hospital base however. For whatever reasons, the government has forced the pace on community care. This being a 'given', we need to ensure that the best mix of home and institutional care is extended to our clients.

Appendix: Useful addresses

Outcome measures
'Bunny' Le Roux
Chief Lecturer, Department of Statistics, Hallam University, Pond Street, Sheffield, South Yorkshire.

Liz Bullock
Senior Physiotherapist, Physiotherapy Department, Mount Vernon Hospital, Mount Vernon Road, Barnsley, South Yorkshire.

Case-weighting
Jon Parker
Social Worker, West and Central Hull Community Support Team, c/o Alderson House, Linnaeus Street, Anlaby Road, Hull, North Humberside.

References and further reading

Ader (1991) *Psychoneuroimmunology*, Academic
Breggin (1993) *Toxic Psychiatry*, Harper Collins
Cambridge Personal Development. *An Introduction to Biodynamic Massage*, Wetenhall Road, Cambridge CB1 3AG
Cartwrights and O'Brien (1976) *Social Class Variations in Health Care, The Sociology of the NHS*, Sociological Reviews, Monograph 22
Chodorow (1941) *Dance Therapy and Depth Psychology*, Routledge
Christ (1990) *Living with Back Pain*, Manchester University Press
Department of Osteopathy, Theory and Methods. *An Outline to Osteopathy in the Cranial Field*, Kirkville College of Osteopathy, Kirkville, Missouri 63501
Feldenkruis (1972) *Awareness Through Movement*, Penguin
Foucault (1967) *Madness and Civilisation*, Tavistock
Foucault (1978) *The Birth of the Clinic*, Routledge
French (ed.) (1992) *Physiotherapy—a Psychosocial Approach*, Butterworth-Heinemann
Goffman (1961) *Asylums*, Peregrine
Goldberg and Huxley (1980) *Mental Illness in the Community, The Pathway to Psychiatric Care*, Routledge
Goldberg and Huxley (1992) *Common Mental Disorders, A Bio-Social Model*, Routledge
Graham (1984) *Women Health and the Family*, Macmillan
Illich *et al.* (1977) *The Disabling Professions*, M. Bowars
Illich *et al.* (1982) *Medical Nemesis*, Bowker
Kapchuk (1983) *The Web that has no Weaver*, Congdon Weed
Kovel (1978) *A Complete Guide to Therapy*, Pelican
Laing (1968) The obvious. In *Dialectics of Liberation* (D. Cooper, ed.), Pelican
Laing (1970) *Knots*, Routledge
Maisel (1969) *The Resurrection of the Body* (including article on the Alexander Technique), Shambhala
Masson (1984) *Against Therapy*, Fontana
Merlean Pontz (1962) *The Phenomonology of Perception*, Routledge and Kogan Paul
Miller and Rose (eds) (1986) *The Power of Psychiatry*, Polity Press
Montague (1971) *Touching*, Perennid Library
Paul *et al.* (1977) *Psychosocial Treatment of Chronic Mental Patients*, Harvard University Press
Peters (1982) *In Search of Excellence*, Harper and Row
Sheldon (1972) *If you meet Budha on the road–Kill Him!*, Sheldon
Smail (1987) *Taking Care on Alternatives to Therapy*, Dent Paperbacks

Smail (1983) *Illusion and Reality—The Meaning of Anxiety*, Dent Paperbacks
Teeguarden (1987) *The Joy of Feeling*, Iona-Japan
Totman (1987) *Social Causes of Illness*, Souvenir
Townsend and Davidson (1982) *Inequalities in Health*, Penguin
Tyrer and Steinberg (1987) *Models for Mental Disorder*, John Wiley
Whitehead (1987) *The Health Divide*, Penguin

6

Practical guidelines for service evaluation

Derek Milne and John Smeaton

Synopsis

The aim of this chapter is to give a practical introduction to the evaluation of physiotherapy services in the mental health field. In order to pursue this aim, the authors have drawn principally on recent research which has appeared in *Physiotherapy*, the most accessible journal, using this to illustrate the main features of evaluation. This should help the reader achieve a better grasp of evaluation methods, improve the ability to understand research articles and be encouraged to participate in and apply the results of service evaluation. This is seen as part of the 'support and guidance' called for by the Chartered Society of Physiotherapy (1992).

The structure of the chapter reflects the traditional headings of a research report, namely 'introduction', 'method', 'results' and 'discussion'. The authors will consider what they regard as the key issues within these sections, including their respective functions, the importance of a 'stakeholder-collaborative' approach, available measurement instruments, and practical research designs. Throughout, the emphasis is on a 'reflective practitioner' model of professional practice, in which research and evaluation can serve a fundamental role in helping us to consider and develop our work (Richardson, 1992). In addition, public services, such as the National Health Service, are increasingly being required to provide evidence of their effectiveness. It is therefore timely to develop as reflective practitioners, given that there is now considerable support and encouragement for such systematic approaches to 'reflection' as research and evaluation. But how do these relate to other topical developments, such as total quality management (TQM) and audit?

What is evaluation?

In many instances, the considerable common ground between the various manifestations of research are obscured by terminology. 'TQM' and 'service evaluation', for instance, may sound quite dissimilar, but they actually have a great deal in common. Both require clear objectives (or standards), emphasize methods by which these should be achieved, incorporate a system for judging success, and specify some way in which this feedback can be used to improve a service. In turn, 'audit' can be construed as an evaluation tool of TQM, one which emphasizes the comparison of results obtained by peers in relation to agreed best practice (Ovretveit, 1990; Parry, 1992).

All forms of research and evaluation are formal methods for answering questions. They usually follow well-established rules governing how the questions are selected and defined, as well as following precise procedures concerning the valid search for an answer. However, 'research' (also known as 'basic research', 'laboratory research' or 'pure research') tends to focus on questions of a theoretical nature and to adopt very rigorous procedures (e.g. control groups). In contrast, 'evaluation' (also labelled 'service evaluation', 'research and development', 'applied' or 'action' research, etc.) starts with practical questions and tends towards more practical procedures. While 'research' is intended to deepen our understanding of nature and reveal 'truths' (e.g. why leaves are green), 'evaluation' focuses on pressing real-life concerns in order to solve problems (e.g. how to improve a client's compliance with therapy). Other differences which can increasingly stretch the common ground are the extent to which findings apply to other settings, the care given to measurement and the extent to which judgement is accepted (Milne, 1987). In summary, therefore, evaluation is the process of judging, by research methods, the extent to which a service achieves its objectives.

Most people, confident that what they are doing is worth while, welcome programme evaluation, but to others, evaluation may appear as a threat. They may feel that they are being evaluated rather than the programme. Perhaps the best way to dispel these fears and ensure that the evaluation is accepted and acted upon is to involve all interested parties from the outset, i.e. a 'stakeholder collaborative approach'. How much collaboration is possible will vary, but practical strategies could include an initial meeting at which the objectives of the research are ironed out. Subsequent workshops can encourage small groups to focus on specific parts of the project. Further meetings can examine drafts of, say, data collection methods or the proposed analysis. In this way political problems can be minimized and evaluation can function as an important method of staff development (Greene, 1988; Lee and Sampson, 1990).

The chapter now considers the main headings of a service evaluation and selects principal issues for comment.

The Introduction

The purpose of this initial section is to tell readers why the evaluation is necessary and to orient them to the topic. The convention is to proceed from the general to the particular, as in having an opening sentence which states the seriousness of the problem to be studied in very broad terms. (A favourable approach, for example, is to cite statistics: 'Health Service clients are receiving a poor service, because practitioners are not sufficiently reflective. A recent survey found that over 90% of physiotherapists in the UK...', etc.). The problem can then be stated in research terms, with the relevant research and theory reviewed. The more rigorous and thorough of introductions will also include a critical review of the most relevant literature. Often this will lead to the clarification of some problems with the prior research, with which the present study will deal. The Chartered Society of Physiotherapy's Information Resource Centre will search indices for a small fee or members may visit the centre and

Table 6.1 Summary of the components of a piece of research, set out in the form of questions which the report should address (After Borchardt and Francis, 1984; Sternberg, 1988)

Introduction

In general terms, why is it important to conduct the investigation?
How will it go beyond previous research?
In what way will this be useful?
Which prior research is relevant?
What do you expect to achieve (objectives) or find (hypotheses)?

Method

Where was the study conducted?
How were the dependent and independent variables measured?
Are the measures reliable and valid?
Who were the participants?
How were they selected?
Which research design was employed?
What was the step-by-step procedure?

Results

Is the presentation purely factual and brief?
Are descriptive and inferential statistics used?
Which statistics were employed and what probability levels were obtained?

Discussion

What were the main findings?
To what extent do they concur with your objectives or hypotheses?
Can you draw any conclusions?
Do you have any reservations to express regarding your methodology?
What are the implications of your findings?

search free of charge (see *Physiotherapy*, April 1993). The research collator of the Association of Chartered Physiotherapists in Psychiatry is also a source of relevant material. At the most particular level, the introduction concludes with some specific hypotheses or objectives. Table 6.1 illustrates these steps and summarizes the remaining sections.

To illustrate, Kerr *et al.* (1991) provide a review of the literature on rising from a chair, which began with the very broad statement that 'standing from a seated position is an activity which most people perform many times daily'. They continue by citing statistics concerning the features of a chair which are regarded as important by health service clients. Lastly, their critical review element (the bulk of the article) provides examples of a detailed examination of previous research, including criticisms of the methods used (such as small sample sizes and poor measurement). Since it is a review article, no hypotheses are evaluated. However, Kerr and colleagues do suggest some objectives for future research.

The Method section

This section typically consists of five subheadings – materials or apparatus, dependent variable assessment, participants, design, and procedure – as considered below.

Materials or apparatus

A good study holds constant the conditions under which the client is assessed (i.e. the 'dependent variable') and treated (i.e. the 'independent variable'). Both should be described in sufficient detail for a reader to repeat the study. For example, if an existing instrument has been used to assess mobility, this should be referenced. If, on the other hand, a new measure has been created, this should be appended or made available. Similarly, the general context of the evaluation and exactly how the physiotherapy was applied should be described.

Dependent variable assessment

There are a number of practical guidelines for assessing a client or service. One is to utilize more than one instrument to measure the thing being evaluated. Sometimes referred to as 'triangulation', this guideline encourages the use of measures of such dimensions as a client's thoughts, feelings and behaviours; or a service's 'effort', 'process' and 'outcome'. Such 'multiple measures' increase our confidence in the findings and provide a richer account than single measures alone. To illustrate, Ernst *et al.* (1990) studied prevention of the common cold by hydrotherapy, measuring the frequency, duration and strength of colds. In addition to assessing different dimensions of a problem, it is desirable to utilize different measurement methods, i.e. to use direct observation, self-report (e.g. self-ratings; questionnaire; diary record), physical measurement, interview and other approaches. Pearson and Jones (1992), for instance, used questionnaires and interviews to study the emotional effects of sports injuries. The questionnaires indicated that many of the 61 injured sportsmen were hostile, confused and depressed, while the interviews clarified the role that physiotherapists could play in raising mood.

There are various sources of such instruments, including journals, colleagues and reference texts. As an example of the latter, the measures which are summarized in such texts as Peck and Shapiro (1991), McDowell and Newell (1987), Hersen and Bellack (1988), Streiner and Norman (1989) or Thompson (1989) may be considered.

A second guideline promotes the measurement of the independent variable, i.e. the service or physiotherapy provided in the study. Unfortunately, published accounts tend to be restricted to rather brief and vague descriptions of what was done. Adherence to the guidelines requires that the therapy or service is also observed and that some check is made on the reliability of that measurement. Meeting these three criteria will allow treatments to be standardized and valid conclusions about their effectiveness drawn (Edwards *et al.*, 1990). Again, multiple measures are desirable, as in assessing the amount of therapy provided, the interpersonal effectiveness of the physiotherapist, and the specific technique that is applied. The psychotherapy literature has some useful examples of such assessments (e.g. Schaffer, 1982).

A third guideline concerns the use of good instruments, i.e. those that are sensitive to change and have known reliability and validity. Reliability concerns the 'reproducibility' or consistency of repeated measurements, and it is clearly desirable that this is high, so that any findings can be attributed to the effects of the therapy rather than error or 'noise' in the measurement process. A number of methods for assessing reliability exist, the two most popular being inter-rater reliability and intra-rater reliability (i.e. the test–retest method). Kilby *et al.* (1990), for example, assessed the inter-rater reliability of the McKenzie approach to back pain assessment. They had two physiotherapists examine 41 clients, finding a very satisfactory level of overall agreement (i.e. 88%), though with some areas of low reliability (e.g. diagnosis averaged 59%). In contrast, Livesley (1992) considered the intra-rater reliability of the hand-held myometer in measuring isotonic strength. She had 20 clients (10 with multiple sclerosis, 10 neurologically normal volunteers) exert maximum force on the myometer on three separate occasions, recorded by one observer. The findings indicated that the myometer was reliable when administered in an identical manner. By contrast, Rose (1991) obtained low reliabilities for four clinical measurements, indicating the need to assess reliability.

'Validity' concerns the extent to which a measure assesses what it purports to measure. Some assessed variables will have high face validity and not require any special attention (e.g. limb movement). Others are less straightforward, as they are inferred from observable behaviour (as in the 'strength' example above). A classic example is pain. Newton and Waddell (1991) assessed the validity (and inter-rater reliability) of lumbar spine mobility in 60 clients, 50 having low back pain. In order to gauge the validity of three assessment procedures (i.e. inclinometer, kyphometer and fingers to floor), the results were compared with X-rays. They reported good results, the best between the inclinometer and the X-ray (a correlation of 0.76).

Another important guideline is to gather both qualitative and quantitative data. Although the former are often seen as 'exploratory' (i.e. serving to define hypotheses for quantitative analysis) and the latter as 'confirmatory' (i.e. 'proving' hypotheses), this distinction is of rather limited value. As Parry (1991) argues, qualitative information can help to give context to an evaluation, including the researcher's reasons for studying a given problem. In addition, qualitative data can provide depth and detail, as in a consumer satisfaction survey in which clients give both ratings and comments. It is therefore not a question of one or the other, but rather of how best to blend the two approaches (Webber, 1991).

A final guideline to highlight concerns the impact of a treatment. This refers to its generalization across time ('maintenance'), settings, people and behaviour. A sound evaluation will at least consider the maintenance of a treatment effect over time, so as to ascertain whether the benefits are transient or enduring. Finlay *et al.* (1990) give an example in relation to physiotherapy provided to 49 elderly people attending a day hospital. They found that the small gains made in mobility by these clients were maintained 1 and 6 months after discharge.

Participants

This part of the Method section should detail the total number of people participating in the evaluation and, if appropriate, the number receiving different treatments. It should clarify how they were selected, so as to indicate whether they should be considered 'representative' or not. (A typical evaluation will not attempt to do more than relate the characteristics of consecutive service users to other research, whereas an experimental research study will aim for random selection of the participants.) Also, a good 'participants' section will say how they came to be involved (e.g. 'one year's consecutive attenders at a routine physiotherapy service were included in the evaluation...'). Finally, the relevant characteristics of the participants (e.g. age, gender, diagnosis, treatment history, etc.) should be set out.

Sometimes this will do no more than help readers to gain an impression of the sample (and hence of how typical they are of their own clients). On other occasions it will allow an analysis of the relationship between participants' characteristics and treatment process or outcome. For example, Nussbaum *et al.* (1990) found that age and gender were not related to the effects of interferential therapy.

Design

Research designs are essentially strategies which reduce the risk that factors other than one's intervention are responsible for the observed changes. Research designs may be classified into three categories: (a) the 'classical' *experimental* approach with its randomization of patients (or 'subjects') into an experimental and a control group; (b) *quasi-experimental* designs, which differ in having non-random allocation to groups and less rigour or control (e.g. trying out a new treatment approach on a group of patients); and (c) *non-experimental* (correlational or *'case study'*) approaches in which there is no manipulation of variables.

Non-experimental designs
In this section, data about phenomena in their natural state, such as activities, attitudes, client need, and quality of life, are collected. As experimental control and variable manipulation are not included, research design issues tend to focus on the development, piloting and application of the measure(s). Questionnaires seem an easy way of data collection, and can be if an existing one can be used, but beware! Rigorous development of one's own questionnaire (i.e. reliability and validity assessment) is not a simple process. Titchen (1987), investigating physiotherapist's attitudes towards continuing education, conducted 30 interviews and then looked at 20 pilot responses before finally sending out her questionnaire.

If truly virgin territory is to be explored and it is felt that a questionnaire might filter out interesting data, then interviewing may be more appropriate. Lynn and Plant (1992) used in-depth group interviews to show that psychiatric nurses had a pharmacological view of the aetiology of abnormal movements in schizophrenia, one which contrasted with the biological focus of the medical literature. Interviews, as mentioned above, can also be used to build up the content of a questionnaire ('item generation' and 'selection').

A basic technique, often overlooked, is observation. This can also be based on existing or specially prepared instruments (Milne, 1987). Observation of videotaped physiotherapy sessions was used by Alderman *et al.* (1992) to time verbal outbursts and assess change in the affective state of a patient with brain injury. This study also used an 'ABA' design (see below).

Quasi-experimental and experimental designs
This section concentrates on the single case design, as this approach can be a realistic way into research for clinicians who are fascinated by their successes and failures but who do not have the time, inclination or resources to consider traditional 'group approaches'.

A recent project in mental health (Douglas, 1988) highlights some of the problems encountered when an experimental/control group study is attempted by busy clinicians in the field. The control group selects itself (they were not prepared to join in the exercise programme), the experimental group suffers from non-attendance and drop-out and extraneous variables affect the two small groups unequally, so that ultimately statistical significance disappoints.

Rather like the clinical psychologists in the 1960s, some physiotherapists are becoming disillusioned with the rigorous between-group approach to research (e.g. the 'drug trial'). This design is totally impractical for the average clinician and does not seem to answer our sorts of questions (Riddoch and Lennon, 1991). As in psychology, attention is turning to the single case design (also known as '$N = 1$' or 'time series' research), a method which, unlike the group design, recognizes the individuality of the patient, an outstanding feature of our work in mental health. The method is also feasible and allows for as much experimental rigour as one has time to devote to it (Hersen and Barlow, 1976).

The single case design and its variants are research designs which have been neglected by UK physiotherapists until recently. A journal survey (Aufdemkampe, 1991) revealed that there were no single case designs published in *Physiotherapy* in 1987, but 16 in *Physical Therapy*. As the Americans appear to have realized, single case research is a practical way of evaluating both the impact of therapy on individual patients and the effectiveness of physiotherapy techniques.

It is important to take a practical look at single case research. Having assembled a battery of measures, the budding reflective practitioner has to decide on a framework for applying them, a design. The design should be feasible; an extension of everyday practice (otherwise the research will never begin). Another vital consideration is control; how confidently can measured changes be credited to therapy rather than natural healing, a depot injection or a wage rise? Put more technically, will the influence of extraneous variables threaten the 'internal validity' of the study? (For more on internal validity see Campbell and Stanley, 1963.)

The approach to control in single case designs is based on an awareness of the respective influences of the treatment variable and extraneous variables by frequent rigorous measurement. This is something the clinician should already be doing.

A simple single case design could be considered, consisting of two phases. Phase A, when the patient is acting as their own control, is when no treatment is given and 'baseline' measurements are taken. Here we are measuring the rate of spontaneous recovery, or at least recovery without physiotherapy (e.g. a chronic patient on the waiting list). For the acute patient whose treatment cannot be delayed, it may be possible to give 'general' treatment during phase A followed by 'general' plus the treatment under scrutiny in phase B, the treatment phase. McCulloch and Kemper (1993) changed to 'treatment plus' faced with a non-healing wound. Because they were already measuring frequently and accurately, they were able to document the changes in the dependent variable (wound size) adequately and publish the results.

There is a chance that improvements (if any) observable in phase B may not be due to treatment but to an extraneous variable (a serious threat to internal validity). At this stage the design is still quasi-experimental. To graduate to 'experimental' status, in some cases phase B could be followed with another phase A, the result measured and then the treatment phase repeated, and so on (ABABAB...). If the improvement continues to be observed in phase B, the probability that this is due to the intervention increases. Using an ABA design, a head-injured patient was given 'general treatment' during a one-week baseline phase (Richardson, 1990). During phase B he also spent periods on a tilt-table. Time spent standing and ankle range of movement improved in phase B. To assess the role of the tilt-table further, a series of simple AB studies on similar patients could be carried out.

Designs like these, where multiple 'things' are being measured (in this case patients), are called, naturally enough, *multiple baseline designs*. Thus we have moved effortlessly from the quasi-experimental single case design to an experimental design for use with small groups. For example, Sime and Sanstead (1985), using triangulating measures of depression and a follow-up interview, examined the effect of aerobic exercise on 15 moderately depressed subjects using a multiple baseline across-clients design. They obtained measures during four phases: baseline (2 weeks), anaerobic exercise (2 weeks), aerobic exercise (10 weeks) and follow-up (measures taken at 6 and 21 months).

If frequent, reliable and valid measurement suggests improvement due to therapy in a series of patients, then the battle is won. If there is a more mixed response, there still remains an interesting study which may indicate why treatment fails in patients with certain characteristics.

The multiple baseline design across treatments is very useful, especially in patients with several treatable problems, as in the following example (Farrell, 1991). After a two-week baseline period (phase A1) a patient with spinal cord compression was taught to transfer. At the same time, baseline measures for walking were taken (phase B1). Backwards walking was taught during the second treatment phase (B2). Improved transfer ability did not generalize to backwards walking which only improved during the second treatment phase; this provided a strong indication that the therapy and not another variable was responsible for improvements.

Single case research can be subjected to statistical analysis (see below) and certainly could be submitted for publication. Publication should mean that the work has relevance to others (generality or 'external validity'). Eventually the following questions would need to be answered regarding treatment generality:

- Will the treatment work with similar patients?
- Will it work for other physiotherapists (e.g. not just the tall attractive ones)?
- Will it work in other settings (e.g. the community)?
- Will it work in relation to other problems/behaviours?
- Will the effects of intervention last ('maintain')?

A single case design may indicate, for example, that reflex therapy reduces anxiety in an acutely anxious patient in the department. Replicating this design with similar patients may establish the generality of this therapy across clients. Further replications involving other therapists and settings (community, etc.) may expand the external validity.

Procedure

Like the Results section, discussed below, the description of exactly what was done, the procedure, should be a strictly 'no-nonsense' section. Enough detail should be included to enable a reader to repeat the study; so getting a third party, naive to physiotherapy, to read through it, is a good idea. A chronological approach should help ensure that relevant details are not omitted. If this section is not comprehensive enough, questions will remain in readers' minds and the findings may not be taken seriously. If the development of physiotherapy treatment schedules for research (Edwards *et al.*, 1990) succeeds, then writing this section should be a lot easier.

The results and analysis section

This is the briefest part of a report, consisting simply of a presentation of the findings. Figures and tables are classic examples of this brevity. There should be no interpretation of results at this point (they belong in the 'Discussion' section). Brevity and conciseness are also pursued by means of statistics. Two forms are generally used: 'descriptive' statistics which summarize the findings in simple and clear terms (e.g. pie charts, percentages, graphs, etc.); and 'inferential' ones that test the probability that the findings were due to chance. In the case of inferential statistics, it is customary to report the name of the test (e.g. 'Student's *T*-test'), the value obtained (e.g. $T = 14.3$), the degrees of freedom (e.g. df = 62) and the significance level (e.g. $p < 0.05$, being the conventional level for accepting that the findings are not due to chance).

Statistics is a specialized field only fully understood by statisticians. An area of multidisciplinary collaboration neglected by most physiotherapists is seeking help from a qualified statistician, which is remarkable considering the worry statistics generate. Universities and polytechnics have statistics departments; seek advice early on while considering measures and design (Maxwell, 1990).

Alternatively, there will usually be someone in one's unit with more research experience than oneself. In the absence of experienced help, some knowledge of the basics will prevent embarrassing mistakes. The clinical researcher needs to understand what is meant by 'significance' and needs to be aware of the sort of data being analysed. Tedious though they seem, these concepts are dealt with first, followed by a rough guide to the practical applications of various statistical tests. Finally, analysis of data from single subject designs is discussed.

Sometimes it is obvious from examining the practical results of a study that a treatment is having a beneficial effect; in such instances it could be said that the results of that study are 'clinically significant'. However, to understand 'statistical significance' it is important to return to hypotheses. A research hypothesis might be: the depression scores of patients following the exercise regimen will be lower than those following the standard regimen only (or the null hypothesis may be stated: that there is no difference between the scores).

A test of statistical significance gives the probability that the data are consistent with acceptance of the null hypothesis. Thus if the probability value is low (below one's stated value of rejection, usually 0.05, i.e. 1 in 20), then the null hypothesis can confidently (19 chances in 20) be rejected and the research hypothesis accepted.

The sorts of statistical tests which may be applied depend, among other things, on the sort of data the measures have produced. Data are classified as follows:

- *nominal data*, e.g. 'phobic': names, symbols, etc. – one 'name' is not greater than another

Table 6.2 Some common non-parametric inferential statistical tests related to questions one might want to ask and to levels of measurement

Type of data	Are two sets of data related?	Is there a difference between two sets of independent data?	Is there a difference between two sets of related data?
Nominal	Cramer coefficient	Chi-square test	McNemar change test
Ordinal	Spearman or Kendall rank-order correlation	Wilcoxon–Mann–Whitney test	Sign test
Interval or ratio	As above	Permutation test for independent samples	Permutation test for paired replicates

- *ordinal data*, e.g. unsatisfied (gap), satisfied (gap), very satisfied: the data can be ranked in a 'greater than' way but the 'gaps' are not meaningful
- *interval data*, e.g. temperature: as ordinal but with equivalent meaningful gaps
- *ratio data*, e.g. degrees of joint movement: as interval but with the added sophistication of an absolute zero.

The sample size and how subjects are allocated to groups are two other factors which determine which class of statistical test is appropriate. Small samples and non-randomization will usually compel the clinical researcher to use 'non-parametric' statistics, a rough guide to which follows.

Table 6.2 considers the type of data one may have and the sorts of questions which may be asked. 'Related samples' are conditions when subjects act as their own controls or when participants are 'matched' for relevant characteristics.

Before continuing, another valuable 'statistical aid' must be mentioned – the computer. Probably the most suitable software package for small projects is the statistically sound and user-friendly MINITAB.

Analysis of single subject designs

The first and essential step is to graph the data and indicate the different phases and any relevant extraneous occurrences. Visual inspection of the graph(s) should be enough to reveal a strong effect (as in Figure 6.1). Purists would

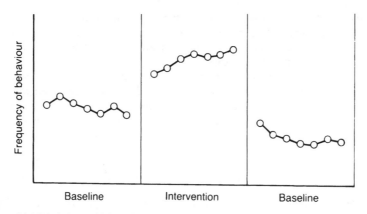

Figure 6.1 ABA design (withdrawal)

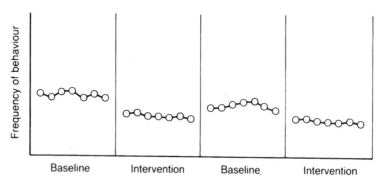

Figure 6.2 ABABAB design (reversal)

contend that if an obvious effect is not demonstrated, the experiment should be repeated or the experimenter should 'admit defeat'. However, imagine that a weak treatment effect is consistently present during all the B phases of an ABABAB design (Figure 6.2). This may not be obvious from visual inspection, but might be revealed by statistical analysis. The split middle technique and the Records test are two of a number of simple, practical statistical procedures that could be applied. For more information see Morley and Adams (1989), Tyron (1982) or Hersen and Barlow (1976).

The Discussion section

The key components are a summary of the main findings, the writer's view as to how these agree with the given objectives or hypotheses, the conclusions, and any implications regarding the methodology used or the theory underlying the project. The following example illustrates these components. The discussion section of a study of the physiotherapy provided in a geriatric day hospital (Finlay *et al.*, 1990) began with a statement of the main finding. This was that 'a small but beneficial gain in mobility after attendance ... was maintained at one and six months after discharge'. These authors went on to note other possible reasons for this finding (e.g. nursing care, OT), as well as possible bias in the assessment (which were made by physiotherapists who were aware of the intervention). These represent implications of the methods they utilized. Finlay and colleagues also highlighted a practical implication of the study, which was the routine use of their mobility index subsequently.

In line with the collaborative approach to evaluation mentioned earlier, any findings and views on their implications should be fed back to all interested parties. At a local level this may involve a meeting and a presentation. To reach a broader audience, publication may be possible in a wide variety of news sheets and journals.

Conclusion

Compared to other specialities, physiotherapists in psychiatry are exploring virgin territory. The potential for research is vast and largely untapped.

Evaluation is challenging, but it is hoped that the authors have shown it is within the scope of practitioners to tackle their problems by combining simple designs with rigorous measurement.

Remember and exploit the collaborative approach. Support for research can come from many directions: psychologists, nurses, psychiatrists, clients, etc.

To promote research, access to information is essential. Superintendents can encourage enquiry and evaluation by giving their staff time to look at the latest journals and time to find or develop good measurement tools.

Finally, a maxim, for those for whom fame is the spur: 'Research is twice blessed, it blesseth the client *and the researcher*'.

References

Alderman, N., Shepherd, J. and Youngson, H. (1992) Increasing standing tolerance and posture quality following severe brain injury using a behaviour modification approach. *Physiotherapy*, **78**, 335–343

Aufdemkampe, G. (1991) Some comments on single case studies. *Physiotherapy Theory and Practice*, **7**, 63–71

Borchardt, D.H. and Francis, R.D. (1984) *How to Find Out in Psychology*, Pergamon, Oxford

Campbell, D.T. and Stanley, J.C. (1963) *Experimental and Quasi-experimental Designs for Research*, Rand McNally, Chicago

Chartered Society of Physiotherapy (1992) Physiotherapy research. *Physiotherapy*, **78**, 356–357

Douglas, J. (1988) The effect of exercise on long-stay psychiatric patients' general behaviour using rehabilitation evaluation. Hall and Baker. Unpublished, available from Association of Chartered Physiotherapists in Psychiatry,

Edwards, S., Partridge, C. and Mee, R. (1990) Treatment schedules for research. *Physiotherapy*, **76**, 605–607

Ernst, E., Wirz, P. and Pecho, L. (1990) Prevention of common colds by hydrotherapy. *Physiotherapy*, **76**, 207–210

Farrell, J.C. (1991) Transfer ability in a patient with spinal cord compression: a multiple baseline design. *Physiotherapy Theory and Practice*, **7**, 39–43

Finlay, O.E., Crosbie, J., Gunning, H.M.A., Beringer, T.R.O. and Gilmore, D.H. (1990) Effectiveness of physiotherapy in a geriatric day hospital. *Physiotherapy*, **76**, 793–795

Greene, J.C. (1988) Communication of results and utilization in participatory program evaluation. *Evaluation and Program Planning*, **11**, 341–351

Hersen, M. and Barlow, D. (1976) *Single Case Experimental Designs*, Pergamon Press, New York

Hersen, M. and Bellack, A.S. (1988) *Dictionary of Behavioural Assessment Techniques*, Pergamon, Oxford

Kerr, K.M., White, J.A., Mollon, R.A.B. and Baird, H.E. (1991) Rising from a chair: a review of the literature. *Physiotherapy*, **77**, 15–19

Kilby, J., Stignant, M. and Roberts, A. (1990) The reliability of back pain assessment by physio-therapists, using a McKenzie algorithm. *Physiotherapy*, **76**, 579–583

Lee, L.J. and Sampson, J.F. (1990) A practical approach to program evaluation. *Evaluation and Program Planning*, **13**, 157–164

Lynn, S.A. and Plant, R.D. (1992) Abnormal motor control in psychiatric patients: operational paradigms (Abstract). *Clinical Rehabilitation*, **6** (Suppl.), 45–46

McCulloch, Jr, J.M. and Kemper, C.C. (1993) Vacuum-compression therapy for the treatment of an ischemic ulcer. *Physical Therapy*, **73**(3), 165–169

McDowell, I. and Newell, C. (1987) *Measuring Health: A Guide to Rating Scales and Questionnaires*, Oxford University Press, Oxford

Maxwell, I.S. (1990) Personal view. Abusing statistics. *Physiotherapy*, **76**, 107

Milne, D.L. (ed.) (1987) *Evaluating Mental Health Practice: Methods and Applications*, Routledge, London

Morley, S. and Adams, M. (1989) Some simple statistics for exploring single case time-series data. *British Journal of Clinical Psychology*, **28**, 1–18

Newton, M. and Waddell, G. (1991) Reliability and validity of clinical measurement of the lumbar spine in patients with chronic low back pain. *Physiotherapy*, **77**, 796–800

Nussbaum, E., Rush, P. and Disenhaus, L. (1990) The effects of interferential therapy on peripheral blood flow. *Physiotherapy*, **76**, 803–807

Ovretveit, J. (1990) *Quality Health Services*, Brunel University, Uxbridge, UK

Parry, A. (1991) Physiotherapy and methods of inquiry. *Physiotherapy*, **77**, 435–438

Parry, G. (1992) Improving psychotherapy services: applications of research, audit and evaluation. *British Journal of Clinical Psychology*, **31**, 3–19

Pearson, L. and Jones, G. (1992) Emotional effects of sports injuries: implications for physiotherapists. *Physiotherapy*, **78**, 762–769

Peck, D. and Shapiro, C. (1991) *Measuring Health Problems: A Practical Guide*, Wiley, Chichester, UK

Richardson, B. (1992) Professional education and professional practice today – do they match? *Physiotherapy*, **78**, 23–26

Richardson, D.L.A. (1991) The use of the tilt-table to effect passive tendo-Achillis stretch in a patient with head injury. *Physiotherapy Theory and Practice*, **7**, 45–50

Riddoch, J. and Lennon, S. (1991) Evaluation of practice: the single case study approach. *Physiotherapy Theory and Practice*, **7**, 3–11

Rose, M.J. (1991) The statistical analysis of the intra-observer repeatability of four clinical measurement techniques. *Physiotherapy*, **77**, 89–91

Schaffer, N.D. (1982) Multidimensional measures of therapist behaviours as predictors of outcome. *Psychological Bulletin*, **92**, 670–681

Sime, W.E. and Sanstead (1985) Prevention and treatment of depression. Study II. In *Exercise and Mental Health* (eds Morgan, W.P. and Goldston, S.E.), Hemisphere, Washington

Sternberg, R.J. (1988) *The Psychologist's Companion*, Cambridge University Press, Cambridge

Streiner, D.L. and Norman, G.R. (1989) *Health Measurement Scales*, Oxford University Press, Oxford

Thompson, C. (ed 1989) *The Instruments of Psychiatric Research*, Wiley, Chichester, UK

Titchen, A.C. (1987) Continuing Education: A study of physiotherapists' attitudes. *Physiotherapy*, **73**, 121–124

Tyron, W.W. (1992) A simplified time-series analysis for evaluating treatment interventions. *Journal of Applied Behaviour Analysis*, **15**, 423–429

Webber, B.A. (1991) Evaluation and inflation in respiratory care. *Physiotherapy*, **77**, 801–804

Part II

7

Touch and handling

Kathryn Poon

Introduction

The act of touching and the feeling of being touched are very powerful experiences. It is well known that patting someone on the back for a job well done gets the desired message across far more effectively than simply congratulating them without the pat on the back. Similarly, a stranger is much more likely to remember you if you have shaken his or her hand as part of the greeting than if you have not. Touch is, in fact, so powerful that we have 'taboos' against it; therefore, when it is used, it has a powerful and direct effect. However, it is also open to interpretation by the receiver who can accept the signals or reject them.

Touch is very much a part of our everyday language. Certain phrases have come to play such an important role in our speech that we use them even though we do not actually mean 'touch' in the sense of physical contact. A footballer could perhaps be described as appearing unable to 'get to grips' with the game, someone who is 'out of touch' could be described as not knowing what is happening around him, an elderly relative may perhaps be described as having a 'touch' of arthritis and there are many more examples of this in the English language (Pratt and Mason, 1981).

Touch can be described as simply the intentional physical contact between two or more individuals (Watson, 1975), but touch is also the earliest and most primitive form of communication and it occurs in several forms: there is instrumental touch, in which an individual is touched to carry out a specific task, e.g. dressing a wound or giving someone a wash; there is 'ritualized' touch, an example of which would be shaking hands; there is 'body language' touch which reflects how much we want to be accepted into the private space of somebody else; and there is expressive touch where the physical touch is not necessarily an essential component of a physical task but may convey reassurance and comfort, e.g. holding a patient's hand (Le May, 1986). Expressive touch in its most intimate form describes the type of touching which would only be used between close friends, or between parent and child.

To achieve a specific aim with a patient, the form of touch will usually be instrumental, i.e. touching for a purpose in order to carry out a specific task; however, it should be done in a very sensitive and caring way which must necessarily involve some aspects of expressive touch. Professional touch is based on a contract of care which must first be established before one can touch.

Without this contract of care, one has no right to touch. Professional touch is based on the need for diagnosis coupled with history-taking and observation. Therapeutic touch consists of using the warmth and energy of one's own hands to create 'tissue relaxation'. It also creates a human response in the patient because when something hurts, there is nothing like human contact to relieve anxiety. The establishment of this contract of care means that most of the boundaries or 'taboos' to touch no longer apply.

Morris states that touch is used mainly to indicate the type of relationship which exists between one person and another (Morris, 1978). He describes different types of touch in terms of indicators or 'body-contact tie signs' and names 14 such signs, some of which include: shaking hands, guiding using pressure lightly on the recipient's body, patting to congratulate or as a greeting, hugging, holding a hand and supporting the body. Each of these body-contact tie signs has its own variations and limits; for example, when shaking hands, there is an opportunity simply to be recognized by and included in the company concerned, but there is also opportunity to show warmth, cordiality, purpose, good faith, to be insistent or to be indifferent, to be accepting or to be demanding. A free hand can also be added to the clasp of the handshake to emphasize meaning (Morris, 1978). In the usual therapist–patient relationship, because the contract of care establishes the use of professional and therapeutic touch, treatments or interventions may involve none, few or many of the body-contact tie signs and could range from perhaps simply supporting the body during an exercise to the use of almost all of the 14 tie signs, depending on the therapist and patient concerned and the boundaries set by each.

Touch as a form of non-verbal communication

Communication can be divided into two main parts, verbal and non-verbal. Non-verbal communication occurs when a number of different non-verbal behaviours are used together to convey a message. Duncan states that non-verbal behaviours include touch, use of space, facial expression, eye contact, body movement, gesture, posture, tone of voice, observation, listening and use of silence (Duncan, 1969). Non-verbal communication, often used subconsciously to express feelings, attitudes and emotions, has the potential of being five times more effective when trying to convey a message than verbal communication (Argyle, 1972).

Frank states that the quality or intent of a message, as contrasted with its content, could be conveyed by: facial expression, gestures and lightness or heaviness of touch and he feels that the recipient responds as much to this intent as to the content of the message (Frank, 1957). If there is disparity between a verbal and non-verbal message, the receiver responds to the non-verbal cues but is confused about the real meaning of the message. Positive feelings are usually expressed verbally, while negative feelings are communicated non-verbally, and when this happens, doubts about the sender's sincerity and credibility are raised and lead to unsatisfactory interactions (De Vito, 1980). The patient's perception of the therapist's feelings can also be altered by good or poor handling (Hargreaves, 1987), something which is very important to the physiotherapy profession if we want to be effective in our practice. Patient compliance is important for successful results and the onus is therefore placed on the physiotherapist's own personality, attitudes and non-verbal skills in order to achieve success, because it is to these that the patient will respond (O'Gorman, 1975). It is important to explain one's actions and intentions at each stage, both verbally and using non-verbal signs and expressions to back these up in order to make the patient feel secure and for trust and confidence in the therapist's abilities to be built up. Such statements as, 'I am going to put my hand on your back – tell me if it hurts', are essential if the patient is to feel secure and not be afraid that something unexpected or painful is about to happen.

Most non-verbal behaviours have been categorized into two main groups: affiliative and dominant. Affiliative behaviours are related to intimacy and are seen as more feminine. These include: touch, close proximity, smiling, friendly tone of voice and eye contact (Exline, 1971). Affiliative behaviours have been found to be more effective in achieving a successful outcome when treating patients, but although a great many affiliative behaviours are demonstrated during our treatments, it has been said that we, as physiotherapists, tend to adopt a more dominant style of behaviour. This might be to maintain professional status (Gallois *et al.*, 1979), but patients are all individuals who each respond to certain approaches in different ways. It is likely that whether or not more dominant or affiliative behaviours are used during therapist–patient interactions will depend more on the individual patient's response to each approach than to which sex the patient happens to be. The amount of time and care taken during such an interaction will be noticed by the patient, as will attention paid to dignity and modesty – something which is absolutely essential if the patient is to feel respected. As physiotherapists, we want to ensure that our patients feel secure, comfortable, supported, accepted and respected. This leads to increased compliance with treatment and, consequently, an increase in the number of successful outcomes.

Sensory healing touch

Touch as a means of healing has been used for centuries. The 'laying-on of hands' is a tradition which goes back at least as far as biblical times and is described as a therapy whereby the healer places his hands on the sick person and they become well again (Pratt and Mason, 1981).

Touch, in the form of massage, is a very ancient form of treatment, which has been used by all cultures throughout the ages, particularly the Chinese, Egyptians and Greeks. As physiotherapists, we use our hands for healing, and for this we need to make full use of the ability to 'feel' and to 'sense' with our hands.

Touch is the first of the senses to develop in the embyro and it plays a very important role both in the birth process itself and in the early life of the individual (Montague, 1977). When the other senses are not wholly effective, we return to the sense of touch to rediscover reality. Clothing is *felt* to determine its quality, fruit is *squeezed* to determine its ripeness and paint is *touched* to test for dryness (Mason, 1985). Touch is, therefore, used by everybody, constantly, as an essential part of everyday life.

Mason describes physiotherapists as having an 'educated pair of hands' (Mason, 1985). We know what oedema feels like, what muscle spasm feels like to the touch, what an inflamed area feels like, what a deformity feels like – we use our hands diagnostically and therapeutically but we are not the only profession capable of this. Other health professionals, the nursing profession in particular, are showing a great deal of interest in 'therapeutic touch', not to mention practitioners of complementary medicine who are taking over where physiotherapists are abdicating these responsibilities in favour of 'assessment', 'management' and 'delegation'. Practitioners of shiatsu and reflexology, as well as osteopathy and chiropractic, all use their hands diagnostically and therapeutically for healing.

As physiotherapists, massage is our central core (Williams, 1986); however, it is not only our central core but our origin. Our founders, the Society of Trained Masseuses, was established in 1894 by a small group of nurses and midwives who practised 'medical rubbing' and were determined to protect their society from the massage scandals that were common at the time. In 1920, the Royal Charter was granted enabling the title of the Society to change to the Chartered Society of Massage and Medical Gymnastics and, in 1942, it became the Chartered Society of Physiotherapy (Jones, 1991). Williams goes on to state that our hands are central to our profession; we are the profession which uses hands and handling skills to assess, we are experts on manual therapy, movement and mobility. Our founders gave us expertise with our hands and that is what they expected us to carry forward (Williams, 1986). However, physiotherapists are not only concerned with massage, touch and physical contact in the form of specialized techniques designed to treat and reduce the symptoms of recognized ailments, but as a form of communication which exists between the therapist and patient as a possible means of reaching those who may feel alienated or disturbed in order to help them understand their world (Pratt and Mason, 1981). Those who are confused and bewildered by what is happening around them, and those who are no longer able to understand the meaning of words, have to rely on tactile and other forms of non-verbal communication. Those who feel depressed or lonely and those who feel that to explain their feelings would be too threatening, challenging or distressing, particularly benefit from the tactile communication of a massage.

Caring therapeutic touch

Before going on to talk about caring, therapeutic touch in detail, it would be useful to consider what can happen to those who are deprived of this more expressive kind of touch, even if instrumental or clinical touch is still given.

Everyone has personal space or a territory which is regarded as their own, and this seems to be a human need which is retained even when someone is very disabled, either physically or mentally, as in the late stages of dementia. Norberg *et al.* (1986) state that when this personal space is invaded by others, the individual exhibits reactions of stress (fight or flight). If, as with severe disability, there are no possibilities for the individual to flee from the situation physically, the last resort will be psychological flight or withdrawal. This kind of withdrawal can occur if the stimulation is inappropriate or in situations of sensory overload as can happen in a very noisy environment (e.g. slamming doors, screaming patients). It can also happen where this valuable personal space is constantly invaded by care-givers for cleaning, feeding and dressing purposes (Norberg *et al.*, 1986).

Care should never be given in this way, i.e. as an invasion of someone's personal space, but should be negotiated even if the patient is unable to communicate verbally. In these cases, the care-givers should look at the expressions on the faces of their patients for signs of discomfort, pain, embarrassment, anger and withdrawal. The correct use of caring, therapeutic touch can reverse this withdrawal if it is introduced in a gentle and gradual way and should be incorporated into the cleaning, feeding and dressing processes themselves.

Therapeutic touch can be used to express caring attitudes of concern, support, protection, acceptance, respect and love (Pratt and Mason, 1981), and tactile experiences can provide feelings of safety and assurance (Mason, 1985), but these feelings or attitudes will only be conveyed if the person giving the touch concentrates fully on the recipient throughout the interaction. Maintaining eye contact for much of the time does act as a good focus for concentration, remembering that if concentration is lost for a moment, the positive, caring feelings will be lost. Being the giver of therapeutic touch can, therefore, be quite physically and emotionally demanding, particularly if little feedback is forthcoming from the recipient. We need to look for the feedback, which does come in many forms and may simply consist of a smile, a squeeze of the hand or even eye contact for a brief moment with someone who otherwise would not initiate any kind of interaction.

Mason states that we, as individuals, use our senses to relate to the outside world as an expression of our integrity or self-image which is subject to change and modification as time, experience and circumstances alter. He goes on to explain that if our integrity is threatened by disease, disability, pain or disfigurement, it may mean that we cannot cope in the world on our own original terms and, therefore, our self-image and the way we relate to the outside world needs to be restructured. Caring, therapeutic touch becomes very important in this restructuring process; it gives us reassurance that we are 'okay', which can eventually lead to the establishment of a new self-image which is both acceptable and realistic. As physiotherapists, we use touch and handling all the time and we need to be sensitive to the way in which the patient's responses change as their perceived integrity shifts and adjusts (Mason, 1985). Disease and disability require emotional as well as physical adjustment. These emotional adjustments may involve grief, confusion, low self-esteem, resentment, anger, depression, resignation and many other reactions, all of which may be expressed verbally but will almost certainly be expressed non-verbally. These non-verbal cues will be picked up by the therapist who must try to deal sensitively with them, perhaps sensing when someone feels uncomfortable and withdrawing a little, and when someone needs a larger dose of caring touch than usual.

Touch, when given in a caring way, can give the individual reassurance and the conviction that he or she is wanted and valued (Montagu, 1971), and in the same way, handling by the physiotherapist with care and interest indicates that the patient has been accepted unconditionally (Pratt, 1978).

Touch and quality of life

As health professionals we are concerned with treatment and recovery, but recovery is not always the expected outcome in the case of a progressive illness such as dementia. This does not mean that a patient with dementia cannot have a very good quality of life and that it cannot be improved further. Indeed, the main reason for physiotherapy intervention with any patient should always be to improve their quality of life in some way, whatever the baseline.

Dementia and communication

Defining and measuring quality of life is a difficult task and one which is demanding more and more research time, especially with patients who have communication difficulties, such as dementia sufferers who may express themselves non-verbally rather than verbally. At present, there are very few definitions and objective measures of quality of life available to use, but one definition, devised by Kitwood and Bredin (1992), describes quality of life in terms of someone's ability to express 12 signs of well-being, verbally or non-verbally, irrespective of their cognitive function or stage in the dementing process. Some of these 12 signs of well-being include: the ability to be assertive, to express a range of emotions, both positive and negative, to be affectionate, to enjoy humour, to show pleasure and to relax. These signs of well-being, if present, will clearly show that someone is doing well as a person (Kitwood and Bredin, 1992). It follows that the way in which someone is touched or handled during a patient–therapist interaction has great potential for improving quality of life by increasing some of the signs of well-being. If someone is able to feel relaxed, secure, comfortable and valued while being handled, they will feel able to assert themselves without fear of repression or ridicule. In the same way, they will demonstrate how they are feeling either by being affectionate, humorous, by initiating contact or showing pleasure in some other way.

Giving someone time when being handled or touched is essential if they are to feel valued as a person. Holding someone's hand and listening to what they have to say is very valuable, but giving someone a hand massage is a more directed way of giving therapeutic touch and maybe more acceptable both to the patient and to the therapist. It takes time to massage both hands and that time is quality individual time which can be used in whatever way the recipient of the hand massage wishes to use it, the aim not being to relieve specific, physical symptoms but to improve the quality of life of someone in a more general but valuable way.

Some elderly people need to talk and be listened to during an interaction and it is important that these people are taken seriously. Difficulties can arise when somebody suffering from dementia is needing to talk; it is particularly important that the therapist uses as many non-verbal skills as possible to encourage speech to continue and feelings to be ventilated even though the actual words used may not mean very much to the listener. Voice intonation and facial expression are essential and should be used appropriately to match the feelings being expressed beneath the words as far as possible. This, together with warm, caring, re-assuring handling, can make a great deal of difference to the way a confused person feels.

Some people like to just relax and feel secure when being handled. Verbal communication may not be necessary, and again, taking the confused person as an example, words may be one cause of them feeling threatened if they do not feel competent to communicate verbally themselves. When giving a hand massage, some people like to just 'switch off' and enjoy the feeling of the massage without having to communicate in any way. Massage, when given in a gentle and caring way as a quality experience, is a continuous flow of non-verbal communication and it has been said that in order for the full communicative quality of the massage to be experienced, it is normally carried out in silence (Pratt and Mason, 1981). This, however, depends entirely on the recipient of the massage, and the need to talk may be greater than the need for silence. A few people tend to fall asleep during massage which generally indicates that they must feel very comfortable and secure in the therapist's presence. Relaxation has occurred, in this case, at both a psychological and physiological level. In fact, during massage and other forms of therapeutic touch and handling there is potential for almost all of Kitwood and Bredin's 12 signs of well-being to be demonstrated.

Boundaries to touch

Referring again to the contract of care, because this will have been established before any use of diagnostic or therapeutic touch in a patient–therapist inter-action, it covers the usual social boundaries to touch, but with those who are unable to express themselves verbally or to understand the meaning of a contract of care, any touch could still be perceived as discomfort and as an invasion of their person (De Wever, 1977). We should try to be very sensitive and attempt to demonstrate and explain our actions non-verbally to these people in order to establish trust and a relationship based on confidence.

Even given the contract of care, there are still individual preferences which must be respected. Some people have had difficult experiences with touch and handling in the past and have only experienced touch in a negative way, perhaps in the form of lack of care and poor handling skills. These people will need very gentle, sensitive and careful handling in order to allow them to experience more positive forms of touch.

A few people simply do not like the feeling of being touched; they find it irritating and are more likely to become agitated if physical contact persists. Facial expression, body language and voice intonation must play a much greater role in interactions with these people.

As has already been described by Norberg *et al.* (1986), if someone's personal space is invaded by others, the fight or flight response will be exhibited and if physical flight is impossible, as in advanced stages of dementia or severe physical disability, the last resort will be a psychological flight (i.e. withdrawal). They then go on to describe how the bedridden patient suffering from the final stages of dementia has a very small territory of his own – his bed – and that he may not even be able to reach his own bedside table. In addition, his bed will often be invaded by the care-givers for cleaning, feeding and so on. In order to feel safe, the patient will withdraw further into himself (Norberg *et al.*, 1986).

A patient in such a position requires particularly careful and gentle handling, as his perception of touch has changed. Even if cleaning, dressing and feeding are carried out in a very caring way, they will often still be perceived by the patient as an invasion of territory or personal space. It will be necessary to introduce gentle, therapeutic touch very gradually with such a patient, to allow for this altered perception of normal touch, before gradually combining the two different forms of touch and handling, i.e. therapeutic touch of an expressive nature with therapeutic touch of a more clinical nature. Some examples might include gentle massage *in situ* before moving and positioning contracted limbs, explanations at each stage even if the patient does not seem to be understanding, watching the face for expressions of pain, moving only one part of the body at a time, moving only in the free range, avoidance of moving into the area of pain, careful use of pillows for support and positioning, use of pauses and frequent use of the patient's name.

Although we are permitted to use diagnostic and therapeutic touch freely as part of the contract of care, we, as individuals and care-givers, have our own personal boundaries and it does not help anyone if we go beyond these and then feel uneasy (Kitwood and Bredin, 1992). Some therapists, as individuals, use touch more freely than others, e.g. one therapist may only use touch when necessary for diagnosis or treatment but another may use it, in addition, for reassurance and comfort. Each therapist is an individual person and should not attempt to use touch more frequently than they are comfortable with. Feelings of uneasiness on the part of the therapist will be communicated to the patient by non-verbal means and will almost certainly detract from the therapeutic process.

Touch for relaxation

Although touch is considered by many to be the most powerful form of non-verbal communication, it has traditionally received the least research attention (Duncan, 1969). Little research seems to have been made into the longer term consequences of touch, and the physiological reactions to touch seem rarely to have been measured.

Traditionally, touching has often been used for reassurance and relaxation in the form of perhaps putting a comforting arm round someone, holding their hand or massaging their shoulders to relieve stress and tension. For a person to feel relaxed, the body needs to change from being in a state of anxiety to being in a relaxed state. When relaxed, the parasympathetic nervous system is dominant and there is a general slowing down of most of the body systems (Keable, 1989), i.e. a decrease in blood pressure, heart rate, blood flow to the skeletal muscles, breathing rate, sweat output and skin conductance. The body can then be described as being physiologically relaxed. However, there is more to the overall relaxation experience than just physiological relaxation. In a study, this time carried out on a group of dementia sufferers in a day hospital, physiological measurements of pulse rate and skin conductance were taken. The pulse rate was taken before and after massage and skin conductance was monitored continuously throughout. In addition, psychological measures were taken before and after massage using a four-point visual analogue scale to try to measure the effect the massage made on the group of individuals in the study on a more subjective level. The results obtained from the physiological measurements were inconclusive in this case, whereas the results from the visual analogue scale showed that the group of patients in the study *felt* more relaxed and comfortable on a subjective and psychological level as a result of the hand massage, i.e. a pleasant, warm, non-threatening experience (Poon, 1991).

Hyperventilation and panic attacks are a more extreme form of anxiety, where the oxygen supply to the brain has been greatly increased as a result of a general increase in respiratory rate often coupled with gasping. There is an increase in heart rate, an increase in sweat production and a generalized erythema. The person may experience 'pins and needles', 'butterflies in the stomach' and may feel dizzy and faint. Panic attacks are very debilitating and can rule the lives of those who suffer from them. The physiotherapist can help by offering touch and massage as a relaxation technique, combined with other forms of relaxation therapy; first, because massage *does* produce physiological relaxation in that it affects the parasympathetic nervous system and alpha rhythms in the brain, which produces a reversal of the physiological symptoms of anxiety, i.e. increase in heart rate and respiratory rate, etc. However, the physical techniques involved in massaging are not sufficient on their own to help someone effectively control a panic attack; relaxation on a more psychological and subjective level is required and this is where the appropriate use of body language and non-verbal communication, that is, the other very important aspects of touch and handling, come into play during massage, e.g. the one-to-one individual time, the feeling of being warm and secure, the feeling of being valued as a person and, as Hargreaves points out, the feeling that the interaction is occurring in a calm and unhurried way (Hargreaves, 1987). Relaxation depends not just on the physical techniques applied but on the *way* in which they are applied, and satisfaction with an interaction between professional and patient has been shown to result not from the actual time taken but from the patient's perception of the time being enough (DiMatteo, 1979).

Touch and the elderly

Elderly people probably rely, more than anyone else, on touch for gathering information about their environment. As a result of sensory deprivation, e.g. deteriorating hearing or eyesight, their need for touch may be very great (Hollinger, 1980), and because the other senses are no longer very effective, touch must be relied upon much more for provision of basic sensory information.

Touch is very effective as a form of non-verbal communication and, therefore, those with communication problems either as a result of a physical disability, e.g. a stroke, or a mental health problem, e.g. communication difficulties associated with a dementing illness, are in very great need of touch. Elderly people often fall into one or both of these categories and therefore their need for touch is greater than those of us without such problems, yet it has been shown that they are one of the least touched groups of all (Goodykoontz, 1979). In a study observing differences in touching behaviour among nurses working in a home for the elderly it was found that men and women who were described as 'severely impaired' were touched less often than those described as 'mildly impaired' (Watson, 1975).

One example is of a lady who had become anxious and restless. The general feeling among her carers was that she needed more stimulation, but the numerous activities they tried with her were not very successful in that she would only show interest for a moment before walking away. When increased frequency and duration of body contact was introduced as another method of approaching her anxiety and restlessness, her day became different. She would still wander around but would be arm-in-arm with a companion. She enjoyed hand and back massages and having her hair brushed very frequently, not to mention lots of spontaneous hugs and kisses in between. As time went on, everyone noticed how much more contented, relaxed and happy she appeared (Kitwood and Bredin, 1992). This is a prime example of the way in which someone's need or problem, in this case, anxiety and restlessness, can be successfully managed using, first, the skilful interpretation of non-verbal communication and, secondly, the therapeutic use of touch.

Those suffering from dementia often have a great deal of insight into their problems for which they are not always given credit, because the rest of us find it difficult to assess exactly how someone with dementia feels. They often know that they are no longer the person they used to be and that they are gradually 'losing their grip' on day-to-day situations. They are desperately in need of reassurance that they are still wanted and valued as people. Caring, supportive touch can reinforce feelings of being wanted and valued as the person they are now, as opposed to how they used to be in the past, particularly if it is given by someone who has only come into contact with them fairly recently, who did not know them before and who will not be tempted to make comparisons with the past. As health professionals, we are in an ideal position to give this kind of reassurance and reinforcement that they are a valued person in the present, not just in the past.

A hand massage, for most people, is a pleasant, warm, non-threatening experience, and a time where they have the therapist all to themselves. Relatives and carers who often sit next to a dementia sufferer desperate to communicate but not knowing how to, can be taught and encouraged to give their relative a hand massage. They are usually grateful for something to do which shows care and concern.

Conclusion

Touch can be used in many different ways within the context of a contract of care established between patient and therapist, particularly those patients suffering from mental illness who are stressed and vulnerable.

Therapeutic touch lies somewhere between instructive or instrumental touch, e.g. guiding a limb, supporting the body, and expressive touch, e.g. hugging, holding a hand, putting an arm round someone. It is essential that care should be taken when touching a patient, to ensure that their dignity is preserved, that pain is avoided where possible and that each person is treated in exactly the same respectful way. It is very difficult for us to assess how much a confused person can understand and it is safer, therefore, to assume that they understand everything.

Caring, reassuring touch and gentle handling can be used for relaxation or for healing and can make someone who is elderly and/or confused and to whom words perhaps do not mean anything anymore, feel wanted and valued, something they may not have felt for a long time. For these people, touch may be their only means of communication – a lifeline.

References

Argyle, M. (1972) *The Psychology of Interpersonal Behaviour*, Penguin Books, London
De Vito, J. (1980) Universals of non-verbal messages. In *The Interpersonal Communication Book*, 2nd edn, Harper and Row, New York

De Wever, M. (1977) Nursing home patients' perception of nurses' affective touching. *Journal of Psychology*, **96**, 163–171

DiMatteo, M.R. (1979) Non-verbal skill and the physician–patient relationship. In *Skill in Non-Verbal Communication – Individual Differences* (ed. Rosenthal, R.), Gunn and Hain, Cambridge, MA

Duncan, S. (1969) Non-verbal communication. *Psychological Bulletin*, **72**, 118–137

Exline, R.W. (1971) Visual interaction: the glances of power and preference. In *Non-Verbal Communication – Readings with Commentary* (ed. Weitz, S.), Oxford University Press, New York

Frank, L.K. (1957) Tactile communication. *Genetic Psychology Monographs*, **56**, 216–245

Gallois, C., Bent, A., Best, M. *et al.* (1979) Non-verbal behaviour in same-sex and mixed-sex physiotherapist–patient interactions. *Australian Journal of Physiotherapy*, **25**, 5–9

Goodykoontz, L. (1979) Touch: attitudes and practice. *Nursing Forum*, **10**, 4–17

Hargreaves, S. (1987) The relevance of non-verbal skills in physiotherapy. *Physiotherapy*, **73**, 685–688

Hollinger, L. (1980) Perception of touch in the elderly. *Journal of Gerontological Nursing*, **6**, 741–746

Jones, R.J. (1991) *Management in Physiotherapy*, Radcliffe Medical Press, Oxford

Keable, D. (1989) *The Management of Anxiety – A Manual for Therapists*, Churchill Livingstone, Edinburgh

Kitwood, T. and Bredin, K. (1992) *Person to Person: A Guide to the Care of Those with Failing Mental Powers*, Gale Centre Publications, Loughton, Essex, UK

Le May, A. (1986) The human connection. *Nursing Times*, **82**, 28–29

Mason, A. (1985) Something to do with touch. *Physiotherapy*, **71**, 167–169

Montague, A.M. (1971) *Touching: The Human Significance of the Skin*, Columbia Press, New York

Montague, A. (1977) *Touching: The Significance of the Skin*, Harper and Row, London

Morris, D. (1978) *Manwatching; A Field Guide to Human Behaviour*, Triad Panther

Norberg, A., Melin, E. and Asplund, K. (1986) Reactions to music, touch and object presentation in the final stages of dementia – an exploratory study. *International Journal of Nursing Studies*, **23**, 315–323

O'Gorman, G. (1975) 'Anti-motivation'. *Physiotherapy*, **61**, 176–179

Perry, J.F. (1975) Non-verbal communication during physical therapy. *Physical Therapy*, **55**, 593–600

Poon, K. (1991) *Hand Massage and Music: The Effectiveness of Each as Forms of Relaxation Therapy with Dementia-Sufferers*, Association of Chartered Physiotherapists in Psychiatry,

Pratt, J.W. (1978) A psychological view of the physiotherapist's role. *Physiotherapy*, **64**, 241–242

Pratt, J.W. and Mason, A. (1981) *The Caring Touch*, Heyden Press, London

Watson, W.H. (1975) The meaning of touch: geriatric nursing. *Journal of Communication*, **25**, 104–112

Williams, J. (1986) Physiotherapy *is* handling. *Physiotherapy*, **72**, 66–70

Neuroendocrine–immune network, nociceptive stress and the general adaptive response

Frank Willard

Introduction

Human beings are faced with protecting their body against the extremely varied and often harsh external environmental conditions. Simultaneously, we also have to maintain a relatively constant internal environment, conducive to the complex chemistry of our metabolism. To accomplish this protection we have developed a sophisticated network of extracellular messenger molecules composed of the secretory products of many cells, chief of which are those in the *neural, endocrine*, and *immune systems*. The components of these three systems, working in a very closely regulated network, called the *neuroendocrine–immune network*, control the movement and behaviour of the body as well as its internal chemistry.

The messenger molecules of the neuroendocrine–immune network, variously termed *neuroregulators, immunoregulators* (or cytokines) and *hormones*, are produced and secreted in normal baseline rhythms which serve to define the homoeostatic condition of the body. The integrated interactions of these three types of messenger molecules tie the neural, immune and endocrine systems into one functional network (Figure 8.1). Alterations in the rhythmical secretion of these messenger molecules are initiated in response to potentially harmful stimuli from either outside or inside of our bodies. These harmful or potentially harmful stimuli were called *stressors* by Selye (1946). The alteration in body chemistry to such stressors defines the *general adaptive response*. As impending threats diminish, feedback regulatory pathways function to re-establish the normal baseline rhythms of messenger molecule secretion, thereby diminishing the general adaptive response.

The protective homoeostatic activities of the neuroendocrine–immune network are responsive to two major types of *sensory* information, *neural* and *immune*. The peripheral nervous system is capable of detecting changes in various forms of energy surrounding and within the body, such as mechanical, chemical and light energy. In response to such stimuli, these sensory neurons release a coded signal of neurotransmitters in the central nervous system to initiate protective reflexes. Similarly, white blood cells (immune cells) sense changes in the antigen body map and, in response, release a coded signal composed of immunoregulators such as the interleukins, a family of small peptide messenger molecules (Arai *et al.* 1990). These immunoregulators

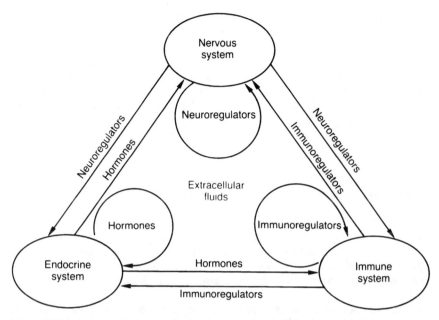

Figure 8.1 Interactions of the neuroendocrine-immune network. Each of these three systems produces messenger molecules called neuroregulators, immunoregulators and hormones. Not only do these messengers influence cells in their respective systems, but they also have effects on cells in other systems. Thus, the three systems truly function as a single, co-ordinated network

co-ordinate the activity of immune cells, as well as other cells to initiate protective immune responses. Both the neural and immune sensory signals lead to alterations in body chemistry as well as in behaviour and cognition. These changes in bodily functions represent significant features of the general adaptive response.

Once a general adaptive response has begun in response to stressors, activity in the central nervous system shifts into a state of increasing arousal, vigilance, and awareness, termed *behavioural adaptation*. Simultaneously, the physiological pathways of adaptation such as gluconeogenesis, the breakdown of complex compounds to form glucose, and the mobilization of energy stores for escape and wound repair processes are activated. Also simultaneously, non-adaptive pathways such as those involved in digestion and reproduction are suppressed. Ultimately, an overall dampening of immune system functions occurs as well as a short-term desensitization of the neural system, termed *anti-nociceptive response*. These responses prevent massive overreaction of the body's defences to the stressor(s). *While in the short term these adaptive responses are very beneficial to the survival of the individual, if excessively prolonged the same adaptive responses can themselves prove to be detrimental to the body* (Cerami, 1992).

This chapter will focus mainly on the adaptive responses initiated by components of the neuroendocrine–immune network in response to noxious or potentially harmful stimuli. Examples of such stimuli are overt or surgical trauma or tissue damage occurring within muscles, bones, joints or visceral organs as a result of misuse or disease. A model will be presented that demonstrates how sensory information from various neural and immune sources converge on a final common pathway in the hypothalamus to influence two major homoeostatic systems: the *autonomic nervous system* and the *endocrine system*. The role of these two hypothalamic systems in the initiation of a general adaptive response will be examined. Primary interest will be directed towards understanding the impact which this adaptive response has on body physiology and psychology. Finally, we will consider what happens when the body experiences prolonged exposure to the substances of the general adaptive response.

Detection of nociceptive information

Nociceptive or painful events are detected by sensory nerves distributed throughout the tissues of the body. There are several classifications of sensory neurons (reviewed in Light and Perl, 1993, and listed in Table 8.1). However, for the purposes of this chapter, sensory neurons can be depicted as dividing into two categories: large type A neurons and small type B neurons (Figure 8.2 and Table 8.1).

The type A neurons tend to have large myelinated axons (Figure 8.2). The peripheral terminals of these axons end in elaborate encapsulated structures. Type A neurons are easily activated, thus they are sensitive to low-energy stimuli. Taken as a group, the type A sensory neurons constitute what has been termed the *A-afferent system*, functioning in discriminative touch and proprioception (Prechtl and Powley, 1990). These neurons give us a constant supply of sensory information concerning our position in space and of the various forms of innocuous stimuli that routinely contact us. Normally, activation of type A neurons does not lead to initiation of the general adaptive response.

Conversely, type B neurons of the dorsal root ganglia have small axons surrounded by little or no myelin. The peripheral ends of these axons terminate in unencapsulated terminals also termed naked endings (Figure 8.2). The small calibre fibres constitute the *B-afferent system* (Prechtl and Powley, 1990). Axons of the B-afferent system are ubiquitously distributed throughout the fascias of the body including the connective tissues surrounding muscle, bone, ligament, tendon and joint capsule, in the meninges surrounding the brain and spinal cord, and in the visceral organs and their suspensory ligaments such as the mesenteries. Neurons of the B-afferent system also provide a sensory innervation

Table 8.1 A classification of sensory axons (From Light and Perl, 1993, by permission of the W. B. Saunders Co.)

	Cutaneous nerve	Muscle nerve	Conduction velocity (m/s)	Diameter (μm)
A-afferent fibres	Aα-Aβ	Group I	72–130 35–108	12–22 6–18
	Aβ	Group II	36–72	6–12
B-afferent fibres	Aδ	Group III	3–30	3–7
	C	Group IV	0.2–2	0.25–1.35

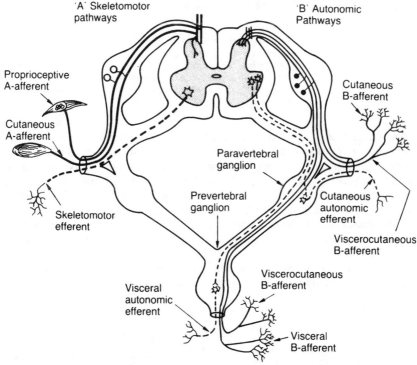

Figure 8.2 Comparison of the A-afferent (left-hand side) and B-afferent (right-hand side) systems. Nerve fibres in the A-afferent system have large encapsulated endings and convey discriminative touch and proprioception. Those in the B-afferent system have naked nerve-endings and convey crude touch, nociception and thermal sense. (From Prechtl and Powley, 1990, by permission of Cambridge University Press)

for the vasculature and lymphatic organs. Many of the B-afferent axons are hard to activate, thus they respond only to high energy containing, or noxious, stimuli. These high threshold nociceptors are silent throughout most of our lives until they are irritated by tissue damage. Activation of type B sensory neurons is contributory to the formation of a general adaptive response. Most importantly, the axons of the B-afferent system can become *sensitized*, lowering their thresholds of activation and responding to low energy containing, or non-noxious, stimuli. In such cases, the patient experiences *allodynia*, a painful reaction to non-noxious or non-painful stimuli.

Two major types of stimuli can activate nociceptive axons of the B-afferent system. Mechanical energy, distorting the tissue and the nerve endings, is thought to open ion channels in the tips of the nerve endings and depolarize the axon (Kandel *et al.*, 1991). In addition, specific chemicals involved in the inflammatory reaction will also interact with receptors on the nerve endings, thereby activating the small-calibre fibres.

Another sensory mechanism for the detection of harmful stimuli in the body is the immune system. When confronted by a change in the antigenic map of the body, such as the presence of a foreign antigen or inflammatory substance,

Table 8.2 A list of immuniregulators

Interleukins (1–7)
Interferons (alpha, beta, and gamma)
Tumour necrosis factor (beta)
Colony stimulating factors
Leukaemia inhibiting factor or neuroleukin
Transforming growth factor (beta)

immune cells and connective tissue cells release messenger molecules termed *immunoregulators* or *cytokines* (Table 8.2). These cytokines are multifunctional, messenger molecules, serving both as intercellular communicators and as growth factors regulating the multiplication and development of many types of cells throughout the tissues of the body (Nathan and Sporn, 1991). The immuno-regulators, such as the *interleukins*, are responsible for co-ordinating the activity of immune cells and connective tissue cells in the response to foreign substances. In addition, these immunoregulators are capable of providing warning signals to the nervous system.

Many of the pro-inflammatory molecules produced by the immune system are capable of interacting with the nervous system at the level of the peripheral nerve

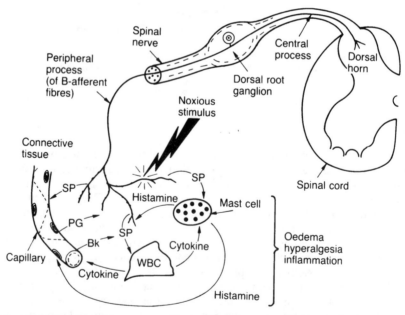

Figure 8.3 Interaction between neuropeptides and immunocytes: production of a feedforward, inflammatory cascade. A terminal of a B-afferent fibre is illustrated ending in connective tissues near a capillary. A noxious stimulus has initiated the release of a neuropeptide, substance-P (SP), from the nerve ending. The SP has triggered the release of histamine from the surrounding mast cells, cytokines from the white blood cells, and bradykinin (Bk) and prostaglandins (PG) from the capillary. These latter substances have triggered the release of more substance-P from the nerve endings, thus a feedforward cycle has been initiated resulting in oedema (swelling), hyperalgesia (sensitivity to touch) and inflammation

terminals (Schaible and Grubb, 1993). The interactions of the cytokines with the small, B-afferent fibres of the nervous system promote the inflammatory process in the surrounding tissue (Figure 8.3). When activated by cytokines, or other pro-inflammatory chemicals such as histamine, bradykinin (Bk), and prostaglandins (PG), or by mechanical irritation, these small sensory fibres secrete several small *neuropeptides* such as substance-P (SP), somatostatin and vasoactive intestinal polypeptide (Payan *et al.*, 1984). The release of these neuropeptides from the peripheral process of B-afferent fibres challenges the traditional concept of sensory neuron organization. Thus, many B-afferent neurons not only detect harmful stimuli and signal the central nervous system, but they also secrete biologically active molecules that regulate cellular activity in the surrounding tissue. Substance-P, a small neuropeptide, is especially notable since it is a very powerful pro-inflammatory compound capable of stimulating the release of histamine from mast cells and several cytokines from white blood cells. In addition, substance-P is an irritant to the very axons that secreted it; conse-quently it can stimulate the small calibre fibres of the B-afferent system, causing them to release more inflammatory neuropeptides. A chemical cascade is thus established, whereby the release of one substance (substance-P) from nerve endings triggers the release of a second (histamine) from mast cells, which in turn increases the production and release of the first (substance-P). The end result of this feedforward pathway within the tissue is swelling (oedema and inflammation) along with increased sensitivity to touch called *hyperalgesia* (Figure 8.3).

Processing of nociceptive information in the spinal cord

As a spinal nerve approaches the spinal cord, it divides into dorsal and ventral roots (Figure 8.4). The individual nerve, its roots and its associated portion of the spinal cord represent a *spinal segment*. Each spinal segment receives sensory information from its spinal nerve. Within the spinal nerve, each sensory neuron has a peripheral process that ends in the tissues of the body, a cell body that is located in a dorsal root ganglion, and a central process that enters the spinal cord. The grey matter of the spinal cord is divided into a *dorsal (sensory) horn* and *ventral (motor) horn*; in portions of the spinal cord, a third region, the *lateral horn*, contains neurons of the autonomic nervous system. The central processes of the B-afferent neurons end in the dorsal horn. Thus, an important function of the dorsal horn is the processing of nociceptive information carried in the B-afferent system.

Several types of neuron are present in the dorsal horn, each type distinguished by the target of its axon (Schoenen and Faull, 1990; Schoenen and Grant, 1990; Figure 8.4–8.6). Neurons contributing axons to the major *spinal cord pathways* or tracts have cell bodies in the superficial and deep portions of the dorsal horn. They send their axons across the midline of the spinal cord to the contralateral side where they enter a pathway called the *anterolateral system* (spinothalamic and spinoreticular tracts) and ascend to reach the brainstem, hypothalamus and thalamus (Figure 8.5). The majority of neurons in the grey matter represent another class of spinal neurons termed *interneurons* (ITN in Figure 8.4 and Figure 8.6). Their axons make up the intrinsic circuits of the spinal cord segment

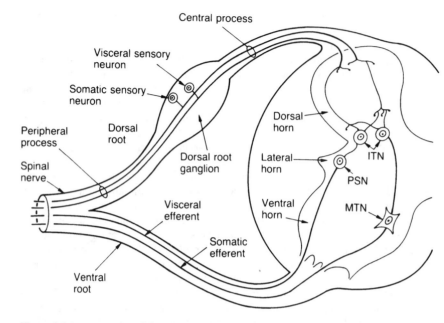

Figure 8.4 A cross-section of the spinal cord and a spinal nerve. As the spinal nerve approaches the spinal cord it separates into dorsal (sensory) and ventral (motor) roots. The B-afferent fibres have a peripheral process that reaches out to the peripheral tissues and a central process that terminates in the dorsal horn of the cord. The interneurons (ITN) of the dorsal horn are the main target of the B-afferent fibres. Axons from the interneurons reach the preganglionic sympathetic neurons (PSN) of the lateral horn and the motoneurons (MTN) of the ventral horn

and terminate in the lateral and ventral horns where they influence the activity in the autonomic and somatic motor systems, respectively.

The interneurons of the dorsal horn contribute to the formation of complex circuits which have important roles in posture and locomotion. Many of these cells are inserted between the synaptic endings of B-afferent fibre system and the motor neurons in the ventral and lateral horns of the spinal segment (Figure 8.4). This group of cells, referred to collectively as the *interneuronal pool*, is also the target of axons that descend to the spinal cord from the brainstem and cerebral cortex (Davidoff and Hackman, 1991). Thus, the interneuronal pool of the spinal cord integrates signals from primary afferent fibres with the motor instructions arising from higher centres of the brain (Figure 8.6). The combined output of these neurons provides the patterns for many complex locomotory (Grillner and Matsushima, 1991; Giszter *et al.*, 1993) and autonomic functions. *In summary, nociceptive information, arising from injury to either somatic or visceral tissues, enters the dorsal horn through the small calibre axons of the B-afferent system. These signals influence the activity of the segmental interneuronal pool, thereby affecting neural activity in both the lateral horn (sympathetic nervous system) and the ventral horn (somatic motor system).*

Nociceptive signals initiate neural reflexes involving the somatic musculature of the body. The most common response to an acute nociceptive event is a withdrawal reflex, thereby helping the individual avoid further injury. Closely

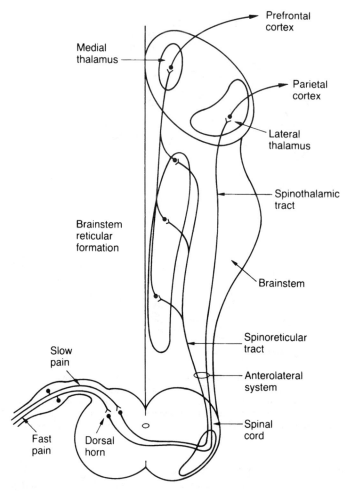

Figure 8.5 Origin and termination of the anterolateral system. Two different axons in the B-afferent system are shown entering the dorsal horn of the spinal cord. One axon, carrying fast pain, is slightly larger and synapses with dorsal horn neurons that, in turn, send their axons to the lateral thalamus. This pathway is involved in localizing pain. The other B-afferent fibre, marked slow pain, synapses on a dorsal horn neuron that sends its axon to the brainstem reticular formation and from there to the medial thalamus. This pathway is involved in the emotion and behavioural components of pain. It is this latter pathway, slow pain, that is effective in initiating a general adaptive response

related, but more complicated reflexes involve escape behaviour and, ultimately, future avoidance of the stimulus. The persistent relay of nociceptive information from inflamed tissues, through the interneuronal pool to the ventral horn, can also alter the tonic activity of its motoneurons, thereby changing the tone in the associated skeletal muscles (reviewed in Schaible and Grubb, 1993). When inflammation involves a joint, this type of response is known as splinting or guarding by the muscles surrounding that joint. Excessive input from joint nociceptive fibres will alter the activity of interneurons at that and adjacent

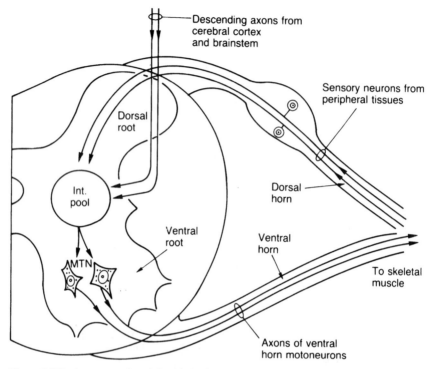

Figure 8.6 The interneuronal pool (Int. pool) of the spinal cord. The interneurons of the spinal cord receive the synaptic endings from the B-afferent fibres and from the axons of neurons in the brainstem and cerebral cortex. The interneurons influence the activity of the motoneurons (MTN) in the ventral horn of the spinal cord and (not shown) the activity of preganglionic sympathetic neurons in the lateral horn. Arrows indicate the general flow of information in these pathways

segmental levels of the spinal cord, resulting in generally increased output from the alpha motoneurons (Schaible and Grubb, 1993). This so-called *facilitated segment* presents clinically as increased tone and spasms in associated skeletal muscles as well as bilateral asymmetry in joint position.

Segmental facilitation has effects on the autonomic system, altering the sympathetic neurons which control glandular and vasomotor activity. Activation of the lateral horn by enhanced nociceptive input to a facilitated segment, such as from an inflamed joint, leads to increased activity of the visceral component of the sympathetic nervous system, ultimately generating a *somatovisceral reflex* (Sato and Schmidt, 1973). For example, neural activation subsequent to inflammation of a knee joint alters the output of the lateral horn in thoracolumbar portions of the spinal cord. This event is observed clinically as an increase in cardiovascular rate, decrease in gastrointestinal function, and an increase in hormones released from the adrenal medulla (Sato et al., 1979, 1984, 1986; Sato, 1992). These alterations in visceral function involve reflexes mediated through endocrine as well as neural pathways. *Thus, dysfunction in the somatic tissues of the body leads to reflexive alteration of function in visceral organs.* The pathway through which this reflex occurs involves the convergence of B-afferent fibres systems from somatic and visceral tissue onto the interneurons of the dorsal horn and their subsequent influence over the visceromotor neurons in the lateral horn of the spinal cord (Sato and Schmidt, 1973; Sato, 1992).

The dorsal horn of the spinal cord gives rise to two major ascending pathways for communicating nociceptive signals to the brain (Figure 8.5). Collectively, these pathways are referred to as the anterolateral system in reference to their position in the spinal cord (reviewed in Bonica, 1977, 1990). The spinothalamic pathway is the newest and fastest conducting member of the anterolateral system. It carries both non-noxious and noxious information from cells in the dorsal horn to the lateral portion of thalamus for relay to somatic sensory portions of the cerebral cortex (Bowsher, 1985). This pathway has an important role in the rapid localization of nociceptive events in the body. The spinoreticular and spino-hypothalamic tracts are the older and more slowly-conducting pathways in the anterolateral system. The spinoreticular tract carries primarily nociceptive information to the brainstem, medial thalamus and hypothalamus. In addition, this information is projected from the brainstem onto medial thalamic areas from which it is sent to the limbic areas of cerebral cortex, a portion of the cerebrum that is instrumental in behaviour and emotions. By influencing nuclei in the brainstem and hypothalamus, the spinoreticular and spinohypothalamic tracts have an important impact on the homoeostatic mechanism that mediate endocrine, immune and autonomic nervous system functions.

Processing of nociceptive information in the brainstem and hypothalamus

Nociceptive information from the spinal cord is processed in the brainstem, thalamus and hypothalamus, as well as several areas in the cerebral cortex (Figure 8.7). The core region of the brainstem, termed the reticular formation (shaded area in Figure 8.7), is a major site for receiving nociceptive signals. It orchestrates control of many visceral functions such as cardiovascular and respiratory rates and the secretomotor activity of the gastrointestinal tract (reviewed in Vertes, 1990). Axons from the spinal cord, ascending in the spino-reticular tract, terminate throughout portions of the reticular formation (see Figure 8.5). These spinal axons exert a strong influence on regulation of visceral functions. It is through the reticular formation that nociceptive informa-tion from spinal nerves reaches the *locus ceruleus* (Figure 8.8), a small cluster of neurons located towards the upper portion of the brainstem (Aston-Jones *et al.*, 1986).

Nociceptive stimuli, such as footshock stimulation, are strong activators of the locus ceruleus (Chiang and Aston-Jones, 1993). Although the locus ceruleus consists of a small cluster of neurons, it plays an important role in the general adaptive response to nociception because each of the ceruleus neurons produces *norepinephrine* (noradrenalin). The ceruleus axons, called adrenergic axons because they contain norepinephrine, are very diverse, featuring multiple branches that reach most areas of the cerebrum, brainstem and spinal cord (Figure 8.8). Thus, the locus ceruleus represents a major source of norepinephrine in the central nervous system.

The locus ceruleus constitutes a prime interest in the adaptive response, since this region of the brainstem is involved in controlling our awareness and arousal

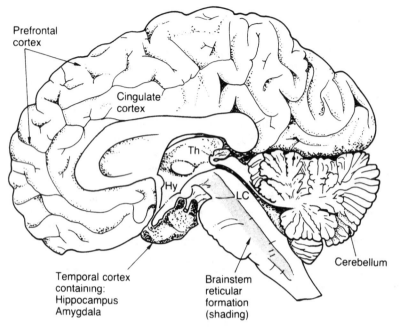

Figure 8.7 Sagittal view of the brain, illustrating some of the major sites for processing nociceptive information. These sites are: brainstem reticular formation (shading), locus ceruleus (LC), hypothalamus (Hy), thalamus (Th), cingulate cortex, prefrontal cortex, and the hippocampus and amygdala of the temporal cortex (After Willard, 1993)

(Aston-Jones *et al.*, 1984). Increased activity of ceruleus neurons is associated with feelings of anxiety. Conversely, the anxiolytic pharmaceuticals are generally effective in preventing the production or secretion of norepinephrine from ceruleus neurons (Gold *et al.*, 1988). The spinal cord connections through the reticular formation to the locus ceruleus provide a means for stimulating the noradrenergic neurons of the ceruleus complex and to initiate a general arousal response in response to nociceptive information from somatic or visceral sources (Figure 8.8).

The hypothalamus, a small region of the forebrain surrounding the lower aspect of the third ventricle, is a major target of adrenergic axons from the locus ceruleus (Figure 8.8). The hypothalamus plays an important role in processing of nociception and is a prime site for initiation of the general adaptive response (reviewed in Willard *et al.*, 1995, in press). The only direct sensory input to the hypothalamic nuclei arises from the visual system (Figure 8.9). This information acts as a circadian clock, providing light/dark signals to regulate, through a complex pathway, the pineal gland (Erlich and Apuzzo, 1985).Other indirect sensory inputs to the hypothalamic nuclei involve somatic and visceral information from the brainstem and spinal cord, as well as olfactory input from the cerebral cortex. Additional input arises from the limbic system involving such forebrain areas as the amygdala and hippocampal formation (Ganong, 1988). *Through these myriad pathways, the hypothalamus is influenced by most sensory information as well as emotional and cognitive processes occurring in the cerebral cortex* (Janig, 1983).

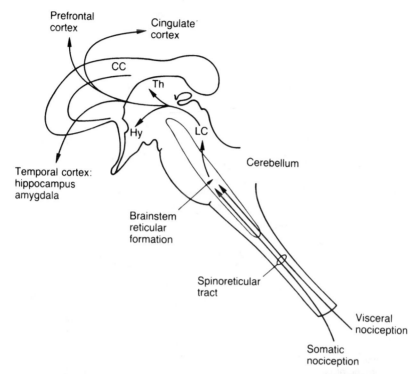

Figure 8.8 Location of the locus ceruleus and some of its connections. The locus ceruleus (LC) is located near the top of the brainstem. It receives axons from the reticular formation which, in turn, has received axons from the spinoreticular tract (part of the anterolateral system) carrying somatic and visceral nociceptive information. The locus ceruleus sends its adrenergic axons to the thalamus (Th), hypothalamus (Hy) as well as to the prefrontal, cingulate and temporal areas of cerebral cortex. Thus the locus ceruleus influences the major sites in the brain that process nociceptive information

Two major efferent systems link the hypothalamus with the homoeostatic processes of the body (Figure 8.9). First, a *neural efferent system* from the hypothalamus involving multiple fibre tracts which descend into the brainstem to influence the activity of the autonomic nervous system. Secondly, a *neurohaemal system* involving neurosecretory cells that produce and release hormones into blood vessels.

The neural output of the hypothalamus influences the autonomic nervous system of the brainstem and spinal cord (Figure 8.9). Through complex brainstem and spinal cord connections, the hypothalamus regulates such parameters as heart rate, blood pressure, gastrointestinal functions, respirations, vascular tone (reviewed in Smith and DeVito, 1984), and even the proliferative functions of cells in the immune tissue (Madden and Livnat, 1991).

The innervation of immune tissue by the peripheral autonomic nervous system also affords the hypothalamus influence over the activity of many immune cells. Adrenergic fibres (fibres containing norepinephrine) of the sympathetic nervous system are present in all of the lymphoid organs such as the thymus, spleen, lymph nodes, bone marrow, tonsils and lamina propria of the gastrointestinal

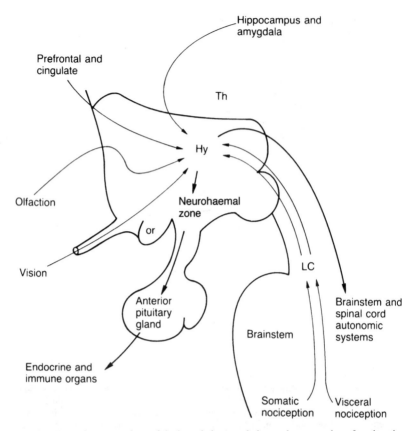

Figure 8.9 The major connections of the hypothalamus relating to the processing of nociceptive information. The hypothalamus receives somatic and visceral nociceptive information from the brainstem and spinal cord. It receives emotional signals from the prefrontal and cingulate cortex and from the hippocampus and amygdala. Two major output pathways from the hypothalamus influence the general adaptive response: the neural pathway into the brainstem and spinal cord to effect the autonomic nervous system and the neurohaemal pathway from the hypothalamus through the pituitary to influence the endocrine system

system (reviewed in Felten and Felten, 1991). Many cells of the immune system have been demonstrated to possess adrenoreceptors and to be responsive to the neurotransmitter norepinephrine which is released from axons of sympathetic nerves. In general, one response of immune cells to norepinephrine is to slow their rate of division and to quicken their rate of differentiation and maturation (Madden and Livnat, 1991; Roszman and Carlson, 1991). The major effect of this reduction in cell division rate is to initiate a general suppression of the immune system's ability to induce new responses. Thus, the sympathetic autonomic nervous system provides protection to the body by preventing the over-reaction of the immune system to harmful or potentially harmful stimuli.

The second major outflow pathway of the hypothalamus is directed to the anterior pituitary gland and, consequently, the endocrine system of the body (reviewed in Ganong, 1988; Figure 8.9 and 8.10). This method of communication with the anterior pituitary involves the production and secretion of releasing and inhibiting factors, termed *hypophyseotrophic hormones* (Figure 8.10), by the small neurons in the hypothalamus. Axons from these small neurons transport the hypophyseotropic hormones to specialized *neurohaemal contact zones* located in capillary beds at the base of the hypothalamus (Figure 8.10). These modified capillary beds are part of a special vascular system, called a portal system, which extends from the base of the hypothalamus to the anterior pituitary gland. At the neurohaemal contact zone, axons form synaptic contacts with blood vessel walls, releasing hypophyseotrophic hormones into the blood. The hypophyseotrophic hormones, usually small proteins with the

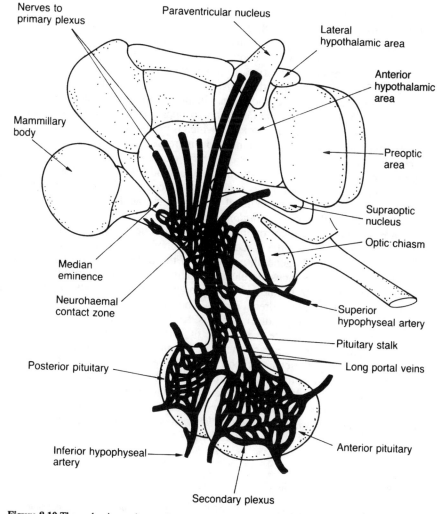

Figure 8.10 The endocrine pathways from the hypothalamus to the anterior pituitary gland. The hypophyseotrophic hormones are produced in the hypothalamus and secreted into a capillary bed in the neurohaemal contact zone. These hormones are removed from the blood in a second capillary bed in the anterior pituitary gland. (From Ganong, 1988)

Table 8.3 The hypophyseotrophic factors produced in the hypothalamus

Hypophyseotrophic factor	Function
Corticotrophin-releasing hormone	Stimulates release of ACTH
Thyrotrophin-releasing hormone	Stimulates release of TSH
Growth hormone-releasing hormone	Stimulates release of GH
Somatostatin	Inhibits release of GH
Gonadotrophin-hormone-releasing hormone	Stimulates release of FSH
Prolactin-releasing hormone	Stimulates release of prolactin
Prolactin-inhibiting hormone	Inhibits release of prolactin

exception of dopamine, control the production and release of the six hormones of the anterior pituitary (Table 8.3).

Several of the hypophyseotrophic hormones have important roles in the general adaptive response of the body to nociception, especially when integrated with the release of norepinephrine from the sympathetic nervous system. With regard to nociceptive stress, the most important of these hormones is that controlling the adrenal gland and the production of the adrenal cortical steroid hormones such as the very important immunosuppressive steroid, cortisol (Table 8.4). *Corticotrophin-releasing hormone*, which is produced in the hypothalamus, is the hypophyseotrophic hormone that increases the release of *adreno-corticotrophin* from the anterior pituitary (reviewed in Ganong, 1991). Adrenocorticotrophin, in turn, stimulates the production and release of the adrenal cortical steroid hormones such as the glucocorticoids from the adrenal cortex (Figure 8.10). This chemical circuit from the hypothalamus to the adrenal gland is called the *hypothalamic–pituitary–adrenal axis*.

The production of corticotrophin-releasing hormone in the hypothalamus is enhanced by signals from the noradrenergic (norepinephrine-containing) axons of the locus ceruleus. In general, activation of the B-afferent fibres by noxious stimuli stimulates the locus ceruleus, thereby enhancing the production of corticotrophin-releasing hormone in the hypothalamus. This leads to increased output of cortisol from the adrenal glands. Thus, as the locus ceruleus and other brainstem structures respond to noxious stimuli such as tissue trauma or inflammation, they stimulate the release of corticotrophin-releasing hormone, thereby enhancing the output of the hypothalamic–pituitary–adrenal axis and ultimately resulting in elevated blood cortisol levels. Many other signals such as visceral pain or emotional trauma can also activate the locus ceruleus and influence the general adaptive response. *This is an extremely important concept in the body's response to stressors; consequently, the hypothalamic–pituitary–adrenal axis has been called the last common pathway from the brain for the manifestation of the general adaptive response.*

Table 8.4 Hormones involved in the adrenal gland

Hypothalamus	Pituitary	Adrenal gland	Example
Corticotrophin releasing hormone	Adrenocorticotrophin	Glucocorticoids Mineralocorticoids	Cortisol Aldosterone

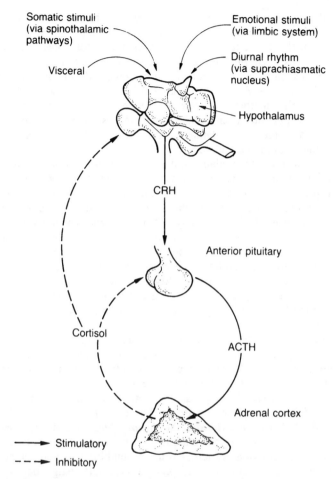

Somatic stimuli
(via spinothalamic
pathways)

Emotional stimuli
(via limbic system)

Visceral

Diurnal rhythm
(via suprachiasmatic
nucleus)

Hypothalamus

CRH

Anterior pituitary

Cortisol

ACTH

Adrenal cortex

——→ Stimulatory

– – –→ Inhibitory

Figure 8.11 The hypothalamic–pituitary–adrenal axis and its controlling factors. Somatic, visceral, and emotional stimuli as well as a diurnal rhythm influence the release of corticotrophin-releasing factor (CRH) from the hypothalamus. CRH increases the release of adrenocorticotrophin from the anterior pituitary gland which increases the release of cortisol from the adrenal cortex. (After Ganong, 1988)

The effects on the body of the adrenal steroid hormones are to create an energy-rich environment facilitating protective and healing pathways. Cortisol, an adrenal steroid, stimulates the breakdown of glycogen and lipids to form smaller, energy-rich compounds such as glucose and free fatty acids. The glycogen and lipids are taken from the body's stores of muscle protein and fats (reviewed in Baxter, 1992). Other activities of cortisol involve the facilitation of norepinephrine. Thus, cortisol enhances the vasoconstriction and pressor response of the vasculature to norepinephrine and epinephrine (adrenaline). Cortisol appears to be necessary for survival in stressful situations and people without its protection, such as those with Addison's disease, risk cardiovascular collapse in the face of excessive stress (Baxter, 1992).

One of the prime functions of cortisol appears to be control of other stress-induced chemicals to prevent excessive reactions (Ganong, 1988, 1991; Munck and Guyre, 1991). For example, one way that cortisol appears to suppress immune functions is by preventing the release of pro-inflammatory cytokines (see Table 8.2) such as the interleukins, interferons, and tumour necrosis factor from white blood cells. Adrenal cortical steroid hormones also block enzymes that degrade cell membranes, thereby preventing the formation of many inflammatory compounds, such as the prostaglandins. Thus, the adrenal cortical steroids prevent some of the damaging effects of prolonged exposure to the pro-inflammatory immunoregulators.

Activation of the hypothalamic–pituitary–adrenal axis also engages the sympathetic division of the autonomic nervous system. Corticotrophin-releasing hormone is produced by neurons in the hypothalamus that also project axons into the brainstem, suggesting a possible direct neural control of the brainstem autonomic nervous system by the hypophyseotropic neurons (neurons that regulate the endocrine functions of the anterior pituitary gland). Physiologically, the increased activity in the sympathetic nervous system is expressed as increased heart rate, blood pressure and total oxygen consumption, with decreased gastric motility. It is clear that there is a very close integration that occurs between the hypothalamic–pituitary–adrenal axis and the autonomic nervous system, leading to the initiation of a general adaptive response (Brown *et al.*, 1985; Brown and Fisher, 1985).

Nociceptive stressors, in addition to activating the hypothalamic–pituitary–adrenal axis, influence other endocrine systems. Increased activity in the *thyroid glands* is detected in certain conditions such as cold stress or exposure to high altitudes. Other endocrine systems, particularly those considered to be involved in non-adaptive processes, are suppressed when confronted with nociceptive stressors. These include the *hypothalamic–pituitary–growth hormone axis* and the *hypothalamic–pituitary–reproductive hormones axis*. Thus, the hypothalamus, acting through the pituitary gland hormones and the autonomic system, has a profound influence on homoeostasis. Critical to an understanding of this process is a knowledge of the factors controlling hypothalamic activity.

Neural control of the hypothalamic–pituitary–adrenal axis

The emphasis so far has been placed on the response of the hypothalamus and neuroendocrine-immune network to nociceptive signals from somatic tissue (Figure 8.12). However, it must be kept in mind that noxious or potentially noxious stimuli from other sources can also influence the chemical balance in this complex network. Multiple neural circuits in the brain and spinal cord are focused on the hypothalamus and specifically on the region producing corticotrophin-releasing hormone. Through these pathways, visceral and emotional stimuli access the hypothalamus as well as somatic stimuli.

Visceral sensory information plays a major role in the control of the hypothalamus through a myriad brainstem circuits (Figure 8.12). Nociceptive stimuli from internal organs are carried in small calibre, B-afferent fibres from the viscera to the thoracolumbar segments of the spinal cord. Thereafter these signals are relayed into the brainstem and hypothalamus through the antero-

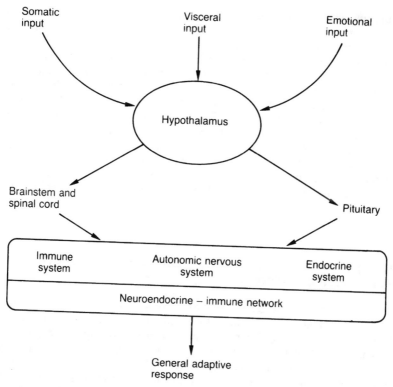

Figure 8.12 Summary of the neuroendocrine-immune interactions in the initiation of a general adaptive response

lateral tracts (see Figures 8.5 and 8.9). This process is similar to nociceptive information from the somatic sensory system. *Most importantly, through these pathways, noxious stimulation of the internal organs initiates a similar response from the hypothalamus (the general adaptive response), as do the nociceptive signals from injury to somatic body parts such as muscles, bones and joints.*

Of particular interest is the major neural influence over the hypothalamus arising in the limbic system of the forebrain (Figure 8.12). The forebrain limbic system can approximately be defined as the medial aspect of the temporal lobe of the cerebral cortex, including the hippocampal formation and amygdala, and the cingulate cortex and prefrontal cortex. These structures are united into a complex limbic circuit by their connections between themselves and those to the thalamus and hypothalamus. The limbic structures were first noted to be involved in processing the moods and emotions by Papez (1937) based on the study of behaviour in individuals who had suffered damaging lesions in this circuit. *Excessive activation of the limbic system, due to emotional stimuli, influences the hypothalamus leading to modulation of the hypothalamic–pituitary–adrenal axis. This mechanism respresents one pathway through which emotions have access to the neuroendocrine-immune network, thereby affecting homoeostasis.*

In summary, it is now apparent that noxious or potentially noxious input from somatic and visceral events, as well as input from emotional sources, form a triad of excitatory drives that increase the endocrine output of the hypothalamic–pituitary–adrenal axis (see Figure 8.11). This axis, sometimes referred to as the stress–response axis, has been portrayed as the *final common pathway for the general adaptive response*. These three diverse, yet convergent sources of excitatory input compound one another's influence. Thus, the input to this axis from somatic and/or visceral dysfunctions may serve to enhance the drive generated by the individual's emotions. Conversely, emotional situations act to exacerbate the influence over the axis of somatic and/or visceral nociceptive events. As such, the model illustrated in Figure 8.12 provides an approximation for conceptualizing the complex and variant physiological and psychological outcomes of somatic, visceral and emotional dysfunction within a given individual.

Dysregulation of the neuroendocrine-immune network: health-related outcomes

Precise regulation of the general adaptive response is necessary to maintain the normal physical and mental health of the individual. The dominant theme of this chapter is that stressors, either external or internal, are capable of shifting the hypothalamic–pituitary–adrenal axis towards the side of increased *cortisol* output from the adrenal gland and increasing the output of *catecholamines* (norepinephrine and epinephrine) from the sympathetic nervous system. The flux of adrenal steroids and catecholamines alters the chemical balance in the neuroendocrine-immune network. Multiple feedback control loops, sensitive to plasma cortisol and other messenger molecules, act to adjust the hypothalamic–pituitary–adrenal axis, returning its level of activity back to the normal, rhythmic homoeostatic condition (Figure 8.13); for example, elevated plasma cortisol and adrenocorticotrophin feed back onto the anterior pituitary to decrease the activity of the adrenal gland. In addition, rising blood cortisol levels feed back to the hypothalamus and hippocampus of the brain to diminish the release of corticotrophin-releasing hormone, ultimately decreasing the production of cortisol from the adrenal gland. *However, it has become evident in recent studies that these feedback control devices are subject to age-related and stress-induced dysfunctions* (McEwen, 1987; Meites, 1991; Stein-Behrens and Sapolsky, 1992).

One possible origin for the age-related disruption of homoeostatic mechanisms may be the loss, through cell death, of specific forebrain neurons involved in the feedback control pathways for regulation of the hypothalamic–pituitary–adrenal axis. Cell death is a normal event in the central nervous system and plays an important role during development. However, physiological and psychological factors, such as stressful stimuli, can damage specific populations of neurons in the primate nervous system (Sapolsky *et al.*, 1990), increasing their rate of cell death, particularly in those neuronal populations that control the hypothalamic–pituitary–adrenal axis. The result is elevated blood levels of cortisol and an increasing tendency to shift toward a general adaptive response. As such, these pathological mechanisms represent contributing factors for the

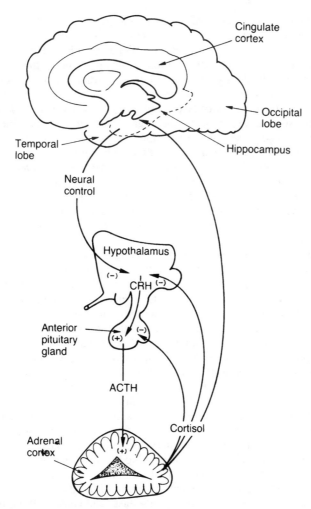

Figure 8.13 The multiple feedback control loops in the hypothalamic–pituitary–adrenal axis. The release of cortisol from the adrenal cortex feeds back to the anterior pituitary to suppress the release of adrenocorticotrophin (ACTH) and to the hypothalamus to suppress the release of corticotrophin-releasing hormone (CRH). Cortisol also feeds back to the hippocampus in the temporal lobe of the cerebrum. Through neural pathways, the hippocampus is capable of suppressing the release of CRH from the hypothalamus

overall decrease in functional properties of the immune system experienced in geriatric populations (Meites, 1990).

Prolonged exposure to inescapable stressors has been demonstrated specific-ally to damage the feedback control systems designed to monitor the activity of the general adaptive response (Sapolsky, 1985; Sapolsky *et al.*, 1985, 1990). Intrinsic to the limbic system are neural pathways that monitor the output of substances such as the adrenal cortical steroids. In response to increased cortisol output, these monitors function to suppress the functions of the hypothalamic–

pituitary–adrenal axis. One of these monitors, the hippocampal formation, contains neurons with membrane receptors for cortisol. Neurons with these cortisol receptors send axons to the hypothalamus where they are capable of suppressing the release of corticotrophin-releasing hormone, thereby acting as a feedback control in the hypothalamic–pituitary–adrenal axis. In some species, such as rats and monkeys, cortisol receptive neurons in the hippocampal formation are vulnerable to prolonged exposure to elevated blood cortisol levels. Thus, chronic stressors, an experimental paradigm of which is inescapable footshock, lead to the demise of neurons in the hippocampal formation, with concomitant loss of control of the hypothalamic–pituitary–adrenal axis. *With a breakdown in the control systems, the shift in body chemistry that was initiated by a noxious physical or emotional stimulus becomes more difficult to reverse, thereby creating a chronic condition of general adaptation, termed* maladaptation.

The chemical messengers of the neuroendocrine-immune network that characterize the general adaptive response are necessary for immediate survival of the individual, yet these same molecules can become deleterious to the body if their production and secretion is prolonged excessively (Cerami, 1992). The chemical cocktail of immunoregulators (see Table 8.2) released into the peripheral tissue by activated immune cells can severely damage vascular walls and, in circulation, can be damaging to liver cells. Particularly, interleukin-1, an important pro-inflammatory cytokine, is destructive to cartilage and to the cells in the pancreas. It has also been implicated in the induction of fever and of anorexia, the inflammation of arthritis and colitis, and the formation of athero-sclerotic plaques (Dinarello and Wolff, 1993). Long-term exposure to such immunoregulators as tumour necrosis factor and interferon leads to wasting of muscle mass and loss of weight, a state called cachexia, typically seen in end-stage cancer patients (Beutler, 1993). Finally, exposure of the nervous system to these pro-inflammatory substances is toxic to neurons. Particularly, these substances, by initiating autoimmune reactions, are destructive to neuroglial (supportive) cells in the central nervous system (Hughes, 1992). Chronic exposure to stress-induced, elevated blood levels of the adrenal cortical hormones influences the activity of the immune system. Examples of such emotional stressors are bereavement, divorce and family care-giving in chronic diseases such as senile dementia (Kiecolt-Glaser and Glaser, 1991). Importantly, the resulting immunosuppression from these stressors can predispose the individual to other secondary disease processes.

Alteration in the output of the hypothalamic–pituitary–adrenal axis affects psychological as well as physiological processes. For example, elevated blood cortisol levels represent a common feature of a cohort of individuals diagnosed with melancholic depression, a disease characterized by such disturbances in personality as increased anxiety, vigilance, obsessionalism, hyperarousal, aggressiveness and feelings of worthlessness (Gold *et al.*, 1988). Physiological profiles of patients with melancholic depression reveal increased production of cortisol and norepinephrine and breakdown in the regulation of these adaptive pathways with a consequent immunosuppression. It has been suggested that this disease represents a malfunction in the neural regulation of the hypo-thalamic–pituitary–adrenal axis, possibly involving the increased activity in the locus ceruleus (Gold *et al.*, 1988). Interestingly, the major depressions such as melancholia appear to develop through a kindling process similar to that which leads to seizure in the cerebral cortex. In this paradigm, episodes of melancholia occur at progressively shorter intervals and with progressively greater intensity in the natural history of the disease. To extrapolate from this observation, it suggests that initial exposure to a stressor does not push the person's regulatory mechanisms irretrievably out of balance. However, repeated exposure to a given stressor or simultaneous exposure to multiple stressors can, in certain circumstances, contribute to a breakdown in the feedback control pathways, leading to chronic dysregulation of the hypothalamic–pituitary–adrenal axis (Johnson *et al.*, 1992).

Stressful life experiences, especially those that are inescapable, appear to be critical factors in dysregulation of the hypothalamic–pituitary–adrenal axis. For example, chronic pain syndrome often manifests itself after the initial trauma has resolved. Individuals with this syndrome are faced with inescapable exposure to intense feelings of pain. Depression and anxiety are common complaints of patients suffering from chronic pain syndrome. A possible explanation of these observations is that the original injury, which led to the chronic pain response, increased the production and release of adrenal cortical hormones and catecholamines. As the chronic pain syndrome developed, the levels of these molecules in circulation were enhanced. This ultimately harms the feedback regulatory mechanisms designed to control the hypothalamic–pituitary–adrenal axis and contributes to the presentation of depression.

Depression is also a common outcome of another inescapable stressor, childhood sexual abuse (Peters, 1988). Specifically, this type of depression frequently presents with anxiety and arousal (Stein *et al.*, 1988), similar to that seen in melancholia. Again, a reasonable explanation of this observation is that chronic elevation of activity in the child's hypothalamic–pituitary–adrenal axis, in response to the prolonged abusive situation, damaged the feedback control pathways, producing a state of chronic general adaptation. As a result of these dysfunctional regulatory pathways, the adult victim of child sexual abuse may experience more difficulty in coping physiologically and psychologically with surrounding stressful situations. *In essence, stressful emotional or physical stimuli initiate a general adaptive response that the adult individual is incapable of controlling, resulting eventually in feelings of depression and anxiety as well as physiological changes in body function.*

It is evident from this discussion that excessive or prolonged activity of the hypothalamic–pituitary–adrenal axis is harmful to many aspects of our lives. Consequently, management of the causative factors such as somatic, visceral or emotional dysfunctions becomes of prime interest in controlling the long-term expression of the general adaptive response. The proposed model of hypothalamic–pituitary–adrenal axis regulation presented in this chapter suggests that somatic and visceral events leading to nociceptive signals could either predispose or be a significant secondary factor to an emotional dysfunction such as some forms of depression or anxiety. As such, the proposed model (see Figure 8.12) provides one mechanism for conceptualizing the close interplay between physical and mental illnesses. It follows from this model that the approach to patients with emotional dysfunctions, such as major psychological illness, should be complemented with a thorough consideration of their physical structure and appropriate treatment of somatic and visceral dysfunctions. This approach should be taken to maximize the ability of the natural restorative forces, inherent in the neuroendocrine-immune network of the body, to return to the pre-illness homoeostatic condition.

Conclusion

This chapter has presented a model to illustrate how noxious or potentially noxious somatic or visceral stimuli in peripheral tissue alter neural activity at the segmental level in the spinal cord producing abnormal, but adaptive, somatic and visceral reflexes. In addition, it has also suggested a mechanism whereby this same nociceptive signal code interacts with emotional stimuli in the limbic forebrain, eventually altering the output from the hypothalamus to the endocrine and autonomic nervous systems. The consequence of these interactions is a shifting of the homoeostatic mechanism within the neuroendocrine-immune network towards the general adaptive response. While this response may be of critical importance in coping with acute stressful conditions, it will become itself a pathological condition in the chronic state. The normal regulatory mechanisms that help ensure a return to homoeostatic rhythms are damaged by prolonged stress, thereby preventing the efficient rebalancing of the system when the stressor is relieved. In this sense, the adaptive response has become the stressor, and the body responds with pathological physiological and psychological processes.

In response to noxious or potentially harmful events, the triad of excitatory inputs to the hypothalamic–pituitary–adrenal axis – somatic, visceral and emotional – appear to exacerbate one another, allowing for the compounding of clinical signs and symptoms. Since it appears that kindling occurs in the neural component of this regulatory network, repeated or prolonged insults are potentially the most dangerous. Thus, the model provides a first approximation of the complex interaction between physical and mental states in the maintenance of homoeostasis and health. Ultimately, it can be concluded from the model that an emphasis must be placed on providing the individual with optimum physical stature as well as emotional balance to best assist them in maintaining a state of well-being.

References

Arai, K., Lee, F., Miyajima, A., Miyatake, S., Arai, N. and Yokota, T. (1990) Cytokines: co-ordinators of immune and inflammatory responses. *Annual Review of Biochemistry*, **59**, 783–836

Aston-Jones, G., Ennis, M., Pieribone, V.A., Nickell, W.T. and Shipley, M.T. (1986) The brain nucleus locus ceruleus: restricted afferent control of a broad efferent network. *Science*, **234**, 734–737

Aston-Jones, G., Foote, S. and Bloom, F.E. (1984) Anatomy and physiology of locus ceruleus neurons: functional implications. In *Norepinephrine* (eds Ziegler, M.G. and Lake, C.R.), Williams and Wilkins, Baltimore

Baxter, J.D. (1992) The effects of glucocorticoid therapy. *Hospital Practice*, **27**(9), 111–134

Beutler, B. (1993) Cytokines and cancer cachexia. *Hospital Practice*, **28**(4), 45–52

Bonica, J.J. (1977) Neurophysiologic and pathologic aspects of acute and chronic pain. *Archives of Surgery*, **112**, 750–761

Bonica, J.J. (1990) Anatomic and physiologic basis of nociception and pain. In *The Management of Pain* (ed. Bonica, J.J.), Lea and Febiger, Philadelphia

Bowsher, D. (1985) Pain: sensory mechanisms. *Handbook of Clinical Neurology*, 1(45), 227–244

Brown, M.F. and Fisher, L.A. (1985) Corticotropin-releasing factor: effects on the autonomic nervous system and visceral systems. *Federation Proceedings*, **44**, 243–248

Brown, M.R., Fisher, L.A., Webb, V., Vale, W.W. and Rivier, J.E. (1985) Corticotropin-releasing factor: a physiologic regulator of adrenal epinephrine secretion. *Brain Research*, **328**, 355–357

Cerami, A. (1992) Inflammatory cytokines. *Clinical Immunology and Immunopathology*, **62**, S3–S10

Chiang, C. and Aston-Jones, G. (1993) Response of locus ceruleus neurons to footshock stimulation is mediated by neurons in the rostral ventral medulla. *Neuroscience*, **53**, 705–715

Davidoff, R.A. and Hackman, J.C. (1991) Aspects of spinal cord structure and reflex function. *Neurology Clinics of North America*, **9**, 533–550

Dinarello, C.A. and Wolff, S.M. (1993) The role of interleukin-1 in disease. *New England Journal of Medicine*, **328**, 106–113

Erlich, S.S. and Apuzzo, M.L.J. (1985) The pineal gland anatomy, physiology, and clinical significance. *Journal of Neurosurgery*, **63**, 321–341

Felten, S.Y. and Felten, D.L. (1991) Innervation of lymphoid tissue. In *Psychoneuroimmunology*, 2nd edn (eds Ader, R., Felten, D.L. and Cohen, N.), Academic Press, San Diego

Ganong, W. (1988) The stress response – a dynamic overview. *Hospital Practice*, **23**(6), 155–190

Ganong, W.F. (1991) *Review of Medical Physiology*, Appleton and Lange, Norwalk, Connecticut

Giszter, S.F., Mussa-Ivaldi, F.A. and Bizzi, E. (1993) Convergent force fields organized in the frog's spinal cord. *Journal of Neuroscience*, **13**, 467–491

Gold, P.W., Pigott, T.A., Kling, M.A., Kalogeras, K. and Chrousos, G.P. (1988) Basic and clinical studies with corticotropin-releasing hormone. *Psychiatric Clinics of North America*, **11**, 327–334

Grillner, S. and Matsushima, T. (1991) The neural network underlying locomotion in lamprey-synaptic and cellular mechanisms. *Neuron*, **7**, 1–15

Hughes, R. (1992) Immune response in the peripheral nervous system. *Seminars in Neuroscience*, **4**, 257–263

Janig, W. (1983) The autonomic nervous system. In *Human Physiology* (eds Schmidt, R.F. and Thews, G.), Springer-Verlag, New York

Johnson, E.O., Kamilaris, T.C., Chrousos, G.P. and Gold, P.W. (1992) Mechanisms of stress: a dynamic overview of hormonal and behavioural homeostasis. *Neuroscience and Biobehavioral Review*, **16**, 115–130

Kandel, E., Schwartz, J.H. and Jessell, T.M. (1991) *Principles of Neural Sciences*, Elsevier, New York

Kiecolt-Glaser, J.K. and Glaser, R. (1991) Stress and immune function in humans. In *Psychoneuroimmunology*, 2nd edn (eds Ader, R., Felten, D.L. and Cohen, N.) Academic Press, San Diego

Light, A.R. and Perl, E.R. (1993) Peripheral sensory systems. In *Peripheral Neuropathy* (eds Dyck, P.J. and Thomas, P.K.), W.B. Saunders, Philadelphia

McEwen, B. (1987) Glucocorticoid-biogenic amine interactions in relation to mood and behaviour. *Biochemical Pharmacology*, **36**, 1755–1763

Madden, K.S. and Livnat, S. (1991) Catecholaminergic action and immunologic reactivity. In *Psychoneuroimmunology*, 2nd edn (eds Ader, R., Felten, D.L. and Cohen, N.), Academic Press, San Diego

Meites, J. (1990) Aging: hypothalamic catecholamines, neuroendocrine-immune interactions, and dietary restriction. *Proceedings of the Society for Experimental Biology and Medicine*, **195**, 304–311

Meites, J. (1991) Role of hypothalamic catecholamines in aging processes. *Acta Endocrinologica*, **125**, 98–103

Munck, A. and Guyre, P.M. (1991) Glucocorticoids and immune function. In *Psychoneuroimmunology*, 2nd edn (eds Ader, R., Felten, D.L. and Cohen, N.), Academic Press, San Diego

Nathan, C. and Sporn, M. (1991) Cytokines in context. *Journal of Cell Biology*, **113**, 981–986

Papez, J.W. (1937) A proposed mechanism of emotion. *Archives of Neurology and Psychiatry*, **38**, 725–743

Payan, D.G., Levine, J.D. and Goetzl, E.J. (1984) Modulation of immunity and hypersensitivity by sensory neuropeptides. *Journal of Immunology*, **132**, 1601–1604

Peters, S.D. (1988) Child sexual abuse and later psychological problems. In *Lasting Effects of Child Sexual Abuse* (eds Wyatt, G.E. and Powell, G.J.), Sage Publications, Newbury Park

Prechtl, J.C. and Powley, T.L. (1990) B-afferents: a fundamental division of the nervous system mediating homeostasis? *Behavioral Brain Science*, **13**, 289–331

Roszman, T.L. and Carlson, S.L. (1991) Neurotransmitters and molecular signaling in the immune response. In *Psychoneuroimmunology*, 2nd edn (eds Ader, R., Felten, D.L. and Cohen, N.), Academic Press, San Diego

Sapolsky, R.M. (1985) A mechanism for glucocorticoid toxicity in the hippocampus: increased neuronal vulnerability to metabolic insults. *Journal of Neuroscience*, **5**, 1228–1232

Sapolsky, R.M., Krey, L.C. and McEwen, B.S. (1985) Prolonged glucocorticoid exposure reduces hippocampal neuron number: implications for aging. *Journal of Neuroscience*, **5**, 1222–1227

Sapolsky, R.M., Uno, H., Rebert, C.S. and Finch, C.E. (1990) Hippocampal damage associated with prolonged glucocorticoid exposure in primates. *Journal of Neuroscience*, **10**, 2897–2902

Sato, A. (1992) The reflex effects of spinal somatic nerve stimulation on visceral function. *Journal of Manipulative and Physiological Therapeutics*, **15**, 57–61

Sato, A., Sato, Y. and Schmidt, R.F. (1979) The effects of somatic afferent activity on the heart rate. In *Integrative Function of the Autonomic Nervous System* (eds Brooks, C. *et al.*), Elsevier, New York

Sato, A., Sato, Y. and Schmidt, R.F. (1984) Changes in blood pressure and heart rate induced by movements of normal and inflamed knee joints. *Neuroscience Letters*, **52**, 55–60

Sato, A., Sato, Y. and Schmidt, R.F. (1986) Catecholamine secretion and adrenal nerve activity in response to movements of normal and inflamed knee joints in cats. *Journal of Physiology*, **375**, 611–624

Sato, A. and Schmidt, R.F. (1973) Somatosympathetic reflexes: afferent fibers, central pathways, discharge characteristics. *Physiological Reviews*, **53**, 916–947

Schaible, H.-G. and Grubb, B.D. (1993) Afferent and spinal mechanisms of joint pain. *Pain*, **55**, 5–54

Schoenen, J. and Faull, R.L.M. (1990) Spinal cord: chemoarchitectural organization. In *The Human Nervous System* (ed. Paxinos, G.), Academic Press, San Diego

Schoenen, J. and Grant, G. (1990) Spinal cord: connections. In *The Human Nervous System* (ed. Paxinos, G.), Academic Press, San Diego

Selye, H. (1946) The general adaptive syndrome and the diseases of adaptation. *Journal of Clinical Endocrinology*, **6**, 117–173

Smith, O.A. and DeVito, J.L. (1984) Central neural integration for the control of autonomic responses associated with emotion. *Ann. Rev. Neurosci.*, **7**, 43–65

Stein, J.A., Golding, J.M., Siegel, J.M., Burnam, M.A. and Sorenson, S.B. (1988) Long-term psychological sequelae of child sexual abuse. In *Lasting Effects of Child Sexual Abuse* (eds Wyatt, G.E. and Powell, G.J.), Sage Publications, Newbury Park

Stein-Behrens, B.A. and Sapolsky, R.M. (1992) Stress, glucocorticoids, and aging. *Aging Clin. Exp. Res.*, **4**, 197–210

Vertes, R.P. (1990) Fundamentals of brainstem anatomy: a behavioral perspective. In *Brainstem Mechanisms of Behavior* (eds Klemm, W.R. and Vertes, R.P.), John Wiley, New York

Willard, F.H., Mokler, D. and Morgane, P.J. (1995) The neuroendocrine–immune network and homeostasis (submitted)

9

Pain, stress and misdiagnosis

Maureen Dennis

Introduction

'Pain is what the patient says hurts' (McCaffrey, 1983). Certain expectations are created when a patient is interviewed by a health professional. Patients want an explanation for and relief from pain. They want to be listened to, believed and reassured that their problem can be alleviated.

In turn, the doctor or therapist wants coherent answers to examination questions and evidence from visual and palpatory examination that an organic lesion exists.

A contractual relationship is thus established and the professional has a responsibility to identify the source of the problem and to alleviate the symptoms. By their questioning and examination, they have already possibly hypothesized concerning the source of the trouble and have predicted a course of treatment which may create a satisfactory outcome.

If the outcome is satisfactory, both patient and health professional believe that the deductions were correct, and the explanation and intervention effective.

The problem

There is a need to consider what occurs when pain and other symptoms are not reduced and what assumptions are made by both patient and therapist after they are confronted with failure.

Doctors and therapists are assumed to be experts, in command of a body of knowledge which enables them to assess and analyse pathology. If an explanation is not found in their specialized area, the patient is sent to another. So rheumatologists will refer to neurologists, orthopaedic specialists to cardiologists or radiologists and the whole game of musical chairs continues within the medical establishment. But at every round of this musical game, somebody does not get a seat, but is pushed to the perimeter. They are the ones who are sent to the community psychiatric nurse, psychiatrist and increasingly the physiotherapist working in mental health. Having played to the rules of the game, they missed their step and lost. There must be some rationalization for their failure to recover – the symptoms must be psychosomatic!

Not only does it increase the anxiety for the patient to have their symptoms labelled 'anxiety induced', but also the therapist may come to have a distorted perception of the patient. The therapist or doctor may project onto the patient some rationalization for the failure to recover. The patient may be said to be 'somatizing', i.e. creating physical illness out of emotional anxiety, or may 'need their symptoms' in order to generate sympathy and support.

How large is the problem?

Fry (1979) warns that doctors in primary care will be faced with a 'mass of apparently unrecognized, undefinable and unfamiliar emotional disorders'. He advises that a wide approach is very necessary to all aspects of the patient and that a 'cure' is rare and 'should not be the overall objective'. Thirdly, he warns the scientifically and academically trained modern physician '(to understand) that emotional disorders cannot be categorized neatly labelled or diagnosed with any accuracy'. He considers that out of a population of 2500, 400 will not receive medical care for their anxiety, 100 will see the family doctor, while only a further 10 will go to the psychiatrist.

As Fry states, 'loss of energy and loss of interest' are features of true depression, which leave patients apathetic about seeking help and unable 'to translate their feelings into medical language'. Physiotherapists should note Fry's comments that a depressed patient often creates a 'feeling of depression, frustration and agitation – in the physician'! He acknowledges that the patient may present only or in addition somatic symptoms, which is where, it might be stated, a minefield of misdiagnosis may occur.

Feighner and Boyer (1991) advise that these 'problem patients' must have a multidimensional diagnosis and that 'isolated symptoms described have no value'.... 'The symptom has a shade of anguish or of affliction ...(and of a) vague diffuse character'. Backache was a frequent symptom, but X-rays reveal only 'irrelevant degenerative malformations'; therefore, in conjunction with other more behavioural symptoms, such as loss of sleep and appetite, it may be masking depression. They do caution, however, that the low mood may be caused by another disease, but advise that 'the more severe the pathological process ... the lesser is the number and intensity of the subjective discomfort'.

The International Classification of Diseases (ICD-10) produced by the WHO found that they could only approximate their definitions of anxiety and depression because of the diversity of cultural attitudes to mental illness. Categories of symptoms could only be standardized after countless interviews and cross-analysis of results, a process which took 10 years. Doctors now have clinical guidelines which define conditions, provide instruction for diagnosis and differential diagnosis of anxiety-related symptoms.

Diagnosis or misdiagnosis?

It can be seen that there is within this area an immense potential for misdiagnosis which can be exacerbated by three main factors:

- initially the failure of communication, especially in history-taking, between doctor and patient, which is perpetuated further between therapist and patient
- the medical cultural doctrine of attributing illness to either physical or mental

causes which leads to a misunderstanding and underestimation of the interplay between the two
- the failure of orthodox medicine to take seriously functional disorder as opposed to pathological disorder, structural displacement as opposed to germ theories.

Structure, it might be said, is related to function and any displacement of any body tissue by trauma, disease or stress can immediately or eventually cause wider dysfunction and a diverse manifestation of symptoms. There is a need for a wider understanding of the complex interaction between the neurophysiological basis of stress (see Chapters 8, 11 and 12) and its effect on body tissue.

A failure of communication: the clinical interview

Pendleton and Hasler (1983) analyse the interaction which takes place when a patient visits a doctor. Pendleton has demonstrated that 20–25% of patients have difficulties in communicating their problems to a doctor, which is probably an underestimation. The problem is examined more fully elsewhere (see Chapter 3), but some salient points are summarized below.

The cultural image which doctors present to their patients may be authoritarian, elitist and unsympathetic. This may be demonstrated by the physical set-up of the clinic, doctor's manner and dress, body language, questioning, cursory physical examination and rapid resorption to a prescription with one eye on the clock. These are demonstrable factors, but there are also unspoken prejudices of class, gender, age and race. We tend to emphathize more with those of our own type and to make assumptions rapidly about those who are different from ourselves.

Both patient and doctor may omit to ask searching questions. The doctors may confine themselves to asking for physical symptoms, i.e. limiting the interview to a biomechanical perspective, while knowing full well that social and emotional factors may be exacerbating those symptoms. Or, conversely, they may advise the patient autocratically that they are stressed and pay scant attention to a patient's precise but diverse descriptions of functional disorder.

Patient satisfaction with an interview is dependent on how much they think the doctor has listened to their problem. It must be remembered, however, that the patient enters the clinic with certain health beliefs which may converge or diverge with the doctor's advice. Whether or not a patient takes advice is also based on their locus of control, i.e. how much they believe they can influence their own state of health. A patient who is ignorant of the effects of accumulative stress on their life may not take kindly to the suggestion that their lifestyle is self-inflicted and eventually harmful. They may feel they are the victim of circumstances rather than the one who chose them.

Women, stress and misdiagnosis
Goudsmit and Gadd (1991) challenge 'the over emphasis and exaggeration of the role of psychological factors in illnesses', especially in doctors' diagnosis of women's symptoms. 'Organic lesions', they claim, may be overlooked because 'doctors' beliefs were based on the reversal of cause and effect', i.e. the physical symptoms may be considered secondary to the anxiety, or 'a consequence of the condition'.

Women have a tendency to describe their symptoms in emotional rather than physical terms, which leads to an undue assumption that they are not only physically vulnerable but emotionally weak. A woman describing her symptoms maybe biasing her history towards a diagnosis of 'stress-induced' by her very choice of terminology. Often, the article states, 'they quote the effect of the symptom rather than the symptom itself'. The shadow of Victorian attitudes which identified hysteria and emotional vulnerability with the 'fragility' of being a nubile woman is still with us. Goudsmit and Gadd quote as an example severe dysmenorrhoea being seen as a consequence of anxiety rather than a cause.

Added to this, in a multi-ethnic society, the cultural gap between male physician and female patient may be aggravated by difficulties with language comprehension, social taboos and downright prejudice.

The cultural dilemma: it's either physical or mental

Doctors can call upon sophisticated technological tests in order to eliminate physical sources of symptoms. It is very difficult to question their judgement when results prove negative. 'Disease may be a medical entity but illness is a social phenomenon' (Suchman, 1970); therefore the patient may also be reflecting the consequences of social impotence, family conflict, intellectual boredom, financial hardship and sexual frustration. However these are sociopolitical factors and not pathological determinants.

Confusion may arise when a patient presents with organic symptoms and with depressive mood of varying pattern. Schiffer *et al.* (1988) take the medical profession to task for inadequate consideration of the physical pathologies which might generate mental illness. The area is complicated by the fatigue and depressive moods that can occur in many as a consequence of metabolic disorders, for example:

Adrenal cortical insufficiency	Cirrhosis
Adult onset diabetes mellitus	Hyperthyroidism
Hypothyroidism	Anaemia
Hypoxia	Congestive heart failure
Renal insufficiency	Aldosteronism
Amytrophic lateral sclerosis	Myasthenia gravis
Systemic lupus erythematosus	Hypokalaemia
Hyperparathyroidism	

These authors take issue with the *Diagnostic and Statistical Manual III* (revised 1987) as to whether a depressive illness 'is caused by or secondary to' a medical illness which would label it an 'organic mood disorder' as opposed to a straightforward depressive disorder. They claim there can be no difference between an 'organic' and a 'nonorganic' depression. They list a mnemonic *dementia* which stands for those causes they consider provocative to depression: drugs and toxins, endocrine, malignancy or metabolic, epilepsy, neurodegenerative, trauma, immunologic and finally atherosclerotic.

A physiotherapist working in the mental field should be aware that there is a strong case for the biological basis for depression, even though it may be aggravated by psychosocial factors.

Functional disorder as opposed to pathological disorder

A structure is only as strong as its weakest part. When undue stress is placed upon that structure, be it emotional or physical, the weakest part will cease to function effectively and symptoms are a manifestation of pathology created by that breakdown.

Butler (1991) questions the possibility of having any one localized structure involved as the cause of a symptom. He states there is a need for a 'multifactorial approach to patient examination and management'. Physiotherapists utilize manual therapies which concentrate on joint structure or facilitative techniques which influences movement created by those joints. What both have in common is the central nervous system. Hence Butler's argument is that physiotherapists must examine the conduction process of that system and discover the adverse neural tensions which it may be experiencing. The focus of treatment must be to release those tensions which will often diminish the 'pain everywhere' pattern of symptoms. He emphasizes that peripheral and central nervous systems are continuous with common electrical and chemical conductivity.

Connective tissue as the basis of structure and the source of symptoms
Butler asserts that non-neural tissues may also experience what he calls 'trophic changes'. The present writer's interest in the importance of connective tissue distortion as a factor in 'psychosomatic diagnosis' was generated because connective tissue is just as pervasive as the neurological system. In fact, the function of connective tissue is to permit the fluctuation of cerebral spinal fluid through the tissues which is essential for the nutrition of nervous tissue as suggested by Upledger and Vredevoogd (1983). Connective tissue, otherwise known as fascia, pervades every structure in the body. Therefore, contraction, torsion or trauma of fascia will in time affect the efficient functioning of every structure which passes through it. It has both a sensory and motor function; it is elastic, but this varies in length and thickness according to the tension placed upon it. Collagen bundles are arranged in a disorganized fashion within it, but 'continuous abnormal tension' will cause the fibres to organize. 'Areas of injury or clinically significant change produce fascial immobility or "drag"'. Sometimes they are not obvious and have to be 'looked for'. Upledger states that among the dysfunctions that fascial drag can cause is dysfunction of the central nervous system which often produces 'bizarre symptoms' typical of the patient who has been labelled stressed.

Bizarre symptoms. What often inadvertently labels patients as 'stressed' is the phraseology they use in an effort to describe the sensory distortions that are experienced by structural displacement. The following are direct quotes from patients treated by the author:

'I get a feeling of indigestion and panic.'
'Dizziness which occurs in busy places.'
'Pressure behind the eyes especially in the evening.'
'Tightness in the scalp when I study.'
'Tingling in both hands when I carry shopping.'
'Intermittent tinnitus and a "tired feeling" in the left eye'
'My hands feel dead and numb but only at night.'
'I get a ringing noise at the back of the head.'

'When I'm worried I get tinnitus in both ears.'

'I get the pain in the neck when I go out in the street.

'The pressure increases on the right side of the head till I feel panic.'

'I cannot tolerate noise and become agitated, which ends up as a headache.'

'I feel discomfort which later in the day becomes pain and it moves from joint to joint.'

'I get a tightness across the whole chest which spreads down my arms.'

We must be more aware that uses of the words 'tiredness', 'tightness', 'pressure', 'dizziness', 'numb sensation', 'discomfort' and others to describe symptoms which are not constant but associated with a different location, time of day or social context, can easily be dismissed as psychosomatic.

Because physiotherapy is a refuge for so many of the non-critical cases which arrive in neurology, these patients are sometimes referred for 'relaxation instruction' or a dose of the powerful placebo effect that is no doubt part of the effectiveness of any therapeutic treatment. Often, owing to the pressure of clinical numbers, very little may have been discussed with the patient.

The need for history-taking of some depth

It is a question of not what question did the doctor ask, but what question was not asked. It is not a question of what tests were carried out, but what physical evidence do the practitioners not see right before their eyes.

It is important to ask the patient searching questions to find out if there have been major or prolonged stress factors in their lives; for example:

- accidents in childhood or adulthood
- major illnesses or causes for surgery in their history
- major prolonged stresses, especially personal or occupational.

Why take this history?

Past stressful/traumatic events create symptoms which appear to recover or rather do not interfere with the patient's immediate functioning. However, more recent stressful/traumatic events, *physical or emotional*, aggravate the earlier symtoms sufficiently to cause them to resurface to interfere with the patient's present functioning. But patients offer only information which they think is relevant to the immediate condition and will omit to mention other contributory events and sometimes symptoms unless specifically asked. The subtleness and seemingly random pattern of these symptoms which have often a sensory, muscular, articular component is provoked by the supporting infrastructure distortions of connective tissue (Upledger, 1991).

Dramatic neurological symptoms, such as loss of sensory function, 'thumping' focal headaches, loss of reflex response or muscular hypertonus, require serious further investigation which doctors would not ignore. However, the present author's concern is for the population which experiences more subtle sensory or motor discomfort in addition to pain, which is often dismissed as psychosomatic.

If greater concern and observation is taken of structural factors governed by the role of soft tissue, an explanation can be offered to the patient for their symptoms. This is not to diverge from the hypothesis of Butler (1991), but to advocate that it is the influence of connective tissue sheaths which affect the nerve fibres they contain. Butler proposes that 'autonomic trunks and ganglia must also be known as symptoms sources'. In addition techniques available to physiotherapists can permit the soft tissue to release its contractures and to adjust to body form which will safely diminish the effect of those symptoms and reduce patient anxiety.

Connective tissue contracts in response to any stressful stimuli, be it due to sudden trauma or chronic emotional stress, pathology or deprivation. We have only to look at the barrel-shaped chest formation of the chronic respiratory patient to see how tissue around the shoulder girdle contracts in response to the extra load it has carried as auxiliary to the diaphragm. Or the deformation resulting from scarring caused by poor tissue healing secondary to an infected wound. These are obvious examples of a process that occurs in more subtle ways within body structure as an attempt to adjust to both emotional and physical stress.

Empirical evidence

In order to discuss these points further, this section will describe the author's empirical experience as a physiotherapist working in psychiatry who received patients from three areas: an addiction unit, an occupational health department of a hospital and the hospital's general outpatient physiotherapy department. They were recommended for relaxation therapy sometimes as a first and sometimes as a last resort.

Patients from the addiction unit
Some patients were withdrawing, and some had been dry for over a year or more and were referred from the community. History-taking revealed a catalogue of physically traumatic accidents sustained in childhood or in working adult life which led to many of the symptoms described above. Social and personality factors also contributed to the pattern of drink dependency, but our opinion was that undiagnosed dizziness, panic sensations, tinnitus, spinal pain, pressure and paraesthesia in varying degrees did not make life any easier.

Patients from occupational health
Staff sometimes sustain injury when they are asked to restrain patients, are randomly struck by confused patients or just simply have an accident. In addition to the local soft-tissue trauma, the body manifested, in some cases, whole body symptoms of pain for many weeks after the initial incident.

Patients from the general outpatient department
These were the most anxious patients because they had been asked to attend the psychiatric hospital if only to see the physiotherapist. These were patients who had been pushed to the perimeter from the 'musical chairs' game of interviews with consultants, referred to earlier. They had failed to respond to 'orthodox' physiotherapy treatments, so their complaints were labelled psychosomatic.

CASE HISTORY 1. An 18-year-old girl was studying for her A-levels. She was referred by the neurologist to outpatient physiotherapy complaining of 'tightness and dizziness' to the right side of the head which spread to the entire scalp. Her jaw was tight and sore and she experienced numb feelings in the right arm and in three fingers of the left. The symptoms were less in the morning but increased in intensity as the day progressed. The doctor had advised that she was studying for too many hours at a stretch for her A-levels and needed relaxation. Her parents, who accompanied her, feared she had a brain tumour.

The unasked question? Any traumas to the head in childhood. Answer: In 1987 she was the passenger in the back seat of a car which was shunted from the rear. She hit her head on the front seat on the right side.

The unobserved symptom. Tenderness at the nuchal line and at the right sternomastoid muscle which extended to the mandibular joints. Also there was restriction of the atlanto-occipital joint and spasm of the left iliopsoas muscle. Yes, the symptoms were exacerbated by studying for A-levels, but they had surely originated in the trauma of a lateral force whiplash injury 4 years ago.

CASE HISTORY 2. A 37-year-old lady was referred, having failed to respond to antidepressant therapy prescribed by the neurologist. He told the patient her symptoms were caused by the presence of her parents-in-law in her home. A physiotherapist referred her for relaxation, claiming that she did not suffer from 'any mechanical pathology, merely poor postural habits and tension'. The tension increased in crowded shopping areas and became such severe anxiety that it was becoming difficult for her to carry out family duties. She had begun to hyperventilate.

History acknowledged in the notes but otherwise ignored. RTA in 1984 when she lost the fetus she was carrying. In casualty they were naturally more concerned about her pregnancy than about her head trauma.

The unobserved symptom. The left temperomandibular joint was very sore and tender and there was a loss of range in both the jaw and the neck.

The ignored symptom. 'Tightness in the stomach' and the spasm of right iliopsoas muscle.

CASE HISTORY 3. A 37-year-old plasterer was referred for relaxation with compounding symptoms associated with the panic attacks that he had experienced since 1980. He was now rehabilitating from alcohol abuse, but had difficulty coping with the tinnitus which arose in both ears whenever he became anxious. He had difficulty with swallowing and a sense of pressure on the right side of the head. His eyes also blurred their focus when he became anxious. He experienced strong mood swings and insomnia.

The unasked question. Have you received any severe trauma to the head? Answer: In 1990 he received a severe blow to the head when he fell from a height of about five feet onto a road.

CASE HISTORY 4. A 30-year-old nurse was struck on the underside of the right jaw by an elderly confused patient. She presented herself very soon after the trauma in a state of anxiety, disabled from work and holding her whole arm to the fingertips in a state of painful tenderness. This soon localized itself to painful joints of symptomology similar to rheumatoid arthritis, which moved from joint to joint. The reaction was dismissed by the doctors as 'pure coincidence' rather than a consequence of her trauma.

What is the relevance of such history-taking?

First there may be distant trauma from which the patient apparently recovers. Sometime later, social and environmental factors which may be adverse or stressful may cause a return of symptoms, but such an interval has passed that the patient does not connect the two events. Alternatively, somebody may have a slowly developing chronic problem due to a stressful lifestyle or self-abuse and neglect. A relatively minor trauma or strain can somehow unleash a list of symptoms out of proportion to the injury, by way of which the body is signalling an incapacity to self-heal and function.

Special note

First it is important that the physiotherapist has a sound anatomical knowledge not only of body parts in isolation but of their interrelationship one to the other, especially of fascial relationships which are so important in the homoeostatic balance of the body:

1. The fascia is longitudinal throughout the body. In certain areas, however, it is horizontal – at the pelvis, at the true diaphragm, at the thoracocervical junction and at the foramen magnum in the skull. Major structures pass through the fascia at each level. Fascial drag at the horizontal level can affect any organs or veins, arteries or nerves which pass through them.
2. Women may have experienced complicated gynaecological histories or surgical intervention, but not in their recent history. Pelvic fascial scarring or torsion caused by difficult birth, surgery, fibroids, prolapsed uterus or obesity can cause not only low backache, but also headaches caused by transmission of tension through the spinal dural membranes (Upledger, 1991).

CASE HISTORY 5. A 43-year-old hospital administrator was referred for low back pain. She had sustained a whiplash injury in 1988 and still experienced occipital headaches occasionally. However, the low back pain was giving her the greater problem. Upon examination, a prominent abdominal scar caused by a Caesarian birth which had taken place 17 years ago was noticed. Examination proved that it was still very adhesive and treatment consisted in gentle soft-tissue massage to the abdominal area. Sufficient release was obtained for the patient to be pain free after one treatment!

3. The powerful effect of any destabilization of the iliopsoas muscle, either bilaterally or laterally, or toxicity of the aponeurotic layer of iliac fascia which covers it. As well as stabilizing the sacroiliac articulation, it interlinks with the true diaphragm and can aggravate respiratory discomfort (Richard, 1986).

CASE HISTORY 6. A 42-year-old man rehabilitating for substance abuse was sent for help and advice regarding his panic attacks. Though not complaining of backache, he had a marked shortening of the right psoas, and a tight bow-shaped thorax with immense tenderness at the base of the sternum. His liver was still slightly enlarged and the abdominal area felt tight. Efforts were made to obtain a psoas release and by gentle connective-tissue massage to release and relax the abdominal fascia. Functionally he felt greater ease with respiration and subjectively felt very much improved.

4. Dysfunction of the temperomandibular joint can have a destabilizing effect on a much wider area, causing post-orbital headaches and neck pain. This can be aggravated by tension in the temporal muscle and masseter muscle at the zygomatic arch (Penn, personal communication).

Trauma to the head or neck can, in time, create subtle symptoms of cranial sensory or motor nerve dysfunction. Especially vulnerable, as in the whiplash condition, is the balance of the occipital condyles on the atlas. If the muscles such as sternomastoid, trapezius, semispinalis capitis, rectus capitis and posterior minor (the only muscle attached to the spine of the atlas) exert a distorting leverage on the cranial base, they can affect the function of all vessels leaving the jugular foramen. This includes not only the jugular veins but the glossopharyngeal, vagus and accessory cranial nerves (Upledger, 1983). Surgical scars on one surface can cause symptoms on the opposite area.

CASE HISTORY 7. A 35-year-old nurse attended for cervical pain C5–7 manifested by acute tenderness in upper right trapezius area (which kept her awake at night) and headaches. Examination revealed a 5-year-old partial thyroidectomy scar and a lower thoracic scar on the left where a malformed kidney had been removed. It was necessary to release the fascial constrictions around both scar areas before any symptomatic relief was obtained.

Head traumas are very common among the population. Distortion at the cranial level is transmitted via the atlanto-occipital joint and the enveloping fascia of the dural tubes to the sacrum. If there appears to be undue emphasis on histories of head injury among those quoted, it must be remembered that the cranium is excessively vulnerable and that many principal structures pass through the basal and jugular foramen, including the 12 cranial nerves, and run parallel in fascial sheaths with many other structures.

Distortions which occlude these structures are certain, with time, to manifest symptoms of pressure, e.g. the passage of the vagus nerve through the jugular foramen, if restricted, can cause symptoms of indigestion and a spasm sensation in the oesophagus (Upledger, 1991).

The physical examination of the patient

Explain what you are looking for. Otherwise an anxious patient will be made more so!

- Observe gait, and general posture from the back and the front. Does there appear to be a torsion to left or right?
- Is the head positioned symmetrically or does it lean to left or right?
- (Undressed) Is one shoulder elevated? Are the anterior sacroiliac spines level or tilted forward? What shape is the thorax and what breathing pattern is demonstrated?
- Are the posterior sacroiliac spines level or is one higher than the other?
- Lumbar flexion – does the spine deviate and rotate as the patient bends forward?

- Palpation of the paravertebrals – is there any sensation of chronic knotted muscular tissues (sign of a chronic lesion) or puffy acute lesion which leaves a red wheal and increased heat and sweat pattern?
- Piriformis spasm – is it evident by a tender bulge deep to the gluteus muscle where it extends from the sacrum to the greater trochanter?
- Are there any operation scars which will exaggerate postural torsion? Palpate for fascial tenderness in the area.
- *In-lying*, is one foot turning out more than the other (caused by piriformis spasm)? (Figures 9.1 and 9.2). Place your thumbs on the inner condyles of the ankle. Is there apparent shortening (due to muscle spasm at the pelvis)?
- Check there is no limitation of shoulder movement then take the patient's hands lengthwise beyond the head and see if the fingertips and transverse wrist creases missmatch, which again indicates psoas spasm (Figure 9.3). This is caused by a reversal of the psoas/iliacus pull which pulls the ilium down on the foreshortened side. It also has an effect on the diaphragm by its fascial interconnections and acts as a spinal flexor.

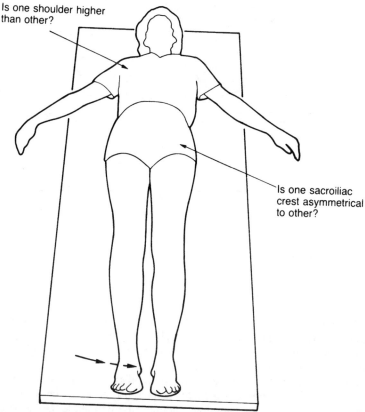

Is one shoulder higher than other?

Is one sacroiliac crest asymmetrical to other?

Figure 9.1 Some indications of torsion caused by 'fascial drag' and muscular torsion. In-lying: Examine for *apparent* shortening caused by psoas spasm (arrow). Stand at the feet and place your thumbs under the medial malleoli. Spasm of this hip flexor cause 1/2–1 in (12–25 mm) shortening of same leg. Also, is one foot externally rotated – an extra indication of spasm? Does the patient lie straight and is there torsion of the whole trunk?

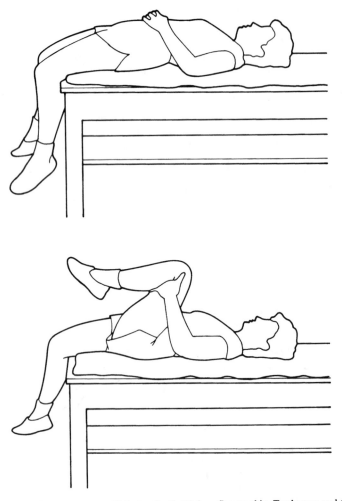

Figure 9.2 Test for psoas spasm. Abduct patient's thighs – flex one hip. Tenderness and tightness can be palpated in the abdomen of the side where the hip is *not* flexed. Repeated stretching and flexing is a gentle way to release psoas.

- Palpate for psoas spasm at the left or right (but warn your patient that you are going to press on the stomach and why!).
- Shoulder flexion will be more evident if one humeral head is higher from the plinth than the other.
- Re-examine the anterior iliac spines to see if there is deviation. Does there appear to be any tightness around the diaphragm caused by fascial drag due to poor respiratory method? Anxious patients are often tender at the base of the sternum.
- Palpate the cervical vertebra and test the atlanto-occipital joint by placing your index fingers in the dip behind the ear lobe with slight pressure.
- Palpate the sternomastoid muscle for any spasm.

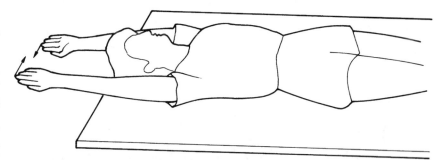

Figure 9.3 Test for atlanto-axial spasm plus psoas spasm. Bring patient's hands to end of treatment couch in fingertip-to-fingertip position (as in prayer). If there is 1/2 in (12 mm) difference in finger length, this is caused by atlanto-axial plus psoas spasm.

- Ask the patient to open the jaw and test sideways glide. Three fingers placed one above the other should approximately fill the buccal space (Figure 9.4).
- Palpate the temperomandibular joint and temporals for any tenderness and tension. Any compression distortion of this joint causes tension in the muscles of the cranium, principally the temporalis and those of mastication.
- Ask the patient to lie on the stomach and palpate the spinal muscles for any spasm, especially along the paravertebrals. Tactile examination will reveal erythematous spots where an underlying lesion persists. Localized sweating may be evident. Recent spasm will feel warm and puffy beneath the examiner's fingertips. At the chronic stage, tissue changes will have taken place. The raised temperature will have diminished and a knotted lumpy sensation will be felt below the skin. Movement in that area will have diminished and a compensatory load will have been diverted to the joints above or below the affected area.

What can the physiotherapist do with this information?

Just as in mental health we have to look at the whole person, in a physical examination we have to look at the total frame and not focus on specific symptoms.

1. Look for symptoms which may appear random. Palpate! For example, the nurse with the traumatized jaw on the right side (see Case History 4) had temporal bone and atlanto-axial dysfunction. This caused tenderness at the insertion of trapezius, and an elevated shoulder. This provoked right ileopsoas spasm, piriformis and hamstring shortening. Her right soleus was very tender, as was the tendo Achilles. She complained of tenderness in the sole of her right foot!
2. *Explain what you have found to the patient.* They are anxious. Involve them in your learning process and do not remain the expert.
3. Understand that, even as wounds naturally heal, the body will struggle to correct tissue imbalances; therefore, it is important to capitalize on those energies. Soft-tissue releases need to proceed articular releases. This does not preclude high-velocity mobilizations but they should be a last resort.

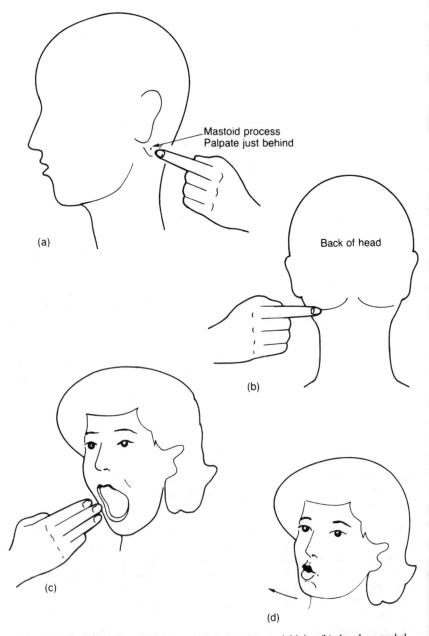

Figure 9.4 (a) Palpate for tenderness and restriction at atlanto-axial joint; (b) also along nuchal line; (c) in addition, examine the jaw using patient's three fingers – can she place them in the mouth or is there restriction? (d) Glide jaw to left and close; glide jaw to right and close – is there unilateral restriction.

4. Allow the patient to lie in a position of maximum comfort that is to fore-shorten these muscles in spasm. With time, relaxation will ease symtoms.
5. Use hands-on techniques which are not invasive but which facilitate comfort, lymph flow and natural tissue release. *Connective tissue massage* is a very positive technique to apply. Just using the warmth of the therapist's hands by positioning and touch can facilitate the release of tissue contraction. Avoid Swedish massage techniques which tend to stir things up.
6. Utilize deep respiration by the patient after soft-tissue work. Osteopaths call this the 'spontaneous release technique' whereby the patient takes a deep breath and holds the breath to build up pressure. This is maintained until released as an explosive breath. The therapist gently works on the affected tissues.
7. Use Shiatsu or acupressure techniques – these are similar to connective tissue techniques and probably assist in the release of endorphins (Kaada and Torsteinbo, 1988). Reflexology is another facilitating, non-invasive technique which may prove helpful.
8. The author has found Craniosacral therapy to be useful in promoting fascial release by encouraging the flow of cerebral spinal fluid throughout fascia. Techniques capitalize on this flow which permit tissue relaxation. This is particularly useful in the area of delicate articular balance around the cranium and neck. Knowledge of cranial nerve function can heighten awareness of sensory and motor dysfunction, e.g. tinnitus or difficulties with swallowing.
9. Ask the patient to report any changes of degree or diversity of symptoms in between treatments. This is important.

Conclusion

The physiotherapist has fine palpatory skills to discover a third opinion – not that of the doctor's, not that of the patient's, but that of the patient's body.

Whatever the intervention chosen, it must be gentle and unhurried with the body positioned in comfort and warmth. Illness is the body's struggle to heal itself and the role of the physiotherapist is to facilitate that healing rather than to intervene in that process.

Chapter 8 shows that the autoimmune reflex response will be modified considerably if there is physical adjustment as well as emotional support.

Catharsis

There is another side to the coin. Physiotherapists must be aware that this approach of gentle touch can have a powerful effect on the patient. Many are under emotional strain and the release of tissue tension effected by touch can cause the release of emotion which is tears. Of course, the patient will have been given an explanation as to intent before even being touched. However, emotions and life experiences are held and sometimes blocked in body tissue and it must be accepted as natural to release this emotion within the safety of a clinical setting. Patients will confide events and emotions that are painful to them. They need to, and it is part of the physiotherapist's role just to be there, to listen and support. It often has a very beneficial effect emotionally and if no further treatment takes place, no matter. Catharsis usually only happens during the first treatment. It is important to let the patient fully recover composure before leaving the treatment area, so they should not be hurried out of the department. If it happens more often, it might be suggested that the patient is clinically depressed and needs further assistance.

Who knows what another human being has experienced? Past domestic violence can afflict many, but it is not so commonly talked about as recent road traffic accidents. Caring relatives may have been handling and lifting dependent family members who have drained them both emotionally and physically for many years, but this can be omitted without comment. A lifetime of occupational overload or tedium can manifest itself in tremendous physical fatigue. These life-draining events may be omitted if the therapist by an officious, authoritative manner does not invite confiding because, to them, the patient's past history does not seem relevant to the present symptom.

On discovery of these factors, it is necessary not to make a quantum leap and assume 'this patient is stressed and if they would only relax, somehow the pain will diminish'. The pain will not go away because it is often based on a true functional disorder. We have to abandon the narrow separate categories of mind and body and realize that an appreciation of the neurophysiological structural basis of the human body permits us to understand something of the complex interaction between emotion and tissue, attitude and structural balance. There is a call for a better understanding of the physical basis of mental illness among doctors. Among the 'well-worried' of our population there is an opportunity for physiotherapists to give more precise assessment, understanding and symptomatic relief. Let us remember we are not the experts. Each patient is unique and has something to teach us if we listen, look and touch with an open mind.

References

Butler, D. (1991) *Mobilisation of the Nervous System*, Churchill Livingstone
Feighner, J.P. and Boyer, W.F. (1991) *Diagnosis of Depression*, Wiley
Fry, J. (1979) *Common Diseases*, MTP Press
Goudsmit, E. and Gadd, R. (1991) All in the mind, the psychologisation of illness. *The Psychologist*, Oct.
Kaada, B. and Tortsteinbo, O. (1988) Increase of plasma B-endorphins in connective tissue massage
McCaffrey, M. (1983) *Nursing the Patient in Pain*, 2nd edn, Harper and Row
Pendleton, D. and Hasler, J. (eds) (1983) *Doctor–Patient Communication*, Academic Press
Richard, R. (1986) *Osteopathic Lesions of the Sacrum*, Thorsons
Schiffer, R.B., Klein, R. and Sider, R. (1988) *The Medical Evaluation of Psychiatric Patients*, Plenum
Suchman, E.A. (1970) Health attitudes and behaviour. *Archives of Environmental Health*, **20**, 105
Upledger, J. (1991) *Somato Emotional Release and Beyond*, D.O. UI
Upledger, J. and Vredevoogd, J. (1983) *Craniosacral Therapy*, Eastland Press
Diagnostic and Statistical Manual III–American Psychiatric Association, 1983

Acknowledgements—The author is grateful to Doug Penn MCSP, DO, who gave invaluable help in introducing this complex subject.

10

Challenging behaviour

Anne Wilson

Introduction

Challenging behaviour is a learned or acquired behaviour that disturbs interactions and relationships with others. People may reject a person because of their
behaviour and the person has problems forming satisfactory relationships. This
makes normal life in the community difficult or impossible, and puts the person
at risk from retaliation from others.

Challenging behaviour is often assumed to be violent, but this is not always
the case. Where there is violence, it might be directed at others, against self (self-
injury) or against objects, e.g. arson. However, the behaviour can also be non-
violent, yet still interfere with normal social functioning; e.g. inappropriate social
behaviours and wandering. These behaviours lead to isolation and alienation.
Causes are varied, but include learning from role models and the environment.
The environment is a major factor in producing frustration, boredom, and in
provoking certain behaviours.

Challenging behaviour can make treatment very difficult, as compliance is
often poor and the behaviour can interfere with the learning process. However,
it must be remembered that people have the right to refuse treatment.
Physiotherapy is not covered under the compulsory section of the Mental Health
Act and treating without the permission of the person, or against their wishes,
constitutes assault (Finch, 1983). Staff attitudes can provoke aggression and
challenging behaviour, and an awareness of the effect of communication and
behaviour on others is important for all health workers to enable them to
minimize difficult behaviour. These skills are particularly important for
those working in psychiatry, accident and emergency departments and in the
community, and will be discussed in this chapter.

Aggression

Media coverage of mental illness often portrays the person as aggressive and
violent. However, everyone has the potential to be violent. There is a higher
incidence of violence in the mentally ill, but this is only slightly higher than in
the general population and could be due to provoking factors such as environment, harassment and compulsory detention. People with mental health problems
might be caught more easily (which would increase crime statistics), but the

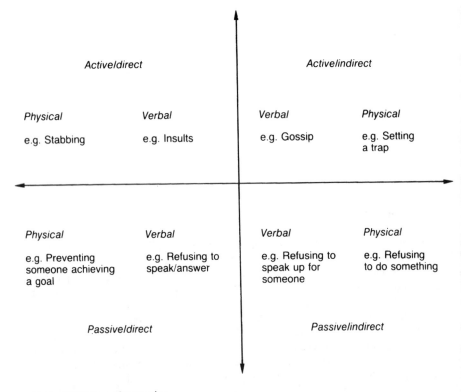

Figure 10.1 Types of aggression

percentage is only a small proportion of the overall crime figures. Psychiatry is open to abuse by using involuntary detention to remove people who do not fit into society (Szasz, 1963).

Aggression ranges from verbal insults to physical violence and is an unpleasant response to something. It is accompanied by an intent to harm and a belief that the behaviour will cause harm, i.e. it is not accidental (Dollard *et al.*, 1939). It can be passive or active and aimed directly or indirectly at a person (Figure 10.1).

Theories of aggression

There are three main theories concerning aggression:

1. The instinct hypothesis (Lorenz, 1966) suggests that aggression is a basic instinct for dominance that ensures that animals or people are properly spaced with a hierarchy that provides group stability. Aggression can be released in socially acceptable ways, e.g. sport.
2. The frustration hypothesis (Dollard *et al.*, 1939) suggests that frustration leads to a state of readiness and always precedes aggression. Frustration is not a reliable antecedent of aggression, but it is a powerful motivator, although the

need to retaliate may be more powerful. Frustration might not lead to aggression if something inhibits it; the aggression can be displaced onto other objects. If an act is interpreted as aggressive or deliberately done, it is more likely to provoke an aggressive response. The initial responses to frustration are affective, followed by higher cognitive functions such as judgements which inhibit or facilitate aggression, e.g. frustration can lead to dejection and resignation rather than aggression.

3. The learned response (Bandura, 1977) suggests that for aggression to occur it must be one of the person's learned responses. Aggression can be learned if it is encouraged, rewarded or achieves a goal, and by copying others.

The act of aggression produces autonomic recovery (aggression catharsis) which decreases arousal and therefore aggression. However, this can reduce social inhibitions which prevent the use of aggression, facilitating its use in future situations.

Some research suggests that releasing frustration in an environment where fear, guilt and anxiety are not produced promotes autonomic recovery and reduces aggression (Green, 1990). Gymnasium facilities provide a safe and acceptable way of releasing frustrations. Aggression appears to be related to arousal levels, and repeated incidents of violence in a particular environment are probably due to the environment itself. A hospital environment can increase arousal, and people who are over-responsive to the environment can become aggressive.

While aggression is thought to be an acquired behaviour, other factors increase its likelihood, i.e.:

- *Personality*. Premorbid personality could be important, making a person more or less likely to choose violence as an option.
- *Genetics*. An extra Y chromosome in men has been linked with antisocial and criminal behaviour, but has not been proved for aggression.
- *Social group*. Peer groups and crowds can respond aggressively to frustration and prejudices, although as individuals they might not be particularly aggressive.
- *Victim behaviour*. The victim can provoke or precipitate violence.
- *Disinhibiting factors*. Drugs, alcohol and anaesthetics can remove cognitive restraints that normally limit or prevent aggression. Alcohol reduces the ability to make complex judgements, but can be used as an excuse to avoid taking personal responsibility for actions. Illegal drugs can lead to a lifestyle related to crime and violence.
- *Environment*. The environment can increase arousal and therefore the risk of an aggressive response. An environment that is too stimulating can become irritating and frustrating, and clients can misinterpret an overstimulating environment, particularly if suffering from hallucinations. Problems in hospital can include overcrowding, lack of privacy or quiet, and can be made worse if the person is unable to leave the ward. A lack of space, or the invasion of personal body space, can be threatening, and aggressive or suspicious people need greater space because of their mistrust. A lack of attention from staff, or inadequate facilities, can produce frustration, and staff attitudes, e.g. bossiness or disrespect, can cause problems.
- *Temperature*. Research suggests that heat increases the likelihood of aggression (Green, 1990).

- *Noise.* High levels of noise increase stress and possibly reduce the ability to cope with frustration.
- *Air pollution.* Noxious odours, tobacco smoke and ozone-related smog increase the number of positive ions in the air which produces fatigue, stress and irritability which can intensify behaviour (Green, 1990). Smoking on some psychiatric wards can be a problem, although many hospitals now operate a no-smoking or restricted smoking policy.
- *Physiology.* This can alter irritability and self-control, e.g. lack of sleep, fatigue and hunger. There can be post-fit irritability with epilepsy (although problem behaviour at the time of the fit is rare). Temporal lobe epilepsy has been linked with psychosis and aggression. Damage to the frontal lobe of the brain can produce disinhibition and egocentric behaviour (propranolol can be useful if there are explosive outbursts). Metabolic problems such as disturbances of endocrine function can facilitate aggression. For example, thyrotoxicosis, hypoglycaemia, excess androgens (testosterone, and the use of anabolic steroids), oestrogen/progesterone balance (particularly at menstruation) and low serotonin metabolism have all been linked with habitual aggression. In youngsters, food allergies and lead poisoning have been suggested as causes of aggression. Metabolic problems can make a person more sensitive to external stimuli that elicit aggression.
- *Mental illness.* Untreated disorders can produce aggression. Schizophrenics can respond to hallucinations and be less able to cope with frustration, while psychopathic personalities can be lacking in normal social inhibitions, and depression and neurosis can be linked to self-injury and destructive behaviour, e.g. arson.
- *Frustration.* This does not always lead to aggression, but deliberate acts of other people are more likely to provoke aggression than accidents.
- *Disease and pain.* These can reduce the ability to deal with frustration and anger, and depression resulting from the problem can overspill into aggression.
- *Gender.* Women tend to be less aggressive than men, but can still be violent.
- *Poor cognitive development.* This is often associated with delinquency and poor self-image, and can produce aggression in people suffering from the frustration of being unable to express themselves. Cognitive impairment in the elderly can result from confusion and dementia, and can lead to aggression. The person might be unable to understand what you are doing to them and perceive an invasion of personal body space as a threat or an assault. There is often no rational or cognitive control over the behaviour which can be totally uncharacteristic. If the confusion lifts to produce lucid periods with insight, the distress and frustration this causes can overspill into aggression.

Warning signs of aggression

Aggressive and tense postures both look very similar, and the body reacts in similar ways: muscles tense, heart and breathing rates increase, and autonomic changes occur such as dry mouth, sweating, etc. It is important when dealing with people to interpret their body language, and to be aware of your own. Tension in yourself can be interpreted as aggression and the person can feel threatened and respond aggressively. Similarly, tension in a client can be interpreted as aggression by staff. Non-verbal communication is important. Look at a person's posture and facial expressions as well as verbal indications of aggression. Be aware of any changes in a person's normal behaviour, e.g. if they become unusually noisy, restless, loud, abusive, quiet or withdrawn (Figure 10.2) and listen to your own intuitions (Lamplugh, 1988).

Aggression is difficult to predict, but the following indicate an increased risk:

- A past history of violent, impulsive or irresponsible behaviour, or the use of a weapon.
- Bruising or signs of injury (including self-injury).
- An inability to cope with stress.
- Difficulties in expressing self-needs.
- Abnormal perceptions, particularly paranoia, hallucinations (especially tactile hallucinations which make a person feel that they have been assaulted), and heightened perceptions (which can lead to overarousal).
- Postnatal depression with attempts to harm the child, delusions of jealousy, and threats to kill herself or her partner.
- Attention-seeking behaviour that is ignored by staff.
- Oversensitivity to correction or instruction.
- Enforced admission or detention in hospital.
- Drug and alcohol abuse.
- Expressing an intention of harming someone, and naming that person.

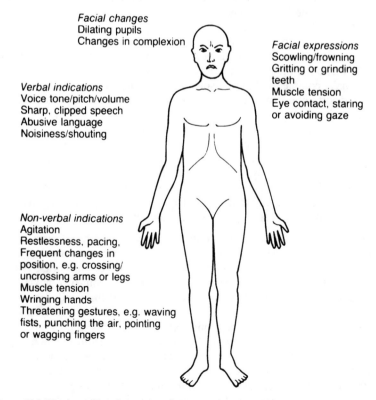

Figure 10.2 Warnings of imminent aggression

with parents and having delusions about them, or having previously
ed them.

esence of a dog in a person's home can be a risk. The person could set
g on you, or if the person becomes angry, the dog is likely to become
aggressive and could attack. If you need to touch the person as part of your
treatment, the dog could attack to protect its owner.

- Domestic disputes in a person's home can be a risk, and it might not be the
  client who is the risk, but the carer.

Dealing with aggression

It is important to recognize the signs of imminent aggression and be aware of
trigger situations. As already stated, be aware of your own posture. Tension can
be interpreted as aggression, while anxiety can make you over-react (Lowe,
1992). Try to keep your voice tone and pitch, etc., as normal as possible and look
relaxed and confident, maintaining a calm approach. Allow the person to express
feelings of anger, but keep yourself detached from that anger to avoid feelings of
aggression in yourself. Focus instead on the person's non-verbal communication
so that you do not concentrate on your own fears.

When assessing a potentially aggressive person:

- Be concerned about that person's best interests even if you do not agree with
  what they say, and indicate that you comprehend.
- Listen to the person and be unhurried.
- Ask questions but do not interrogate or challenge.
- Introduce yourself and explain the purpose of the interview. If necessary repeat
  the information as they might not absorb it first time.
- Do not make comments about personality or be judgemental.
- Allow opportunities for the person to withdraw from any confrontation
  without losing face.
- Position furniture to enable you to get out easily.
- Do not argue against hallucinations or delusions: they are real to the client,
  but do not reinforce them. Remember, you could be part of the person's
  delusional hallucinatory system, and could be seen as a threat.
- In a person's home, you have no legal or moral right to stay if asked to leave.
- If you are visiting someone at home, always leave a note of where you are and
  report back after the visit. If you are in any doubt, do not go alone.

If a person is verbally aggressive, indicate that you have heard them without
being drawn into the argument. This gives you the chance to acknowledge what
they have said, and state your point, e.g. 'I know you're furious but I'd like you
to put that walking stick down'. Self-disclosure reduces your own anxiety, e.g.
'I feel afraid'. This enables you to take charge of your feelings and also conveys
honesty, which can facilitate open communication. A person can simply
be unaware of the effect their body language has on others, and by saying that
you find it threatening, you are giving feedback on the person's behaviour, and
allowing that person to change it without losing face. Accepting or asking for
appropriate criticism, without reacting as if it is an accusation, makes you feel
less defensive. It gives the person an opportunity to express their feelings, and
the information can be used constructively. In your statements, be specific and

brief. Always allow the person time to calm down and collect their thoughts. It might not be possible to talk rationally until the person has cooled down.

Stand sideways on to the person, rather than square on, as this is less threatening. If a cat is threatened, it arches its back and raises its fur to make itself look bigger and more threatening. Similarly, standing square on, particularly with hands on hips and feet apart, makes you look bigger and more threatening. You are also presenting a bigger target to hit, and vulnerable areas such as the face, throat and abdomen are unprotected. If you stand with one foot in front of the other and the back foot slightly turned to the side the trunk rotated sidways and the arms loose, you are less threatening, less easy to hit and able to move away easily. Never stand with your hands in your pockets or your arms folded. They need to be free to defend yourself if necessary. Standing up from sitting could be threatening; standing over someone is. Avoid leaning over a person as it is easier for them to hit out or pull your hair. Do not get too close or touch the person without saying what you intend doing. Most people need space and it is threatening to invade someone's body space. However, moving in very close makes it more difficult for the person to hit you. Stand to the side of the person rather than directly in front. It is less threatening and it is also more difficult to hit or kick out to the side. Do not turn your back on someone, e.g. to put their shoes on. It is easy for them to pull your hair.

It is important not to get trapped in a corner. Try to keep clear of walls and stay near to an exit. Do not let yourself get blocked in. If you are visiting someone at home, sit near the door. If there is any risk, leave immediately. If you are in any doubt, visit in twos, and warn other staff that there is a risk. In the department, you might want to put a large piece of equipment or furniture between yourself and the other person, and try to remove any potential weapons such as sticks, crutches, weights, scissors, etc. If you are threatened, try to establish dialogue and personalize the communication by using the person's name (if you don't know it, ask), tell the person who you are and what you want. You can try to divert their attention, e.g. 'Shall I make a cup of tea', or introduce some humour (it is difficult to be angry and laugh), but ensure that the humour is not seen as an insult or a threat and does not make the person feel they are being laughed at. If the person is armed, do not approach but ask them to put the weapon down. If they are about to throw something, shouting a command such as 'Stop!', or 'Put that down!' can startle a person into complying and allows time to initiate dialogue, but ensure you are out of range. Never attempt physically to stop a person from throwing something. Even an unarmed person should not be tackled if you are alone, unless you have no other choice. If violence occurs, get any other clients out of the area and, where possible, retreat. Retreat might not be practicable or possible if others need your protection (see legal aspects, below). If you can escape, call for help, and always watch the person. Never turn your back. You might need to adjust clothing so that it does not restrict your ability to move. At the same time, ensure that your posture is non-threatening, and that you are not vulnerable should the violence be directed at you.

If violence is aimed at property, use your judgement as to whether or not you should try to control it. Do not try to control violence if you are alone, or if it would place anyone (including yourself) at risk. If you are physically attacked, continue talking, try to diffuse the situation and call for help. Deflect any blows and try to retreat or restrain the person. If you cannot break away or are overpowered, protect your airway and vital organs by curling into a ball and covering your head with your hands.

Remember, do not get physical. Break away or retreat. Only restrain if necessary. The aim is to prevent aggression, facilitate the release of pent-up emotions and enable the person to deal with their feelings. Following an incident, the person should be allowed to express fears and anger, and talk through their reactions. It can be useful to set limits of acceptable behaviour. The constructive use of rules gives guidelines on what will and will not be accepted.

Breakaway techniques

Breakaway techniques are based on large circular movements, using strong muscle groups against weaker ones. Speed and surprise are important; training and regular practice are essential.

If a person gets hold of you, continue talking and avoid escalating the situation. Ask the person to let go. If they do not release you, call for help and try to break away.

The choice of breakaway technique depends on the form of attack:

- *Hand grips.* Pull against the person's thumb using a circular movement to twist away and, if necessary, use the other arm to assist.
- *Punching.* Wave your arms to distract and to block punches.
- *Hair pulling.* Immobilize by putting your hand on your assailant's and pushing it down onto your head. Pressure on the knuckles will release the grip.
- *Pinching.* Push the fingers onto your skin to immobilize and release.
- *Biting.* Move into the bite (pulling away will tear the skin). Pressure at the sides of the mouth will open the jaws.
- *Strangulation from behind.* If the hands are around your throat, turn your head to the side to ease the pressure on your airway, and apply leverage to the little fingers or pressure to the nailbed to release. If the arm is around your neck, turn your head to the side. Then pull down on the hand and pull up on the elbow, twist your body and step out backwards.
- *Strangulation from in front.* Bring your arms up through the middle of the person's arms and swing out in a circular motion; *or* turn sideways and step away, and circle your arms over theirs to break the grip.

Blankets can be effective in smothering attacks with weapons. If a weapon is used, always keep your eye on it.

Restraint should only be used if you have been trained in the correct use of techniques and can use them confidently with team support. Each area has its own policy on dealing with violence, and staff should be familiar with their local guidelines. Head and neck holds should never be used, nor should primary blood flow be occluded. After any incident, there should be a debriefing session for staff and patient to explore antecedents, behaviour and feelings. As a physiotherapist it is important to get involved in the training of breakaway techniques and methods of restraint. Physiotherapists have much to offer on the prevention of injury in the instruction and performance of these techniques.

Legal aspects

Under the Health and Safety at Work Act, managers and employees have a duty to ensure safety at work. This could include a policy of using two people to visit a client, or setting up a procedure to highlight training needs. All violent or potentially violent incidents should be recorded so that safety measures can be monitored and improved.

The law allows the minimum of force to be used to avoid injury to the client or others, and in self-defence against potential or escalating violence. You should retreat where possible, but bear in mind that you have a duty of care to the client. Non-action which results in injury to the client or others could be seen as negligent. Intervention could include: trying to diffuse the situation, distracting the person, raising the alarm or sending someone for help while you monitor the situation. Physical intervention might not be a realistic option.

Ask yourself the following questions:

1. Under criminal law:
   – If you don't act will a crime occur?
   – If force is used, is it reasonable?
2. Under the mental health legislation:
   – Are you acting in good faith?
   – Are you exercising reasonable care?
   – Is the necessity of your action proven and the method appropriate?
3. Under civil and common law:
   – Is retreat reasonable or is action necessary?
   – If you do not act, could you be negligent?
4. Under professional and ethical considerations:
   – What is your local policy?
   – Will your action be judged as reasonable by the public?
   – Does it safeguard the person or is it detrimental?

Even if you act in self-defence, you could be liable for prosecution for criminal offences (e.g. assault) unless the force used was justified, reasonable and not out of proportion to the risk of harm.

Coping strategies

The client needs to become more aware of their aggression, what triggers it and how to deal with it. It is important to give the person opportunities to express feelings of anger and find ways of dealing with them. Normal coping strategies include:

- mental and physical activity such as hobbies, exercise
- self-nurture activities such as having time to relax
- expressing emotions through crying, talking, painting, writing
- confronting the problem and working through it.

People need to be able to use a variety of ways of dealing with stress and frustration. This can be difficult in a ward environment. A person might be angry for a valid reason, but need to control that anger or find an appropriate outlet. The physiotherapist can teach relaxation to deal with stress and reduce the body's arousal. When aggressive feelings become strong, the person can use other techniques; talking to someone and expressing feelings verbally can help the person to regain control. Positive thinking can help a person to remain in control, for example by saying to themselves: 'I can cope', 'I don't need to get angry' or 'Well done, I kept my cool'. Distraction techniques can allow the person time to calm down and reduce tension. Some examples are: SOS (sigh out slowly) breathing, counting to ten, changing your focus and studying an object in minute detail. Leaving the situation by going for a walk or going and sitting somewhere quiet can reduce aggressive feelings, as can reading a book, listening to some music or doing something energetic. The silent scream (which is the act of screaming without vocalizing the sound) is a good way of releasing tension.

Training in assertiveness can help a person to express their needs without becoming angry or manipulative. Assertiveness allows the person to recognize their rights and the rights of others and enables them to take responsibility for their feelings and accept the consequences of their actions. Releasing aggression in a safe, constructive way is important and the physiotherapist can be involved in the planning of exercise programmes. Exercise is associated with improved self-esteem, can lift depression and promotes social interaction. A non-competitive programme enables the person to release aggression in a constructive and acceptable way (Hayden *et al.*, 1986; Moses *et al.*, 1989).

When treating potentially aggessive people, remember that their attention span can be short and they might be unable to take in all that is said to them, which can produce frustration. Repeat or write down instructions. Misunderstandings can escalate into violence. Make your requests easy to understand and agree treatment goals and plans with the patient.

A person can object to undressing or being touched (particularly if they are suffering tactile hallucinations), and their wishes must be respected. Beware of asking too many questions which can seem like an interrogation. Use open questions and gentle prompts where possible. Equipment can seem threatening if the person is suffering from ideas of reference. You might need to treat them somewhere else. Be guided by the person's requests and allow them as much control over the situation as possible. If you are unsure or feel uncomfortable with the person, have a nurse escort during the activity as people are very sensitive to any anxieties shown by staff.

Self-injury

Suppressed anger can be turned inwards producing feelings of depression and poor self-worth which can result in self-injury behaviour. Self-injury includes cutting, burning and head-banging. It is distressing for staff and cannot be ignored because of the risk of damage. Bizarre mutilation and life-threatening cutting can result in challenging behaviour from a person responding to hallucinations, but most self-injury is not life threatening. It is commonest between the ages of 16 and 24 and is three times more likely in females than in males – the true incidence is unknown as many cases go unreported.

Often the person is attractive. They may have had some experience in the nursing or paramedic field. There is often a history of trauma at school, trouble with the police, family violence, excessive punishment, abuse or parental deprivation. Self-esteem is frequently low and the person might express a dislike of her body, or suffer from an eating disorder (such as anorexia or bulimia) which could be linked with a distortion of body image (Crown, 1984; Hawton and Cowen, 1990). Nearly half have used drugs and alcohol to excess. Simpson (1975) reported mutilation in connection with sexual problems. The problems cited include confusion of sexual identity in 66% of cases, as well as high levels of promiscuity or a complete lack of sexual encounters. Few seem to enjoy satisfactory sexual relationships and there is often a negative reaction to menarch, while irregular periods and ammenorrhoea are not uncommon, and cutting often increases around menstruation (Crown, 1984; Hawton and Cowen, 1990). These people find difficulty expressing feelings, or experience feelings of emptiness, tension and occasionally depression. Self-injury behaviour can be learned from others and used to gain attention or manipulate others. Some people use self-injury to relieve pain. Head-banging, cutting or burning provides a controlled pain which is separate from their normal pain. It can also provide stimulation if a person is understimulated and bored. However, it is usually tension-reducing behaviour, with the anger directed at self (Crown, 1984; Faulk, 1988; Hawton and Cowen, 1990).

Tension can be precipitated by rejection, frustration, perceived damage to self-esteem, loss of a meaningful person or problems within a relationship. There is a sudden irresistible urge to harm without a perceived ability to resist, and feelings of being out of control, increasing anxiety, agitation and anger. Tension becomes intolerable. The person might realize they are going to cut and feel some relief. They become self-engrossed and withdrawn, might feel empty and numb, and pass into a state of depersonalization (Hawton and Cowen, 1990). They often go somewhere quiet and make several cuts, usually to the wrists and forearms, which are superficial but draw blood. Drawing blood appears to be important. It might be seen as necessary to re-establish the boundaries between inside and out, so that the person can return to reality. People often cut until there's 'enough blood', but do not normally feel pain at the time of cutting, only relief. The person might even express a lack of awareness of cutting, 'I see I've cut myself'. There might be feelings of guilt or disgust afterwards.

Self-injury behaviour is difficult to manage and cannot be ignored. It is important to accept the person while not accepting the behaviour (Carl Rogers calls this unconditional positive regard; Rosenhan and Seligman, 1984).

Different approaches to treatment include isolating the person and not tolerating the behaviour. However, this can provoke destructive behaviour. Individual attention may help by allowing the person to talk through the problem, but this can be difficult if the person refuses to talk. Staff might give medication to reduce tension, and structured behaviour management can be used to discourage self-injury and encourage appropriate behaviour. Results vary. People often improve in hospital, but deteriorate at home, although this might be related to the aftercare available. Behaviour appears to improve with age and over half are well or much better after 5–6 years (Nelson and Grunebaum, 1971).

Excessive restrictions (such as not allowing a person to leave the ward unescorted) do not appear to inhibit the self-injury behaviour but can precipitate further cutting as each restriction is removed. It can help to give firm consistent limits of what is acceptable and what will not be tolerated. Nurturing the positive aspects of personality works well, and assertiveness techniques can improve self-esteem and communication, particularly when expressing emotions, so that self-destructive phases are avoided. It is important to analyse the behaviour and establish which factors increase and which decrease the likelihood of self-injury, thus building up a picture of the behaviour. Tension-reducing techniques can be useful, e.g. relaxation, impulse control (see aggression) and distractions previously suggested; also, flicking an elastic band on the wrist which causes pain but not damage. The person should be encouraged to go to the key worker if tension becomes intolerable. Physical contact can improve self-esteem, and exercises such as yoga and tai chi improve body image and body awareness. The person needs to be made aware of the effect of their behaviour on others (they are often unaware), but paying attention to the injury itself could reinforce the behaviour, so the wound itself should be dressed with the minimum of attention. Medication can help underlying problems such as psychosis or temporal lobe epilepsy, but is not otherwise helpful. Help must be directed at enabling the person to control their feelings and each person must be assessed and managed as an individual, with a consistent team approach.

Violence to property

This behaviour can include throwing or smashing objects and arson. Three out of every eight fires are deliberately set and the reasons include:

- suicide attempts
- political reasons
- responding to hallucinations
- revenge or spite
- when under stress
- for attention, excitement or out of boredom.

People in the last two categories are commonly male and between the ages of 18 and 25, often with a history of psychiatric illness. There is usually a period of increasing tension and restlessness which becomes out of control following a trigger, e.g. a quarrel. Tension is reduced by setting a fire which is unplanned and often set where it will be easily seen, e.g. on stairs or in the hall. Afterwards, the person feels a sense of satisfaction and calm. Alcohol can reduce inhibitions sufficiently to lead to fire-raising and there is no motive other than an irresistible desire to create and watch a fire. If there is a motive, it is often out of proportion to the effect of the fire. Fire is a destructive force which allows a person to destroy something passively. This can be useful and symbolic (e.g. burning an ex-partner's love letters), but it can remove feelings of responsibility for the destruction. Fire-raising is a difficult problem to manage. Crown (1984) suggests using behavioural techniques such as stimulus satiation, e.g. giving a person matches to strike during a set period of time and asking them to strike the matches until the end of the set period. The person becomes bored with the matches and the behaviour decreases.

These people are at risk in the community and could place others at risk. Using fireproof furniture where possible and restricting smoking and matches to designated smoking areas is essential. It is important to assess the behaviour, and it can be helpful to teach ways of controlling and releasing tension and expressing feelings.

Inappropriate social behaviour

'Normal behaviour' depends on society's ideas of what is 'normal', and changes with time. At one time, premarital sex and homosexuality were classed as deviant, but are now accepted as normal. Normality is a matter of personal opinion; what one person accepts another does not, and extremes of behaviour are likely to be labelled abnormal, whereas a lack of that behaviour can be labelled normal.

Inappropriate behaviour includes asocial behaviours which are embarrassing or offensive but not violent, such as undressing in public, and antisocial behaviours which constitute a criminal act, including sexual disorders such as exhibitionism, voyeurism and paedophilia. Exhibitionism and voyeurism are usually carried out by people who are insecure and inadequate. Treatment might include psychotherapy, behavioural techniques and ways of improving self-esteem and self-confidence. Exhibitionism can occur as a result of reduced inhibition in early dementia, and with temporal and frontal lobe damage. Paedophiles are rarely violent, but are unable to form satisfactory adult relationships and might need to feel powerful. Psychotherapy and behavioural techniques can help. However, it can be difficult to treat these people as the subject evokes strong feelings in staff.

Some people have inappropriate behaviours which make it difficult for them to be accepted by and integrated into the community. Some inappropriate behaviours are the result of institutionalization. For example, undressing in front of others might have been the norm in a hospital where there's little privacy, but is not appropriate in a supermarket. Single sex wards can produce a tendency towards homosexual behaviour and difficulty relating to members of the opposite sex. Lack of privacy can lead to the acceptance of behaviours such as masturbation in the ward, which are unacceptable in public. Sometimes it might only be necessary to set acceptable limits for behaviour within given situations. Inappropriate behaviour can result from hallucinations, e.g. laughing at the voices or acting upon them. Behaviour modification techniques are effective ways of dealing with inappropriate behaviour by giving the person a motive for changing the behaviour and providing an appropriate behaviour for them to use.

Wandering

Confused and demented people can be restless, irritable, withdrawn or wandering, with personality traits that are exaggerated or reversed (Page, 1992). The person might be agitated and confused over time and place, etc. This can often lead to wandering. For example, a female patient may say she needs to go home to cook her husband's tea. Wandering can occur with any mental health problem where concentration is poor or the person is confused. Aimless wandering can become part of institutional behaviour and is responsive to structured behaviour programmes. It is important to keep sessions short and to allow the person to move position, e.g. from the bed to a chair.

Institutional behaviour

Being treated as a patient in hospital has an effect on people. There is often segregation of sexes. There might be lack of privacy, space and freedom which can produce frustration and lead to aggression. On admission to hospital, people are pushed into the 'patient' role (D'Arcy, 1984). Responsibility is taken away from them. They do not have to make decisions, work or deal with bills, etc. The patient is expected to conform to this role, and being accustomed to hospital facilities and the lack of responsibility can encourage people to stay in a safe environment. A large number of people are long-stay, i.e. more than two years. Due to the nature of the illnesses, the most common being schizophrenia, the person might be responding to hallucinations and delusions, which, combined with the effects of institutionalization, can produce inappropriate behaviours (McGrath and Bowker, 1987).

These behaviours can be copied, particularly if they receive attention from staff. Staff attitudes can perpetuate problems, e.g. 'He can't help it', or by giving attention to shouting, aggression, etc., while normal behaviour goes unnoticed. Odd speech can inappropriately be encouraged by asking the person to repeat it or by laughing at it.

The negative symptoms of schizophrenia, such as withdrawal and poverty of speech, can be made worse by ward conditions which might encourage a person to become monosyllabic or mute due to the lack of opportunity for meaningful speech on topics of interest to the person. A lack of visitors can make this problem worse. Relatives and friends might be reluctant to visit, being put off by the ward, lack of privacy, pestering from other clients and the stigma of mental illness. The person's emotions could be flattened, leading to a lack of social sensitivity, or they might withdraw to protect themselves from distressing relationships or overstimulation. Within this environment it is easy for staff to become complacent and run the ward for the benefit and ease of the staff, rather than provide the best environment for the person. For example, 'herding' increases efficiency, but removes choices and individuality, leaving little scope for initiative. Personal possessions might be few, lost or stolen and this can produce hoarding behaviour, with the person being reluctant to leave his possessions or constantly returning to check them. Authoritarian attitudes can result in the person accepting everything without question. This reduces decision-making abilities and leaves the person vulnerable to exploitation and abuse within the community.

Normal behaviour becomes abnormal if it is: (a) performed excessively, e.g. checking that a door is closed is normal; checking it repeatedly is not; (b) performed in an inappropriate place, e.g. undressing for the doctor to examine you is normal; undressing at the supermarket is not.

Modifying behaviour

Behaviour can be modified by *classical conditioning* where a stimulus becomes linked to a response, e.g. Pavlov's dog. This is not a reliable way of learning, as it is gradually extinguished if the pairing does not continue. *Operant conditioning*, where the appropriate behaviour is rewarded, has a better chance of changing behaviour (Skinner, 1971). Long-stay patients respond well to operant conditioning, where the appropriate behaviour is rewarded by a desirable consequence (i.e. is reinforced) and inappropriate behaviour is followed by undesirable consequences (i.e. is not reinforced or is punished).

As long as inappropriate behaviour is not punished, client autonomy is preserved as the person is able to choose which behaviour to use. Inappropriate behaviour will restrict a person's life in the community, whereas appropriate behaviour will enable a person to integrate into the community and is likely to be reinforced by verbal approval. Behaviour modification techniques are designed to extinguish inappropriate behaviour and replace it with appropriate behaviour which will allow the person to function socially.

Inappropriate behaviour can be: (a) a handicap to the person, e.g. behaviour which restricts their adaptation to the environment and needs to be replaced with appropriate behaviour; (b) deficiencies in skills which needs retraining.

Techniques should only be taught if there is a reasonable expectation that the person can acquire the skills upon which the change in behaviour depends, and that they will reduce distress or allow the person to live a less restricted life.

In theory, behaviour modification techniques should not be used without the person's consent, but in practice this might happen if the behaviour puts the person at risk, or severely restricts their life. However, this does raise ethical concerns, especially regarding the use of aversive stimuli, punishment and deprivation for unacceptable behaviour – these should only be used with the person's consent. The programme should be discussed with the person, the main carer and the staff implementing the programme. All the parties should agree that the programme is tailored to the person's needs, so that the person knows what is expected of them. Diagnoses are often not beneficial or often accurate and labels can be difficult to remove. Each person should be assessed individually, looking at their strengths and weaknesses. The behaviour should be assessed using ABC:

A: Antecedents. What happens prior to the behaviour? Changing this might change the behaviour. Look at the environment. Where are they? Who else is there and what were they doing?
B: Behaviour. What actually happens? It is not enough to say the person was violent. What exactly did they do? For example, they threw a chair across the room at the wall six times over a period of five minutes.
C: Consequence. What happened as a result of the behaviour? Did they gain attention or were they left alone?

It is important to measure the baseline. It's not enough to say that Mr Jones attended twice for treatment last week. How often should he have attended? Was he late? Did he leave early? If he did not attend did something prevent him from attending, e.g. another appointment? When planning a programme, look for positive reinforcers (any stimulus that increases the likelihood of a response). Attention is often a positive reinforcer. Negative reinforcers can increase a behaviour by avoidance, and attention can, for some people, be a negative reinforcer.

Reinforcers include:

- *Social reinforcers*, e.g. attention and verbal approval. Problems can occur if a person becomes dependent on approval.
- *Material things*, e.g. cigarettes, food. These can produce problems of satiation.
- *Privileges*, e.g. money, cards, tickets. These have the advantage of being easily recordable. The person can choose what they want to buy (which further reinforces the behaviour) and it can be used for different people. There are no problems of satiation and there is some educational value for counting and budgeting. However, it is artificial and the value of tokens might not be appreciated by some people.

Satiation is where there is too much of a reinforcer: the person becomes satisfied and the behaviour decreases. Overusing a reinforcer can reduce its strength or even make it neutral or aversive. Incompatible behaviours are things that can be done instead of the problem behaviour, but cannot be done at the same time as it, and result in the same reinforcement. Some reinforcers are stronger than others. Find out what works for each person. Ask likes and dislikes. Use requests and complaints, and observe behaviour. For example, a person attending for treatment might want to use the gym. This could be used as a positive reinforcer for attending for his appointments on time. Some reinforcers are more appropriate than others, e.g. tokens for work behaviour, social reinforcers for social behaviour. Motivation is important. According to Maslow's hierarchy of needs, people will try to satisfy basic needs such as hunger first. Then they can go on to develop and achieve their potential. Reinforcers help to motivate people to achieve their potential which improves self-esteem. Setting small achievable goals helps reinforce behaviour.

Punishment

Punishment includes aversive stimuli, e.g. smacking, verbal reprimands, withdrawing privileges (such as putting people into pyjamas) and seclusion. It has tended to be overused, as it is an easy option for staff to choose. Because of ethical issues, punishment such as smacking should never be used, and practices like putting people into pyjamas also raises ethical problems. Verbal reprimands are only temporarily effective in stopping behaviour. Once the punishment is withdrawn, the behaviour reverts to its previous level. It is effective in stopping the behaviour immediately, which is why it has been so often used, but it does not eliminate the behaviour. It also produces emotions in both the punisher and the recipient which is not conducive to learning. It does not teach the appropriate behaviour, but can easily escalate into violence. A person might learn to avoid a situation so as to avoid reprimands. Time out (i.e. removing a person from a situation) gives no opportunity for positive reinforcement, but can be useful if the person finds the environment too stimulating or if the person is screaming or violent, and to ignore the behaviour would disturb others or put them at risk. It is not appropriate if the person has omitted to do something.

The success of behavioural programmes relies on a consistent approach from all involved with the person, and can be measured in terms of achieving the behaviour, extending it to other situations (i.e. generalization) and gradually removing reinforcers (i.e. weaning).

Weaning should be gradual. Sudden withdrawal of reinforcers can produce extinction of the behaviour, unless accompanied by an increase in natural reinforcers, e.g. social reinforcers and privileges. Weaning can include:

- Reducing the size of the reinforcer.
- Using tokens for other behaviours, so that the overall amount earned is the same.
- Delaying reinforcement by accumulating rewards and presenting them as a lump sum, which teaches the person not to expect immediate payment.
- Reducing the frequency of reinforcers. This includes: *linking and chaining*, where consecutive behaviours are needed before the whole is reinforced; *random schedules* where the person does not know if the behaviour will be reinforced or not. With *fixed ratio schedules* the behaviour is reinforced after a set number of responses, e.g. after every three correct responses. However, people can learn to anticipate this and behaviour tails off between reinforcements. *Variable ratio schedules* reinforce the behaviour after an average number of responses (e.g. after an average of x number of responses, but can be reinforced after w or y number). People cannot anticipate and behaviour is

more likely to be maintained. This behaviour is very difficult to extinguish once learned. It is the principle behind fruit machine payouts.

Extinction can be useful to reduce inappropriate behaviour, e.g. by moving away from the person, by ignoring the behaviour or showing no interest in it. The person looks for other ways to gain attention. The behaviour will initially increase, but if ignored, will eventually decrease. Some behaviour cannot be ignored (e.g. self-injury), so it is important to show the person an appropriate alternative behaviour.

Paradox appears to work where there is high resistance and involves asking the person to perform the behaviour you want to eliminate. This might produce *compliance-based paradox* where the person tries to obey and realizes it is silly or unreasonable, or *defiance-based paradox* where the person opposes the instructions. Research suggests that it works better than ignoring or reprimanding the inappropriate behaviour, and insight is not necessary for it to work (Wood and Chamove, 1991). The inappropriate behaviour is requested, e.g. 'Show me how you do that again'. This does not appear to be interpreted as a positive reinforcer.

Functional equivalent training teaches an equivalent behaviour to the inappropriate one. Assessment is essential to establish what maintains the behaviour, and the equivalent behaviour must provide the same consequences. Using communication (i.e. functional communication training, FCT), the person is taught to ask for information on their behaviour (e.g. 'Am I doing this right?', 'Is this OK?') to produce positive reinforcement. If the person needs attention, they can be taught to ask for it in a way that produces a positive response, until it becomes automatic to request attention rather than to use the inappropriate behaviour. This behaviour provides an acceptable alternative which has a high probability of being reinforced with attention. It is a technique which works well if the inappropriate behaviour is maintained by social attention (Duand and Carr, 1992).

Both paradox and FCT are compatible with self-advocacy as the person can choose alternatives, and with FCT the person initiates the intervention.

Strategies for Crisis Intervention and Prevention (SCIP) is a new non-aversive approach to the management of problem behaviours, developed in New York at the office of Mental Retardation and Development Difficulties.

The SCIP strategies taught, provide an alternative to other methods available in England. SCIP methods do not cause pain or panic and are designed to enable staff to work through episodes themselves, having given consideration to all other possibilities of defusing the situation. the aim is to encourage the client to take control of there own behaviour.

Currently there is no nationally approved training. SCIP training is being recognised by some authorities but it is essential that all participants develop their own policies and have sought consent from their organisation before SCIP is implemented.

The physiotherapist might come across some of these techniques on the wards and it is important to be aware of them and to work with other staff to create a consistent environment which reinforces appropriate behaviours. Challenging behaviour can severely restrict a person's life, and reduces the chance of integration into society. It can cause problems in daily living and makes the formation of meaningful relationships difficult.

Working as part of a team, the physiotherapist has a valuable role to play in the assessment of challenging behaviour and in working towards assisting patients to take responsibility for their behaviour and in helping to improve their quality of life.

References

Balter, R.J. and Rosenthal, G. (1978) *Behaviour and Rehabilitation – Behavioural Treatment of Long-Stay Patients*, Wright, Bristol

Banchura, A. (1977) *Social Learning Theory*, Prentice Hall, New Jersey

Cheshire Social Services *Guidance to Staff on Violence by Clients, Policy Practice and Procedure*, Crown, S. (1984) *Contemporary Psychiatry*, Butterworths, London

Dallard, J., Doob, L.W., Miller. N.G., Momrer, O.H. and Sears, R.R. (1939) *Frustration and Aggression*, Yale University Press, Connecticut

Darcy, P.T. (1984) *Theory and Practice of Psychiatric Care*, Hodder and Stoughton, London

Durand, V.M. and Carr, E.G. (1992) An analysis of maintenance following functional communication training. *Journal of Applied Analysis*, **25**(4), 777–794

Faulk, M. (1988) *Basic Psychiatry*, Blackwell Science, Oxford

Finch, J. (1983) Consent to treatment. *Nursing Mirror*, 23 March, p. 37

Frazer, R., Fadim, J., McReynolds, C. and Cox, R. (1987) *Motivation and Personality, Abraham Maslow Revised*, 3rd edn, Harper and Row, London

Friedman, H.S. (ed.) (1990) *Personality and Disease*, Wiley Interscience,

Green, R.G. (1990) *Human Aggression*, Open University Press, UK

Hawton, K. and Cowen, P. (ed.) (1990) *Dilemmas and Difficulties in the Management of Psychiatric Patients*, Oxford University Press, Oxford

Hayden, R.M., Allan, G.J., Camaione, D.N. (1986) Some psychological benefits resulting from involvement in aerobic fitness from the perspective of participants and knowledgeable informants, *Journal of Sports Medicine*, **26**, 67–76

Lamplugh, D. (1988) *Beating Aggression – A Practical Guide for Working Women*, Weidenfield Paperbacks, London

Lorenz (1966) *On Aggresion*, Harcourt, New York

Lowe, T. (1990) Characteristics of effective nursing interventions in the management of challenging behaviour. *Journal of Advanced Nursing*, **17**, 1226–1232

Lowe, T. (1992) Characteristics of effective nursing interventions in the management of challenging behaviour. *Journal of Advanced Nursing*, **17**, 1226–1232

McGrath, G. and Bowker, M. (1987) *Common Psychiatric Emergencies*, IOP,

MacMahon, (1990) The psychological benefits of exercise and the treatment of delinquent adolescents. *Sports Medicine*, **9**(6), 344–351

Moses, J., Steptoe, A., Matthews, A. and Edwards, S. (1989) The effects of excercise training on the mental well-being in the normal population: a controlled trial. *Journal of Psychosomatic Research*, **33**, 41–67

Nelson, S.M. and Grinebaum, H. (1921) A follow-up study of wrist-slashers. *American Journal of Psychiatry*, **127**, 1345–1349

Page, S. (1992) Aggression in Alzheimer's disease. *Nursing Standard*, **6**(24), 37–39

Richards, D. and McDonald, B. (1990) Behavioural psychotherapy, a handbook for nurses. Heinemann Nursing

Rosenham, D.C. and Seligman, M.E.P. (1984) *Abnormal Psychology*, Norton, London

Simpson, M.A. (1975) The phenomenalogy of self-mutilation in a general hospital setting. *Canadian Psychiatric Association Journal*, **20**, 429–433

Skinner, B.F. (1971) *Beyond Freedom and Dignity*, Knopf, New York

Szasz, T. (1963) Law, Liberty and Psychiatry: An Enquiry into the Social Uses of Mental Health Practices, Macmillan, New York

Wood, V.E. and Charmove, A.S. (1991) Paradox, reprimand and extinction in adults with a mental handicap. *Journal of Mental Deficiency Research*, **35**, 374–383

11

Stress management

Stephen T. Heptinstall

Introduction

The science 'stressology' has become very popular over the past decade. The word 'stress' is as much a part of our modern vocabulary now as 'compact disc' or 'hamburger'. It is seen in general terms to be reflective of the negative aspects of twentieth century life; otherwise, most people would find it difficult to give a more specific definition. Lader (1979) comments that the term 'stress' has become 'a convenient, non-technical shorthand term which communicates our ignorance not our knowledge'.

It is true to say that, despite a great deal of scientific research on the subject, stress has not yet been precisely defined.

There are four questions which 'stressologists' are attempting to answer: What is stress? Why and when is stress harmful? Why do some people cope better with it than others?, and finally, What are the skills necessary to cope with stress?

The aim of this chapter is: (a) to explore the work done in each of these areas, and (b) to give the reader a better appreciation of this field and how important it is to incorporate aspects of stress management in their work.

Researchers and scientists view stress in three ways – that stress is a stimulus, is a response, or is a combination of the two. The latter of these viewpoints is known as the transactional model of stress and is proving the most popular of the three concepts. It was first developed in the 1970s by the American psychologist Richard Lazarus. In the view of Lazarus, it is a person's interpretation of an event that makes it stressful, not the event itself, which remains 'neutral' until given meaning.

Stress arises when the perceived demands made upon an individual outweigh that individual's perceived ability to cope with them. This occurs in situations seen as threatening and harmful as well as challenging (Figure 11.1). It is important to note that not all stress is bad and detrimental. Due to our unique interpretation of any event, the same situation may be distressful, unstressful or eustressful, depending on how one sees it, e.g. performing in front of an audience, or a parachute jump. Although many of the physiological alterations will be the same, our psychological reactions to each view will be very different, with only the first proving harmful if stress continues unabated. It is also important to note that it is not always the predominance of one stressor that causes suffering (although this does occur), but rather a build-up of less significant stressors over time.

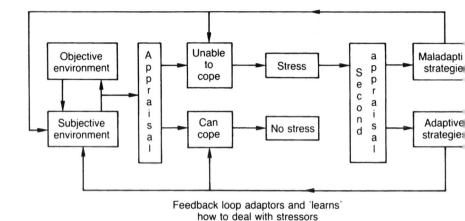

Feedback loop adaptors and 'learns'
how to deal with stressors

Figure 11.1 Diagrammatic representation of the stress process, highlighting the nature of stress coping

Effects of stress

It would appear that stress manifests itself in three ways – physiologically, psychologically and behaviourally.

Physiological effects

Hans Seyle was one of the first doctors to look seriously at the physiological changes that take place in an organism during periods of stress. he discovered there was a patterned physiological sequence which occurred in response to a stress stimulus. In 1944 he published his findings and called this sequence of changes the general adaptation syndrome (GAS). This syndrome can be divided into three stages – the alarm reaction, the resistance stage and the exhaustion state.

Alarm reaction
During this stage a body's defences are mobilized against a potential 'stressor' (Figure 11.2). Adrenaline and noradrenaline, from the sympathetic branch of the autonomic nervous system, and cortisol are released, causing a chain of various 'internal' changes to occur and maximize a person's ability to react.

The various effects of these increased chemicals concentrations are as follows:

1. Adrenaline and noradrenaline:
    – increased alertness and decision-making ability
    – dilated pupils, acute hearing
    – saliva production reduced
    – increased heart beat and force of contraction
    – increased respiration rate and bronchodilatation
    – redirection of blood flow to striated muscle
    – gut activity slowed, blood supply reduced
    – mobilization of fat and glucose from liver and fat stores
    – spleen contracts, increasing red blood cells in the bloodstream

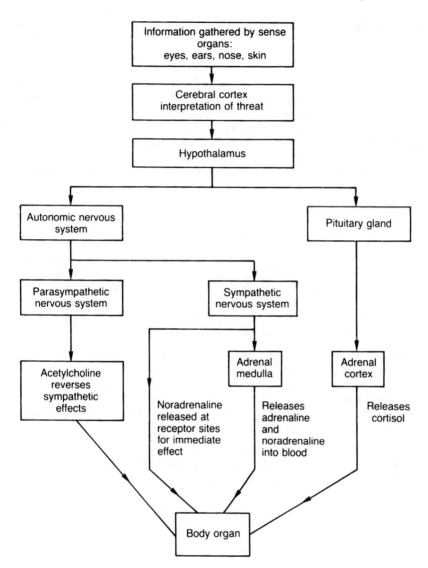

Figure 11.2 The alarm response

- kidneys reduce urine formation
- clotting factor of the blood increased
- reduced blood flow to skin and increased sweating.
2. Cortisol:
    - reduces allergic responses and reactions
    - mobilizes glucose and fats from body stores
    - enhances immune activity
    - sensitizes organs to noradrenaline and adrenaline
    - reduces inflammation
    - aids in wound healing.

All these alarm reactions can manifest themselves as short-term physical stress symptoms (Figure 11.2).

Resistance stage
Here, the organism adapts to the stressor, although neurological and hormonal changes continue. If the stress does not abate, Seyle believed that disease would eventually occur. Normal levels of cortisol enhance immune activity, but prolonged excessive levels actually suppress the immune system. Continued stress also raises the blood cholesterol levels. Scientists have recognized tentative links between stress and the onset of certain medical conditions. These include, chronic heart disease, gastrointestinal problems such as ulcers, irritable bowel syndrome, as well as rheumatoid arthritis, asthma, cancer and diabetes.

Exhaustion state
The capacity to resist stress is finite and eventually breakdown results. According to Seyle, this can take the form of depression and even death. This stage is characterized by the activation of the parasympathetic division of the autonomic nervous system. Function drops to an abnormally low level in a vain attempt to compensate for the high levels of sympathetic activity that preceded it.

Newnham (1990, unpublished) highlights many examples of the physical effects of prolonged psychological stress:

• A large number of widows die within 5 years of the bereavement of their husbands, most of these with cardiovascular disease.
• In males there is a higher incidence of heart attack following divorce or loss of a close friend.
• In neoplasia, the aetiology is unknown, but more and more evidence points to a stress element in its onset.

According to Newnham, long-term psychiatric patients are often heavy smokers and yet these patients rarely get cancer or bronchial problems. He argues that this may be due to the fact that this group exhibit strong emotional outlets which helps control their stress. Could it be, then, that smokers who have poor outlets for emotional discharge are more susceptible to cancer, with prolonged stress acting as the catalyst in its onset?

'A sorrow which is not vented in tears may make other organs weep.'

Psychological effects

Many studies have outlined the psychological effects of stress and some of the short-term effects are listed in Table 11.1. However, little evidence exists that stressful events by themselves cause long-term psychological disorder.

Dohrenwend (1979) outlines three factors she believes that, when present together, make an individual more susceptible to stress-induced psychological problems. They are:

• the presence of physical illness or injury
• an undesirable life event
• loss or lack of social support.

Behavioural effects

Understandably, there are behavioural consequences to the physical and psychological effects of stress. Absenteeism from work is one of the most obvious of these. Some government papers have claimed that up to 60 million working days are lost each year in the UK due to stress-related illness.

Alcohol abuse is another behavioural consequence of stress, as people turn to drink in an attempt to cope better with their problems. Studies have shown that high levels of alcohol consumption are more common in people with stressful occupations. A list of common behavioural responses to stress are shown in Table 11.1.

Table 11.1 Examples of physical, psychological and behavioural signs of stress

Physical	
Weakness and lack of energy	Difficulty breathing
Tight, tense muscles	Sudden palpitations
Stiff movements	Cold extremities
Lack of co-ordination and balance	Flushes
Dizziness and headaches	Emotional sweating
Blurring of vision	Tremors
Dry throat	Indigestion, flatulence, etc.
Tight chest	Skin rashes
	Hair loss
	Weight loss
Psychological	*Behavioural*
Anxiety	Disturbed sleep pattern
Depression	Increased absenteeism from work
Poor self-esteem	Increased use of stimulants, e.g. caffeine,
Negativity	tobacco and drugs
Poor body image	Alcohol abuse
Generalistic	Antisocial behaviour, e.g. vandalism, violence
Fatalism	Low productivity
Inadequacy and defeatism	Decreased self-care
Fear	Sexual problems
Anger	Increased pain/illness behaviour
Overmagnification of problems	Social isolation/withdrawal

Stressors

Seyle refers to a stressor as being the stimulus which causes a stress response to occur. Although individual perception is crucial to the stress equation, common stressors have been recognized.

People suffer the direct effects of climate, micro-organisms, terrain, chemical and physical forces and also through their interaction with other human beings, e.g. overcrowding, marital problems.

Two main factors influencing the severity of stress are its predictability and duration. The less predictable and/or longer it is endured, the more severe stress will be.

All individuals respond and cope differently to stressors, and some are more successful at coping than others. Researchers talk of a person being 'vulnerable' to stress and have identified some key factors that might make a person more susceptible (Cooper *et al.*, 1988). These are:

- the number and nature of life events an individual encounters
- personality variables
- the number of existing coping strategies an individual employs.

Number and nature of life events

In 1967, Holmes and Rahe published their Social Readjustment Rating Scale (SRRS), shown in Table 11.2. They developed this scale after lengthy research which concluded that events causing life adjustment are a key ingredient of stress. However, this scale has suffered repeated misuse by individuals attempting to predict future ill health. The fact is that the scale only measures one aspect of a person's vulnerability. Someone may score over 300 (seen as the critical number on the SRRS) and not become ill as a consequence.

Lazarus has taken a different view of how events in one's life may help to cause stress. He argues that it is in fact the routine daily problems (hassles) that more readily cause stress. He produced the Hassle Scale in an attempt to measure these. As a predictor of psychological health, the Hassle Scale has been shown to be more accurate than life events like the SRRS (Kanner *et al.*, 1981).

Personality variables

Researchers have identified 'personality types' which appear to be more 'stress prone' than others.

Type A – coronary-prone personalities

Cardiologists Friedman and Rosenman first coined this term in the 1950s. They recognized character similarities in many of their patients recovering from heart attacks and associated conditions.

Type As may be described as individuals that are agitated, hard-driving, hurried, impatient and hostile. They are often poor listeners, over-competitive and over-ambitious. Perfectionists in an imperfect world, they invariably suffer the effects of their 'self-maintained' stress. This results predominantly in heart disease and associated problems (Friedman and Rosenman, 1974).

Locus of control

Conceptualized by Rotter (1960), someone with an internal locus of control is said to believe they have control over most situations and outcomes of their life. In contrast, someone with an external locus of control believes they have little influence over events and that most outcomes are determined by fate.

Many studies have explored the importance of control and its links to stress. They indicate that when a person perceives they have control over situations and surroundings, that person is less vulnerable to stress. Hence, a person who has an external locus of control is more likely to suffer from stress than someone who demonstrates an internal locus of control.

The hardy personality

This theory was developed by Kobasa (1979). There are three key attributes of this kind of personality:

Table 11.2 Rating scale of Life events – the Holmes and Rahe Social Readjustments Rating Scale*

Rank	Life event	Mean value
1	Death of spouse	100
2	Divorce	75
3	Marital separation	65
4	Jail term	63
5	Death of close family member	63
6	Personal injury or illness	53
7	Marriage	50
8	Fired at work	47
9	Marital reconciliation	45
10	Retirement	45
11	Change in health of family member	44
12	Pregnancy	40
13	Sexual difficulties	39
14	Gain of new family member	39
15	Business readjustment	39
16	Change in financial state	38
17	Death of close friend	37
18	Change to different line of work	36
19	Change in number of arguments with spouse	35
20	Mortgage over £30 000	31
21	Foreclosure of a mortgage or loan	30
22	Change in responsibilities at work	29
23	Son or daughter leaving home	29
24	Trouble with in-laws	29
25	Outstanding personal achievement	28
26	Spouse begins or stops work	26
27	Begin or end school	26
28	Change in living conditions	25
29	Revision of personal habits	24
30	Trouble with boss	23
31	Change in work hours or conditions	20
32	Change in residence	20
33	Change in school	20
34	Change in recreation	19
35	Change in church activities	19
36	Change in social activities	18
37	Mortgage or loan of £30 000 or less†	17
38	Change in sleeping habits	16
39	Change in number of family get-togethers	15
40	Change in eating habits	15
41	Vacation	13
42	Christmas	12
43	Minor violations of the law	11

* Reprinted from Holmes, T.H. and Rahe, R.H. (1967) *Journal of Psychosomatic Research*, no. 11, pp. 215–218, with kind permission from Pergamon Press Ltd.
† NB. The figure for the mortgage has been adjusted.

- that the individual expresses positive commitment to all aspects of their life
- that the individual believes they can influence events around them
- that the individual accepts change as part of life, meeting it with willingness and a sense of challenge.

It is argued people high in 'hardiness' are less likely to fall ill as a consequence of stress.

The identity disruption model
This is a more recent attempt to relate personality factors to stress, which was developed by Brown and McGill (1989). They contend that it is only life events which make an individual change what they think about themselves that cause stress rather than the events themselves. The more life events which do this, the greater the risk of developing illness.

They also suggest that positive life events (like those in the SRRS) only have negative health effects on people with low self-esteem. This is because positive events lay outside their sense of identity.

Coping strategies

Lazarus and Folkman (1984) define coping as 'constantly changing cognitive and behavioural efforts to manage specific external and/or internal demands that are appraised as taxing or exceeding the resources of the person'.

They outline several factors on which coping ability depends. These are: healthiness; positive self-belief; good problem-solving and social skills; the presence of social support and having good material resources, i.e. money.

The way an individual deals or copes with stress becomes an integral part of their overall 'vulnerability' to it (Cooper *et al.*, 1988).

Stressful encounters are dynamic and complex, rather than static and unitary. They are constantly changing and unfolding, so that the outcome of one stressful event alters the subsequent appraisal of new events (Brannon and Feist, 1992).

A person who chooses maladaptive coping strategies to deal with a stressor is both unsuccessful in relieving their immediate stress, but also does not learn how to adapt to the same stressor in the future (see Figure 11.1). A person with a good array of adaptive coping strategies is more able to deal with potential stressors than someone with only maladaptive, limited or no knowledge of such strategies.

All these factors offer explanations as to why some people are affected more readily than others by stress. However, all are still undergoing research and are in no way firm conclusions.

Assessment

Essential to stress management training is effective assessment. Due to the diversity of stress presentation, this can be a difficult and time-consuming process.

Meichenbaum (1985) lists specific objectives for the assessment phase of training. These include:

- establish a collaborative relationship with the client and with significant others if appropriate
- discuss the client's stress-related problems and symptoms
- collect information in the form of interviews, questionnaires, self-monitoring procedures, etc.
- assess the client's expectations with regard to effectiveness of the training programme and formulate treatment plans establishing, short-, intermediate- and long-term goals.

- educate the client about the transactional nature of stress and coping and consider the role that cognition and emotions play in creating and maintaining stress.

Having counselling skills is a useful asset during assessment and training, but is not an essential prerequisite.

As long as the physiotherapist is approachable, accepting, remains objective but shows a real desire to understand, is empathic and trustworthy, an effective relationship can develop.

Below is an overview of items to include during assessment.

A. The interview
1. *Time.* Allow up to 1 hour.
2. *Environment.* Private room free from interruption. Have a whiteboard available to underline important points. A clock on the wall facing you, but behind the client, prevents offputting glimpses at a watch.
3. *The welcome.* Very important. The therapist should be open and friendly without being uncomfortably informal. Shake hands to help communicate warmth and acceptance.
4. *Interview introduction.* Give a brief overview of session structure and make clear time available for discussion at each meeting.
5. *Investigation of present problems*
   (a) Encourage the client's own description. Use open questions: 'What things have led you to seek help from us?'
   (b) Ascertain some degree of distress: 'How serious is the problem?'
   (c) Ask about specific stressors.
   (d) Question about onset-related factors: 'What else was occurring in your life at the time?'
   (e) Discuss the consequences of stress, i.e. on sleep, appetite, etc.
   (f) Investigate in detail any particular physical, psychological or behavioural symptoms.
   (g) Find out the duration, frequency and severity of symptoms (visual analogue scales may be used here).
6. *History of the problem*
   (a) 'How long have you had this stress?'
   (b) What is its course? 'Is it getting better or worse?'
   (c) Question-related previous history: 'Has it happened before?' 'How did you cope with it then?'
7. *Current coping methods*
   (a) Discuss coping strategies adopted to deal with the stressor. Question to find out whether they are adaptive or maladaptive.
   (b) Investigate the use of comfort zones and/or comfort rituals, e.g. the client is able to relax when alone in the bedroom or when walking the dog.
   (c) Ask about support networks: 'Is there anyone you feel supports you, someone you can talk to and confide in?'
   (d) Question whether the client has any hobbies, interests, takes part in any sort of social activities, uses religious belief to cope.
   (e) Ascertain the client's 'perceived' degree of control over their present situation (a visual analogue scale may be used here).

8. *Other professionals /problems*
   (a) 'Are there any other disciplines involved at present or have been so at any time during this period of stress?'
   (b) Find out about relevant medical or psychiatric investigations: X-ray, CT scan, etc.
   (c) Question generally about previous medical and psychiatric history.
9. *Current medication*
   (a) List all currently taken medication, including caffeine, alcohol, nicotine and self-medication.
   (b) Note relevant previous medication.
10. *Other relevant details.* This may include selective, detailed questioning about:
    (a) Status
    (b) Home dynamics, i.e. family relationships.
    (c) Work dynamics, e.g. type of position, workload, etc.
    (d) Other responsibilities, e.g. financial, social, etc.
11. *Client expectations*
    (a) Of treatment: 'What do you expect from our session?' 'What would you like to happen?'
    (b) To change: 'Are you prepared to change should doing so enable you to cope better with stress?'
12. *Ending*
    (a) Recap on main points raised. Highlight positive aspects of the discussion and attributes of the client.
    (b) Encourage client questioning and their collaboration in analysing the information shared.
    (c) Plan next session briefly; give reading or homework, e.g. stress diary to supplement next meeting.

B. Self-rating questionnaires
This is a time-effective way of gaining information and can be very helpful as a subjective marker with which to gauge progress. There are many types of questionnaire available, measuring all aspects of stress, i.e. anxiety, depression, pain as well as specific stressors.

According to Kirk (1979) it is only worth while using questionnaires supported by substantial validational data. Content validity is particularly important and refers to the extent to which the questionnaire adequately measures the relevant area.

If self-report questionnaires are to be used, it is worth implementing them after initial interview so that some specificity can be made.

C. Observation and physical assessment
During interview and subsequent interventions there are various observations the physiotherapist should make. These include:

1. *Appearance.* Is the client well groomed or untidy and dirty. Do they take pride in their appearance? Do they look tired and ill?
2. *Posture.* Is it slumped, depressed, restless, open or withdrawn? Is there muscular tension, eye contact?

3. *Movement*. Is there lassitude, clumsiness, inhibition? Or is it hurried, nervous, fidgeting? Are there any functional difficulties?
4. *Autonomic disturbances*. Flushing, sweating, sighing, breathing difficulties, dizziness, pallor, swallowing.
5. *Apparent sadness*. Reflected in speech, facial expression, etc.
6. *Concentration difficulties*. Does the client demonstrate difficulty collecting their thoughts, leading to confusion etc.?
7. *Thoughts*. Are they of worry, pessimism, hostility. Are there any signs of hypochondriasis?
8. *Phobia*. Representing feelings of unreasonable fear in specific situations, i.e. buses, supermarkets.

The physiotherapist may wish to use established observer rating psychophysiological scales to help provide measures for this part of the assessment, e.g. the Clinical Anxiety Scale (CAS) (Snaith *et al*., 1982), the Hamilton Rating Scale for Depression (HAMD) (Hamilton, 1967) or the Montgomery–Absberg Depression Rating Scale (MADRS) (Montgomery and Asberg, 1979).

The physical assessment should follow the basic guidelines of musculoskeletal examination with the physiotherapist looking for areas of excessive muscle tone, tightness, joint limitation, muscular weakness and limitation of function, as well as autonomic disturbances in cardiovascular, respiratory and gastrointestinal systems.

They should also look closely at the reflexes, testing postural, as well as weakness and disinhibition within primitive and inter-uterine reflexes which can reflect dysfunction in the central nervous system. According to Blythe (1980), a weakened central nervous system is often misdiagnosed as emotional/stress problems.

On occasions, the physiotherapist will be faced with someone who presents with a common triad of stress symptoms, but does not agree or recognize the existence of these as being a consequence of stress. Often, in these cases, the assessor will glean some information from interview, but again mostly from their observations of physical, psychological states and behaviour.

There are many reasons why a client may take this standpoint; some of the most common are:

1. *Denial*. This is a coping mechanism employed by a client to protect themselves from a stressor(s). Denying its/their existence helps them to cope. Dealing with this type of presentation is discussed later.
2. *Distrust* – of either the therapist, the situation, or the path they have been directed upon by other disciplines that has led them to this interview. Here the physiotherapist must decide whether they can work slowly to build trust and develop a therapeutic relationship, or to refer their treatment to someone else with whom the client may feel more comfortable.
3. *Lack of understanding*. The client does not recognize stress because he cannot identify a particular stressor and/or does not understand how stress can affect a person. A reason for the former may be due to the build up of less substantial, less recognizable stressors over a long period of time which has eventually caused suffering. Without being educated to look for this chain of stressors, many will not recognize it. Regarding the second point, a moderate percentage of people will not easily connect the physical, psychological and behavioural aspects of self and how one can affect the other. Here, education

is the priority. The client should first be taught to understand the nature and effects of stress, having the opportunity then to reconceptualize their situation and symptoms. This client group is often resistive to accept their symptom as stress based, even after formal teaching. However, if you can get them to agree there is a possibility that stress could be involved to some degree, then a 'what have you got to lose?' approach often makes them more amenable to try management techniques.

According to Lazarus (1987) initial assessment can be used to derive 12 determinations:

1. Are there signs of 'psychosis'?
2. Are there signs of organicity, organic pathology or any disturbed motor activity?
3. Is there any evidence of depression, suicidal or homicidal tendencies?
4. What are the persisting complaints and their main precipitating events?
5. What appears to be some important antecedent factors?
6. Who or what seems to be maintaining the client's overt and covert problems?
7. What does the client wish to derive from therapy?
8. Are there clear indications or contraindications for the adoption of a particular therapeutic style?
9. Are there clear indications as to whether it would be in the client's best interests to be seen individually, as part of a dyad, triad, family and/or in a group?
10. Can a mutually satisfying relationship ensue or should the client be referred elsewhere?
11. Why should the client be seeking therapy at this time?
12. What are some of the client's positive strengths and attributes?

One should also add: Is there evidence of denial, mistrust or lack of understanding?

To aid the physiotherapist in analysis and intervention planning, the information gathered during assessment can next be categorized into six groups. Each group is subheaded: Behaviour, Affect, Sensation, Imagery, Cognition, Interpersonal, and Drug/Biology. These are easily remembered by using the acronym BASICID. These groups help form a problem checklist which serves as a working plan that specific treatment approaches can be matched against (Table 11.3). This forms part of what is called a multimodel approach to stress management.

Although the therapist uses their experience to indicate what interventions may be helpful, the client should also be given the opportunity to choose any technique they may want to use. For example, if a client has a strong belief that hypnosis would be beneficial, then this should be considered (Palmer, 1993). Meeting client expectancies seems to lead to more positive outcomes (Lazarus, 1973).

During interview, information may be divulged or stressors identified that the physiotherapist is not trained to deal with, e.g. sexual abuse, marital problems. Likewise a particular technique may be indicated that the therapist also has little experience in. In these cases the client should be referred to another therapist who is trained to meet those needs, such as a psychologist or a marriage

Table 11.3 Modality profile (or BASICID chart)

Problem identified	Possible intervention
1. Behaviour	
(a) Sleep disturbance	(a) Sleep hygiene
(b) Avoidance of people at work	(b) Relaxation – Bensonian
	(c) Assertiveness training
2. Affect	
(a) Anxiety attacks	(a) Demo health anxiety cycle and breathing exercises
3. Sensation	
(a) Rapid heartbeat	(a) Relaxation
	(b) Vagal innervation technique
4. Imagery	
(a) Images of physical abuse	(a) Imaginal exposure – refer to psychologist
5. Cognition	
(a) Must perform well	(a) Cognitive restructuring
(b) Not as good as others	(b) Dispute irrational beliefs
6. Interpersonal	
(a) Passive in relationships	(a) Assertiveness training
7. Drugs/biology	
(a) Aspirin for headaches	(a) Relaxation training
(b) Lack of exercise	(b) Encourage lifestyle change; give fitness programme

guidance counsellor. This does not mean the physiotherapist must then discharge their client. They may continue to work alongside the new therapist complementing 'their' input and focusing on other aspects of the person's stress.

Having a wide 'theoretical' knowledge of various stress management techniques is therefore helpful. It enables the physiotherapist to make judicious decisions about where and how a client will best be served.

Stress management techniques

Lazarus and Folkman (1984) described two types of coping:

1. *Problem-focused coping.* Designed to manage the problem causing the distress, e.g. counselling, problem-solving techniques.
2. *Emotion-focused coping.* Designed to regulate emotions of distress, e.g. relaxation training, diversion techniques.

Meichenbaum (1985) argues that an effective stress management programme should nurture skills in both these areas. he also describes three phases which effective stress management should pass through:

1. *The conceptualization phase.* This is where the therapist strives to establish a working relationship with the client. The client is also educated to better understand the nature and effects of stress, reconceptualizing it in transactional terms.
2. *Skills acquisition and rehearsal*, during which the client develops and rehearses a variety of coping skills.

3. *Application and follow-through.* Using follow-up appointments after a course of treatment, the physiotherapist can help minimize relapse and boost strategy effectiveness.

Using a multi-modal approach to stress management, the physiotherapist maximizes treatment specifity. Coping strategies that can be taught in physiotherapy include:

1. Behavioural techniques
   - reviewing lifestyles
   - assertiveness training
   - modifying type A behaviour.
2. Simple cognitive strategies
   - constructive self-talk and cognitive reappraisal
   - thought stopping and mental diversion
   - problem solving
3. Body awareness training
   - self observation
   - posture
   - movement
   - touch
   - exercise.

Behavioural techniques

Reviewing lifestyle

Much has been written on the subject of 'reasonable living patterns'. Belloc and Breslow (1972) list several practices that highly correlate with 'good health'. They are:

- sleeping 7–8 hours daily
- eating breakfast
- never or rarely eating between meals
- being about the prescribed height-adjusted weight
- never smoking cigarettes
- moderate or no use of alcohol
- regular physical activity.

Research also indicates that an individual who has social support and perceives himself as being in control of most life situations is less likely to fall ill as a consequence of stress.

With the physiotherapist acting as a collaborator with the client, these factors should be investigated. If any is absent, then lifestyle changes should be considered which might facilitate them.

Other areas of lifestyle which the client/therapist may wish to review are:

- life demands and responsibilities
- activity levels – exercise, sports played, etc.
- diet/nutritional intake
- social habits – smoking, drinking alcohol, caffeine, other self-medication

- ways of relaxing – adaptive and maladaptive strategies, use of comfort zones and rituals
- distractions – hobbies, interests, club membership, evening classes
- time management
- bedtime rituals and sleep patterns
- support systems – family, friends, etc.
- spiritual beliefs, attitudes, practices.

Assertiveness training

During interaction, many people create unnecessary stress for themselves through lack of assertiveness (Davies *et al.*, 1988).

Assertiveness training can reduce stress by teaching the person to become objective, stand up for their legitimate rights and avoid manipulation. A person's legitimate 'rights' include:

- the right to make mistakes
- the right to set one's own priorities
- the right for one's own needs, opinions and convictions to be considered as important as those of others
- the right to refuse requests without having to feel guilty about it
- the right to express oneself as long as one does not violate the rights of others
- the right to change one's mind
- the right to judge oneself, behaviour, thoughts and emotions and to take responsibility for the consequences of them
- the right to feel and express pain
- the right to ask for help or emotional support
- the right to be the final judge of one's own feelings and accept them as legitimate.

Assertiveness training can be divided into seven steps:

1. Understanding what assertiveness style is.
2. Recognizing situations of non-assertiveness.
3. Devising a working plan for change.
4. Learning to communicate assertiveness through body language.
5. Learning how to listen.
6. Managing workable compromises.
7. How to avoid manipulation.

A person is said to behave assertively when they stand up for themselves, express their true feelings, and do not let others take advantage of them. At the same time they are considerate of other's feelings, acting in their own best interest with regard to others, but not feeling guilty or wrong about it.

There are six elements a person can include in a script for change:

(a) Look at your rights, be clear what you want.
(b) Arrange a time and place to discuss your concerns with the person(s) you are in disagreement with.
(c) Define the problem situation as specifically as possible.
(d) Describe feelings so that the other person has a better understanding of how important an issue is to you.

(e) Express your request in short, clear sentences and be specific.
(f) Reinforce to the other person what you want with positive consequences, e.g. 'It will save the company money' or 'We will have more time together'.

These points can easily be remembered using the acronym LADDER (Davies *et al.*, 1988).

Assertive body language includes:

- using direct eye contact, maintained for an appropriate length of time
- erect, yet relaxed posture
- fluent and smooth use of voice, with a positive and strong tone
- use of congruent gestures and facial expression to add emphasis to any communication
- standing in comfortable proximity to those in conversation with.

'Brainstorming' tactics can help manage workable compromises with people whom the client disagrees. This can take the form of listing all possible solutions to a conflict and then systematically working through it with collaborative discussion. The aim should be to look for a compromise which both parties can live with rather than be totally satisfied with.

There are a number of techniques which can be taught to help the client resist another's manipulation. These include:

1. *The broken record.* Repeating a concise request or refusal over and over again.
2. *Content-to-process shift.* Shifting the focus of a discussion from the topic to an analysis of what is going on between the two parties, e.g. 'You appear to be getting annoyed?'
3. *Defusing.* Putting off a discussion in the face of rising anger.
4. *Assertive delay.* Putting off the response to a challenge until one is in control to deal with it accordingly.
5. *Assertive agreement.* Acknowledging criticism with which you agree without apologizing.
6. *Clouding.* Repeating criticism factually without promising to change, e.g. 'You are right, I am late'.
7. *Assertive enquiry.* Prompt criticism in order to find out what is really bothering another person.

One way of aiding fluency in assertiveness skills is to rehearse them through role play. the client re-enacts problem situations in a controlled environment, guided and supervised by their therapist. Over time they develop competency and increased self-belief about using these techniques. Eventually the client incorporates the taught 'new behaviours' into their personal repertoire of behaviour and 'forgets them', but is perceived as more assertive. The new behaviours can then be said to have become a part of the person (Burnard, 1991).

Modifying type A behaviour

There are a number of ways a type A individual can attempt to manage their own 'stress-inducing' characteristics. Friedman and Rosenman, the originators of the type A concept, devised a number of drills (which others have modified) to help these patients combat the negative aspects of their behaviour. These drills include:

- restraining being the centre of attention and attempting instead to listen to others
- attempting to control 'obsessional time directed' behaviour; learning to occupy time constructively and patiently when waiting
- developing 'reflective thinking'; taking some time during the day to review its content
- learning to tackle one task at a time and not taking immediate action all the time
- developing outside interests from work; playing games for fun and not to win
- avoiding diary clutter, by not making unnecessary appointments and deadlines
- learning to protect time and say 'no'.

Friedman and Rosenman also tried to help the type A person see how his behaviour affects his relationship with others. Indeed, leading researcher R. Williams argues that it is the 'cynical hostility' which is sometimes an aspect of type A behaviour that is in fact the toxic element of their personality. He contends that people who mistrust others, think the worst of humanity and interact with others based on their cynical hostility are harming themselves (Williams, 1989).

Drills which focus upon this aspect of behaviour include:

- accepting mistakes in oneself and others
- making oneself aware of the impact one has on others; attempting to stem unnecessary hostility
- trying to reward people for their efforts; also attempting to be more relaxed and positive towards them
- taking time off to develop social relationships.

Looker and Gregson (1989) advocate family involvement with management. Encouraging relatives to be both monitors and motivators of drill adherence.

Simple cognitive strategies

Habitual cognitive coping strategies often develop in people meeting repeated or continuing stress. These are complex and individualistic, but some occur frequently and have been identified. These are called defence mechanisms because they protect the individual's self-esteem and defend them against excessive stress.

All defence mechanisms involve self-deception in the form of denial (repression of memories or actions that may cause stress) and disguise (masking from ourselves our true motives).

There are some occasions when doing nothing and not thinking about stressful events can be a more adaptive response than any other action. This is especially true in circumstances where a person has no control. Denial can act as a means of self-protection, allowing the individual to pace their exposure to a stressor (Meichenbaum, 1985). It is only when such mechanisms become dominant modes of problem solving that they may be maladaptive.

The therapist must be cautious not to force confrontation with a stressor when a client is employing denial and/or disguise as a coping strategy to deal with that stressor. Rather, training should focus upon peripheral complaints and work slowly towards the real problem at a pace dictated by the client.

Cognitive therapy helps bring to a client's attention the impact of thoughts and feelings on their stress levels. There are a number of simple cognitive strategies which the physiotherapist can learn and teach to their clients, supplementing the more tangible physical techniques used. These include, constructive self-talk and cognitive reappraisal, thought stopping, mental diversion and problem solving.

Constructive self-talk and cognitive reappraisal

In almost every minute of a person's conscious life they are engaged in self-talk. These are the internal sentences with which a person describes and interprets their world. If self-talk is rational, positive and optimistic, an individual functions well. If it is irrational, negative and pessimistic, the person experiences emotional disturbances and stress.

Ellis developed a system to attack irrational thought patterns and replace them with realistic, positive statements (Ellis and Harper, 1961). He called this system 'rational emotive therapy'. He based it on the theory that emotions have nothing to do with actual events. In between the event and the emotion is realistic or unrealistic self-talk. It is the self-talk that produces the emotion, self-talk that produces the stress response. A person who can learn to substitute unfounded negative thoughts with more constructive self-talk can help to control potential stressors through this cognitive reappraisal. Examples are given in Table 11.4.

Table 11.4 Constructive self-talk

Situation	Irrational monologue	Constructive self-talk
A friend cancels a date	He does not care for me – no one does	I know he's under a lot of pressure right now –I'll do something by myself
Recovering from a heart attack	I almost died. I'll die soon. I'll never work again	I didn't die – I made it through. The doctor says I'll be able to work soon
Preparing to make a public address	I'm going to blow it. I'm going to lose my voice	This ought to be a challenge. I'll take a deep breath and enjoy it

Thought stopping and mental diversion

These two techniques were described in detail by Quick and Quick (1984). Thought stopping means recognizing potentially damaging thoughts and halting them immediately. This can be done effectively by visualizing the word 'Stop' in neon lights or on a road traffic sign. The individual can then use mental diversion techniques to switch their attention away from the negative thoughts. These techniques include:

- mental games – doing puzzles, crosswords or other word games, reciting a poem, singing and counting backwards

- environmental focus – concentrating on a specific detail of the surroundings, e.g. a car number plate, guessing what people passing may do for a living
- using a bridging object – this could be a photograph of a loved one or a particularly good holiday, perhaps a souvenir from such a holiday; looking at the object generates positive anxiety-reducing thoughts
- physical activity – having a task to do takes a person's mind off worrying thoughts.

Problem solving

A final component of cognitive therapy worth considering is 'problem solving'. Hawton and Kirk (1988) outline what they believe to be the aims of problem-solving skill training. They are to:

- assist clients to identify problem causes of dysphoria
- help them recognize the resources they possess for approaching their difficulties
- teach them a systematic method of overcoming their current problems
- enhance their sense of control
- equip them with a method of tackling future problems.

An eight-step procedure can be followed to help the client attain this skill:

(a) Identify what the problems are and which should be tackled first.
(b) Brainstorm – collect all relevant data relating to the problem and analyse.
(c) Collaborate to list all possible solutions to the problem. Agree realistic goals from this.
(d) Develop an action plan – the steps necessary to achieve the goals.
(e) Implement action plan.
(f) Review – including all difficulties encountered. Continue or redefine problems and goals.
(g) Develop new action plan if necessary.
(h) Review again, redefine or conclude outcome. Work on other problems.

Body awareness training

No scientific research has yet resolved how the mind and the body appear to coexist and interrelate (Granville-Grossman, 1983). However, state of mind does affect the body and vice versa, even though the exact nature of the interaction remains unknown.

F.M. Alexander, founder of the Alexander technique, called it the 'psychophysical' unity of self and believed that every physical activity has a mental component, and every mental activity has a physical component.

Taking this further, it is not difficult to recognize that 'the way we use our bodies is an expression of our state of "being", our thoughts, feelings and patterns of cognitive and effect, tension, etc.' (Skelly, 1993). When we are stressed our bodies react defensively, curling in upon oneself, with fluency, efficiency and ranges of movement becoming restricted.

The aim of body awareness training is to help the client realize this relationship and appreciate how psychological state can effect physical state and vice versa. With this knowledge the client can then be guided in the formulation of strategies aimed at alleviating stress effects through physical means.

Physiotherapists entering into a programme of body awareness training should:

- encourage the art of self-observation and sensory awareness
- modify static and dynamic postures which are or may cause strain
- teach how movement and activity can aid physical fitness, self-esteem and interaction
- use touch to help the client identify problem areas and encourage 'hands-on' self-help techniques; also to help them become aware what an important dimension of communication touch is and how to use it positively to make contact with others.

Self-observation

A simple seven-step technique can be taught which helps nurture self-awareness in the client. It encourages them to listen to what their bodies are saying and find out how they react physically to stress.

A seven-step self-analysis technique
Each of these techniques should be performed standing in front of a mirror with a chair available:

1. *Posture*. First, encourage the client to look at body posture, noting symmetry and also differences between the two sides of the body. also whether weight-bearing is balanced between both feet.
2. *Body tension*. Ask the client to 'tune in' to the subtle sensations being relayed back up to their brain from the body. Focus upon any areas of tension and see whether these correspond with postural asymmetry. If so, move until tension is less and observe this new position.
3. *Joints*. Slowly work through moving the major joints of the body noting any limitation due to stiffness or tightness.
4. *Contact points*. The client should now attempt consciously to release muscular tension, e.g. visualizing it draining like liquid out of the limbs can promote this. Over time a sensation of increased pressure through weight-bearing or contact points may occur. The client should use this as a positive guide to effectiveness, when attempting to relax in various positions.
5. *Balance*. The client should now notice how their body segments balance upon each other when standing on both legs; then standing on one foot, alternating from right to left. Again, shifts in muscle tone and increased areas of tension should be noted as well as balance skills upon a smaller base.
6. *Breathing*. Standing back on two feet in as relaxed a posture as possible, the client now concentrates upon their breathing. They should first watch the movement of their chest and then notice the sensations of inspiration and expiration. After passive observation, the client then braces back both knees and notices whether any changes in respiration take place. If so, the same exercise should be done again, attempting to maintain a steady rate of respiration.
7. *Movement*. The last stage is to observe how gross movement affects the body. From standing, the client goes to sitting. They monitor any increase in body

tension prior to transfer initiation. They should also notice any alteration in breathing pattern.

Another area of self-observation is how a person reacts to their surroundings. Many people habitually overreact to external stimulus, i.e. the telephone or doorbell ringing. The client should note how they react to such stimulus. If there is a tendency to 'jump' at these noises, a pause, concentration upon steady, comfortable breathing should precede their further attention. This technique helps the client become more acutely aware of low-intensity cues that can signal a stress response.

Each activity of life requires different levels of muscle tone. According to Park (1989), many people use a ridiculous amount of tension to perform the most delicate actions, e.g. writing. Combine this with the tension that stress creates and a person can quickly become fixed in a state of habitual hypertonia.

Clients should be taught how to be selective about muscle activity, releasing excessive tone in muscle groups not required for specific activity, e.g. releasing tension in shoulder elevators while playing the piano.

Posture

When looking at posture, the physiotherapist is advised to take heed of the observations of Wells (1971): 'In view of the great variety of human physiques and individual differences in structure, due either to hereditary or to early environmental influence, there can be no single detailed description of good posture.'

Both static and dynamic posture can only be judged on the basis of how well it copes with the demands made upon it.

Though the eye of a trained physiotherapist may see potential postural problems due to positional or movement malpractice, they should resist 'imposing' changes upon their client. Rather they should seek the client's co-operation and willingness to change after discussing assessment findings with them. Through education and objective self-analysis, the client learns what is good posture for them.

Some changes to furnishings or use of support aids may be beneficial, e.g. the McKenzie lumbar roll, especially prior to body reconditioning. Ergonomic considerations are also very important and should be applied to a client's work practices and home life, if at all possible.

Movement

Movement efficiency, i.e. 'movements that achieve their objectives with the minimum of effort and cumulative strain', should be taught as part of an ergonomic approach. This involves changing from top-heavy movement patterns (constant use of upper limbs and spine) to more base movement patterns (increased use of legs, lowering and balancing of the centre of gravity).

Top-heavy movements cause excessive postural fixation which in turn causes adaptive shortening of muscles (Crosier, 1990). It also decreases tissue extensibility and stiffens the joints. As a result of these changes, teaching new movement patterns without first conditioning the body to accept them can lead to injury. Therefore, conditioning exercises must precede all movement re-education, e.g. stretching tightened structures and strengthening weak musculature.

One of the most valuable aspects of conditioning movements is that they teach the client how to assess and know what is good safe movement. Other forms of posture- and movement-related therapy worthy of note are the Alexander technique and the Feldenkrais approach.

Touch

Touch is an integral part of most physiotherapists' work and can be used to great effect when teaching body awareness. It can help to locate and treat areas of tension and pain, with an immediacy other techniques do not possess. It can also help the physiotherapist communicate with the client at a more personal level, allowing the building up of a more therapeutic relationship.

Good stress management is all about promoting self-sufficiency to tackle stressors. Hence, care must be taken that any 'hands-on' intervention does not result in therapy dependency. Self-help techniques (in massage, acupressure, passive stretching, etc.), with supportive others' involvement when possible, should be introduced and encouraged.

However, many clients new to physiotherapy and body awareness training may initially dislike or feel threatened by touch. In these situations it is in the interest of the client that the therapist invests time attempting to break down defensive barriers and help them become used to 'caring touch'. Only then can the client begin to appreciate how satisfying and effective touch as a form of communication is; by increasing a person's ability to communicate with others, you improve their chances of being able to manage stress.

Massage is one of the most basic 'hands-on' techniques one can use. There are many different types of 'therapeutic' massage, each of which places a different emphasis on different elements of the therapy.

Common techniques used by physiotherapists for massage are those developed by Swedish doctor Per Hendrick Ling in the nineteenth century. These affect the body, mechanically and physiologically, reducing 'psycho-physical' tension through the pleasurable manipulation of various tissues. This type of massage is easily taught and can also be used as a medium to increase communication between families and friends and as a sense of support. The techniques used, e.g. stroking, kneading, picking up, etc., transpose easily into self-help techniques.

Vagal innervation is another very helpful self-help technique which clients who suffer from acute panic attacks can use. Tachycardia is a trigger symptom of panic flare; increased vagal innervation lowers the heart rate, which can avert 'full-blown' attacks occurring. This technique consists of exerting pressure on the sternum with the hand, massaging gently, which stimulates the baroreceptors and lowers the heart rate. According to Sartory and Ocajide (1988), this technique is quicker at reducing the symptoms of panic attack than breath control exercises. It also engenders a greater measure of perceived control over panic.

There are other forms of massage which claim to be more intuitive and holistic in their approach than Swedish techniques. One such claim is made by 'biodynamic' massage, which was first developed by Boyesen, a psychologist in the 1920s. She used it with verbal psychotherapy to attain a deeper level of communication with her clients.

Biodynamic massage is not just 'body work'. Boyesen argues that the human body is composed of energies in a constant state of vibration. Heat, movement, thoughts and emotions are all different forms of energy vibration that can be worked for therapeutic purpose through massage.

Unique to this form of massage is the theory of 'psychoperistalsis'. Boyesen was of the opinion that the gastrointestinal system 'digested' not only food but also emotional experience. By massaging the abdomen, tension trapped within the intestines can be released. Digestive tract rumblings are a sign of release and are listened for through a stethoscope during treatment.

Other types of touch-related interventions which claim to have stress-relieving qualities include shiatsu, aromatherapy, reflexology, connective tissue manipulation, myofascial release and rolfing.

Exercise

Physical fitness appears to be not the only benefit of formal exercise. It contributes to psychological well-being by decreasing both clinical and non-clinical depression, reducing anxiety and buffering against the harmful effects of stress (Brannon and Feist, 1992).

The reasons for such psychological uplifts are unclear. One popular theory is that exercise releases increased levels of endorphins into the bloodstream. Endorphins are known to produce analgesia and euphoria, which elevates mood and may help counter the effects of stress. However, recent studies have cast some doubt over this hypothesis (McMurray *et al.*, 1984).

Another explanation for the stress-reducing effect of exercise is the enhanced feeling of self-esteem which often follows it. People who regularly exercise often have better feelings about their body shape and physical health. In this way perceived 'physical' well-being boosts psychological well-being.

Studies indicate that aerobic exercise offers the most health benefits, including decreasing symptoms of stress. However, research also suggests that long-term commitment to exercise is low, with a recidivism rate of approximately 70%.

It is clear from this that encouraging a client to maintain any exercise regimen is difficult, despite its benefits. An individual must be interested and motivated towards formal exercise if there is any hope of adherence. The physiotherapist should never force a programme upon a hesitant or resistive client.

Mahoney (1975) offers some useful guidelines that can be used to sustain compliance to an exercise programme. They are:

- self-monitoring – a diary system which records improvement
- goal-setting – which should be moderate, realistic and with target dates for review
- feedback – to discuss problems and progress
- development of a reward system – some tangible or intangible reward
- modelling – of appropriate behaviours from interaction with others who can observe, teach and encourage
- cognitive engineering – the client is encouraged to visualize the positive results of adhering to exercise programmes and the negative consequences of failure.

Martin and Dubbert (1982) suggest that self-set goals are more effective than external set goals. If possible, let the client set their own; only question what you feel to be unrealistic, unattainable goals.

All exercise should be enjoyable. The physiotherapist can optimize this by prudent guidance of the client towards activities which complement their personality, i.e. extreme type A individuals often exercise in the same way as they live life – as if they were responding to a challenge. They set overambitious aims and compete vigorously against themselves and others (Friedman and Rosenman, 1974). This can cause them as much stress as it is supposed to alleviate. In this case, the client should be encouraged to participate in less competitive activities, e.g. Tai Chi Chuan (Jin, 1992).

Exercise increases a person's perception of 'self' – the way one moves, balances, uses flexibility and strength to manipulate their surroundings and pass through it. It gives an individual the opportunity to interact and communicate with others and can also act as a distraction from stressors.

Dance movement therapy has elements of all these latter points. According to Stanton (1991) this approach uses movement as a 'medium through which one may gain contact with conscious and unconscious processes and emotions. It can also assist the client in gaining insight into how he/she builds and maintains relationships with others'.

Alleviating inpatient stress

Alleviating inpatient stress involves the physiotherapist taking a more holistic approach to the treatment of people admitted to hospital who may require physiotherapy. Upon entering hospital, individuals are bombarded by potential stressors. Not only do they have the burden of illness and/or injury, but subtle depersonalization takes place as the person becomes 'patient', is categorized by their complaint and placed on the ward. In most hospitals, but certainly where traditional 'Nightingale' bed rows still exist, personal privacy is eroded. Wards are noisy, and they expose people to 'ugly' sights and even death (Bentley *et al.*, 1977). Control over one's own body, routines and surroundings are lost (Taylor, 1979) as responsibility for welfare is handed to nursing and medical staff.

The 'patient' is made to fit in with established ward timetables and rules, isolated from the support of family and friends. Furthermore, physical examinations can be embarrassing and unpleasant. Research suggests that surgical procedure is the most stressful routine hospital event.

Contanch (1984) recommended a number of general changes that hospitals could make to improve health care. These include:

- offering health education
- encouraging self-responsibility
- offering treatment alternatives.

A few basic considerations by the physiotherapist can help a person cope much better with hospital admission and may help speed rehabilitation. These include:

1. If possible, written information should be sent to the individual prior to admission. This should outline entry procedures, e.g. what to bring and what

to expect from assessments and treatment during their stay. If physiotherapy is required, then this should be outlined also.
2. The physiotherapist should try to develop a therapeutic relationship with their clients. This does not have to be time consuming – a few extra minutes can make a difference. Most physiotherapists are time pressured, but should strive to strike a balance between quantity and quality. This can be done in a number of ways:
   (a) Listening to what the person has to say without allowing presumptions or judgemental thoughts to cloud one's mind.
   (b) Being aware of one's own body language – making sure you are not conveying the wrong signals. In general terms, the therapist's posture should be open, relaxed and confident but not aggressive. They should also respect the client's personal space.
   (c) Use of non-procedural touch, e.g. a handshake, pat on the back, etc. In a study done by Fisher (1989), 87% of inpatients questioned found non-procedural touch soothing and comforting.
3. The physiotherapist should respect the patient's privacy and wishes, allowing them to direct their own treatment as much as possible, e.g. times of your visit.
4. Information relating to physiotherapy must be communicated at a pace that suits the client. The therapist should also avoid confusing terminology. Two-way communication must be encouraged, so that misunderstandings and fears are recognized and can be allayed.
5. Treatment details may be shared with relatives, so they are encouraged to help decrease the client's stressors, e.g. bringing them books, letters, practising relaxation techniques, etc.
6. Simple palliative coping strategies can be taught, e.g. distraction, relaxation, etc., combined with repeated encouragement. If applicable, some group work may be possible where modelling can take place, e.g. learning by watching others perform. This can also create a sense of camaraderie, where people in similar positions become a support for one another.
7. Stress-reducing techniques may be administered on the ward, e.g. massage or reflexology, and taught to relatives as part of self-help techniques.

References

Belloc, N.B. and Breslow, L. (1972) Relationship of physical health status and health practices. *Preventative Medicine*, 1, 409–421

Bentley, S., Murphy, F. and Dudley, H.A.F. (1977) An objective analysis of the noise background to surgical care – S.R.S. Abstract. *British Journal of Surgery*, 64–822

Brannon, L. and Feist, J. (1992) *Health Psychology – An Introduction to behaviour and health*, 2nd edn, Wadsworth, Belmont

Brown, J.D. and McGill, K.L. (1989) The cost of good fortune. When positive life events produce negative health consequences. *Journal of Personality and Social Psychology*, 57, 1103–1110

Burnard, P. (1991) Coping with stress in the health professions – a practical guide. In *Therapy in Practice 21*. Chapman and Hall, London

Contanch, P.H. (1984) Health promotion in hospitals. In *Behavioural Health: A Handbook of Health Enhancement and Disease Prevention* (eds Matarazzo, J.D., Weiss, S.M., Herd, J.A., Miller, N.E. and Weis, S.M.), Wiley, New York

Cooper, C., Cooper, R.D. and Eaker, L.H. (1988) *Living With Stress*, Penguin, London

Crosier (1992) Back care – a brief introduction (unpublished)

Davies, M., Eshelman, E.R. and McKay, M. (1988) *The Relaxation and Stress Reduction Workbook*, 3rd edn, New Harbinger Publications, Oakland, California

Dohrenwend, B.P. (1979) Stressful life events and psychopathology: some issues of theory and method. In *Stress and Mental Disorders* (eds Barrett, J.E., Rose, R.M. and Klerman, G.L.), Raven Press, New York

Ebner, M. (1962) *Connective Tissue Massage: Theory and Therapeutic Application*, E. and S. Livingstone, London

Ellis, A. and Harper, R. (1961) *A Guide To Rational Living*, Wilshire Books, North Hollywood, California

Fisher, L.M. (1989) A scale to measure attitudes about non-procedural touch. *Canadian Journal of Nursing Research*, **21**(2), 5–14

Friedman, M. and Rosenman, R.H. (1974) *Type-A Behaviour and Your Heart*, Knopf, New York

Granville-Grossman, K. (1983) Mind and body. In *Handbook of Psychiatry 2: Mental Disorders and Somatic Illness* (ed. Lader, M.A.), Cambridge University Press, Cambridge

Hawton, K. and Kirk, J. (1989) Problem solving. In *Cognitive Behaviour Therapy For Psychiatric Problems: A Practical Guide* (eds Hawton, K., Salkowskis, P.M., Kirk, J. and Clark, D.M.), Oxford University Press, Oxford

Holmes, T.H. and Rahe, R.H. (1967) The social readjustment rating scale. *Journal of Psychosomatic Research*, **11**, 215–218

Ivancevich, J.M. and Matteson, M.T. (1988) Promoting the individual's health and wellbeing. In *Causes, Coping and Consequences of Stress at Work* (eds Cooper, C.L. and Payne, R.), Wiley

Jin, P. (1992) Efficacy of tai chi, brisk walking, meditation and reading in reducing mental and emotional stress. *Journal of Psychosomatic Research*, **36**(4), 361–370

Kanner, A.D., Coyne, J.C., Schaefer, C. and Lazarus, R.S. (1981) Comparison of two modes of stress measurement: daily hassles and uplifts versus major life events. *Journal of Behavioural Medicine*, 1–3

Kirk, J. (1989) Cognitive behavioural assessment. In *Cognitive Behaviour Therapy for Psychiatric Problems: A Practical Guide* (eds Hawton, K., Salkovskis, P.M., Kirk, J. and Clark, D.M.), Oxford University Press, Oxford

Kobasa, S.C. (1979) Stressful life events, personality and health. An inquiry into hardness. *Journal of Personality and Social Psychology*, **37**, 1–11

Lader, M.A. (1979) Emotions, physiology and stress. In *The Cardiovascular, Metabolic and Psychological Interface* (eds Elsdon-Dew, R.W., Wink, C.A.S. and Birdwood, G.B.F.), Academic Press, London

Lazarus, R.S. (1973) Multi-modal behaviour therapy, treating the B.A.S.I.C.I.D. *Journal of Nervous and Mental Disease*, **156**, 404–411

Lazarus, R.S. (1987) Multi-modal approach with adult out-patients. In *Psychotherapists in Clinical Practise* (ed. Jacobson, N.S.), Guildford Press, New York

Lazarus, R.S. and Folkman, S. (1984) *Stress, Appraisal and Coping*, Springer, New York

Looker, T. and Gregson, O. (1989) *Stresswise – A Practical Guide For Dealing With Stress*, Headway, Hodder and Stoughton, Sevenoaks

McMurray, R.G., Sheps, D.S. and Guinan, D.M. (1984) Effects of naloxone on maximum stress testing in females. *Journal of Applied Physiology*, **56**, 436–440

Mahoney, J.J. (1975) The behavioural treatment of obesity. In *Applying Behavioural Science to Cardiovascular Risk* (eds Englow, A.J. and Henderson, J.P.), American Heart Association, Dallas

Martin, J.E. and Dubbert, P.M. (1982) Exercise applications and promotion in behavioural medicine: current status and future directions. *Journal of Consulting and Clinical Psychology*, **50**, 1004–1007

Meichenbaum, D. (1985) *Stress Inoculation Training*, Pergamon Press, Oxford

Newnham, J. (1990) Not all in the mind (unpublished)

Palmer, S. (1993) Multi-modal assessment and therapy. *Stress News*, **4**(4), 8–13

Park, G. (1989) *The Art of Changing – A New Approach to the Alexander Technique*, Ashgrove Press, Bath

Peck, D.G. and Shapiro, C.M. (1990) *Measuring Human Problems – A Practical Guide*, John Wiley, Chichester

Quick, J.C. and Quick, J.D. (1984) *Organisational Stress and Preventative Management*, McGraw-Hill, New York

Rotter, J.B. (1966) Generalised expectancies for internal versus external control of reinforcement. *Psychological Monographs*, **80**, 609

Sartory, G. and Ojalide, D. (1988) Vagal innervation techniques in the treatment of panic disorder. *Journal of Behaviour Research Therapy*, **26**(5), 431–434

Skelly, M. (1993) The importance of attitudes, touch, posture, body use and body language (unpublished)

Stanton, K. (1991) Dance movement therapy: an introduction. *British Journal of Occupational Therapy*, **54**(3), 108–110

Taylor, S.E. (1979) Hospital patient behaviour: reactance, helplessness or control? *Journal Of Social Issues*, **35**(1), 156–184

Wells, K.F. (1971) *Kinesiology – The Scientific Basis Of Human Motion*, W.B. Saunders, London

Williams, R.B., Jr. (1989) *The Trusting Heart: Great News About Type-A Behaviour*, Times Books, New York

12

Relaxation training

Stephen T. Heptinstall

Introduction

Relaxation training is a very effective treatment intervention and one in which physiotherapists can play an important part.

What is relaxation and how can one teach it to another are at first glance daunting questions which threaten complicated, lengthy answers. Faced with mountains of paperwork dealing with the subject, many taking tentative steps into this area may quickly turn and run, overwhelmed by it all.

Next, one may ask why should physiotherapists involve themselves with relaxation training when other professionals, e.g. occupational therapists and psychologists, already count it as part of their work?

The aim of this chapter is to draw together concisely the main points of relaxation therapy, help the physiotherapist understand why it should be part of their repertoire of skills, and then not be discouraged in the pursuit of its acquisition.

What is relaxation?

A clear, concise definition of relaxation is difficult to find. Rosa (1976) describes the relaxed state as: 'Total physical immobility and relaxation of the skeletal muscle with a regulating effect on the sympathetic nervous system. This is accompanied by a feeling of diminished consciousness of the external world, drowsiness, passivity and focusing of attention on feelings of internal well-being.' This is a good attempt at description, although total immobility and relaxation of skeletal muscle only occurs after death.

He goes on to describe some of the cognitive changes reported to occur in relaxation as 'passive concentration' or focusing of attention and awareness of inner experience, where 'spontaneous mental activity is reduced, being replaced by observation of bodily and mental sensations'.

Wilson (1983) described relaxation as 'not so much the opposite of anxiety, but rather as its complementary state'. Keable (1985) also argues this important point, that relaxation is 'more than mere cessation of effort in a negative sense, rather it is a positive change and refinement of activity. Stoyva and Anderson (1982) describe it as a switch from an active mode of coping with stress to a rest mode of coping.

Table 12.1 Some comparisons between the stress response and the relaxation response

	Alarmed	*Relaxed*
Adrenaline/noradrenaline	More	Less
Cortisol	More	Less
Respiration rate	Faster	Slower
Heart rate	Faster	Slower
Blood pressure	Increased	Decreased
Blood flow to skeletal muscles	Increased	Decreased
Blood flow to external genitalia	Decreased	Increased
Muscle tone	Increased	Decreased
Muscle action potential	Increased	Decreased
Stomach acid	More	Less
Gastric motility	Slower	Faster
Blood cholesterol	More	Less
Blood glucose	More	Less

Relaxation is an important part of human function. Without it, one is imbalanced and open to injury. Research indicates that relaxation induces physiological effects opposite in nature to those induced by a stressed state. Specifically, that relaxation produces decreases in sympathetic nervous system activity and a corresponding increase in parasympathetic activity. The combined and intergrated actions of the autonomic nervous system, the endocrine system and the brain cortex result in a generalized 'trophotropic' or relaxation response. Table 12.1 lists some of the general effects.

Teaching someone to 'relax' who has forgotten how to do so, helps decrease the physical effects of tension, gives the client back some controllability of body and mind, and helps reduce maladaptive coping behaviour, e.g. alcohol abuse. It may not resolve their stress directly, but can help them to cope in positive manner.

Why physiotherapy in relaxation training?

All this still leaves us with the question: why do physiotherapists need to be involved in relaxation therapy and training?

As we have already outlined, relaxation has many physical effects. As physiotherapists we are well qualified to evaluate these. Our observation and tactile skills, combined with carefully nurtured physiotherapy intuition, also make us well placed to administer such a treatment intervention, being able to recognize when it is appropriate and its effect.

In an aroused, anxious state a person holds their muscles tense, contracting everything in order to cope better with a sense of insecurity or fear. As physiotherapists, we will recognize this in their closed posture and feel it in their tight muscles.

A nervous person hangs onto their breath, breathing in but not letting go, holding onto it as they hold onto all their movements keeping them within a restricted range. Again the physiotherapist will see the limitations and lack of fluency in the way this person moves.

Relaxation training with other interventions, e.g. body awareness techniques, can help open up the posture with a release of tension and increase fluency of movement. It can bring about better breathing, feeeing the voice and expression.

Having stress management skills (of which relaxation therapy is one) allows the physiotherapist to become more holistic in their approach to clients – not working solely on an impaired malfunctioning body system, but rather on the whole person, with the aim of mobilizing the body's own healing powers to restore it to a state of equilibrium.

The cause or effect of injury and illness should always be seen as having three components, which are physical, psychological and behavioural. All three should be taken into consideration when planning treatment and should be dealt with to a greater or lesser degree on its application. This is a more 'holistic approach', treating the person as a whole and in a balanced way, rather than for a single problem.

These three components of injury and illness also act as a doorway through which treatment can be introduced. By taking the 'physical' route, a physiotherapist often does not meet the same stigma attached to psychological or behavioural approaches made by a psychologist or psychiatrist. However, the physiotherapist can apply treatment which overlaps these sensitive areas, e.g. relaxation training, helping to bring about improvement where otherwise there may have been resistance.

Relaxation training

Relaxation training is never taught solely or in an isolated fashion, but it is incorporated into a wider regimen of intervention. Although the order in which stress management coping strategies are taught varies, many therapists begin with relaxation training. It is seen as one of the simplest and easiest to use of all interventions (Blanchard and Andrasik, 1985), is readily learned by most clients and has a good deal of face validity, i.e. belief by the client about its possibility for success (Meichenbaum, 1985).

Many people gain relaxation just through planning and being part of enjoyable, distracting activities away from a busy routine. Highlighting this may be the only input a trainer needs to do, pointing out possible comfort zones (places where one feels relaxed) and comfort rituals (relaxing activities like walking the dog). However, others will need more formal training in relaxation techniques, being unable to switch to a rest mode alone.

There are many types of relaxation techniques taught and programmes that they follow. Techniques can be divided into two groups: those which focus upon physical relaxation, e.g. Jacobson or Mitchell methods; stretching techniques and those which hope to produce mental quieting, e.g.. guided imagery, visualization, autogenic training and meditative techniques.

Burnard (1991) outlines some of the uses of relaxation training, which are to:

- decrease anxiety
- assist in stress management
- promote sleep
- reduce pain or the perception of pain
- alleviate muscle tension

- warm or cool parts of the body
- decrease blood pressure
- slow the heart beat
- combat fatigue
- reduce or prevent the physiological and psychological effects of stress
- serve as a coping device or skill
- enhance the effectiveness of pain relief measures.

Burns (1981) has also listed a number of advantages of relaxation training:

1. Stress-related problems such as hypertension, tension headaches, insomnia, etc., may be eliminated or ameliorated.
2. Overall improvement in performance of vocational, social and physical skills may occur as a result of reduced tension levels.
3. Relaxation can be an aid to recovery after certain illnesses and surgery.
4. An important psychological consequence of relaxation is that the individual's level of self-esteem and self-assuredness is likely to be increased as a result of much improved control of stress reactions.
5. Interpersonal relationships may expect to improve. During high levels of tension, cognitive distortions resulting in the adoption of untenable positions are more likely to arise. The relaxed person in difficult interpersonal situations will think more rationally. Also, a relaxed person, through modelling processes, may have a notable calming effect on an emotionally upset person.

There is a wide body of research which supports the benefits of relaxation training. It has been found to be an effective part of treatment in a number of clinical areas; for example:

- diabetic control (Lammers *et al.*, 1984)
- treatment of asthma (Millis and Schonell, 1981)
- alcohol abuse (Ritson, 1992)
- sexual problems (Glantz and Himber, 1992)
- pain (Miller and Kraus, 1990
- cardiac rehabilitation (Tomes, 1990)
- insomnia (Nicassio and Buchanan, 1981)
- substance abuse (Dodge, 1991)
- hypertension (Patel and Marmot, 1988)
- tinnitus (Kirsh *et al.*, 1987)
- anxiety (Eppley *et al.*, 1989)
- panic attack (Beitman *et al.*, 1987)
- migraine and headaches (Prima *et al.*, 1979)
- Raynaud's disease (Surwit, 1981)
- irritable bowel syndrome (Blanchard *et al.*, 1987).

Although relaxation programmes differ, Stoyva and Anderson (1982) have recognized many common features, including:

- usually some emphasis on muscular relaxation
- regular and frequent practice
- the individual being encouraged to use relaxation in everyday stressful situations

- the client being given some cognitive procedure for producing mental quieting
- they all emphasize 'passive attention', seen as being the opposite of a striving or effort response.

Some attention to breathing and/or breath control also forms part of most techniques and treatment regimens.

Most people are suitable for relaxation training, but there are some exceptions, according to various sources. Bird and Wilson (1982) argue there are a number of mental illnesses that do not respond well to relaxation training. These include depression, psychosis, recurrent headaches and people on tranquillizers. Clark (1989) talks of relaxation-induced anxiety in clients with fear of loss of control, who find aversive the feeling of 'letting go' which accompanies relaxation. He also highlights how relaxation techniques which focus upon the body can lead panic patients to notice sensations they misinterpret and perpetuate their symptoms further with.

However, much of this would seem extreme by therapists such as Ricketts and Cross (1985) who believe everyone can benefit from a basic knowledge of relaxation and training. Certainly the boundaries are not clear and it would seem that the safest way to measure whether relaxation training will be of benefit is to make an individual assessment of every client.

Breath control

For centuries, breathing exercises have been an integral part of mental, physical and spiritual development in Far Eastern countries. In relative terms, it is only recently that the West has recognized the importance of proper breath control.

Most relaxation techniques pay some attention to breathing as a focus to produce mental quieting and/or as a technique to produce physiological calming. Assessment of the client's breathing, followed by teaching of an awareness exercise (see below) with modification if indicated, is usually done prior to administering a specific relaxation technique. A client is usually asked to monitor their breathing periodically during most techniques, maintaining a steady, calm, controlled rate.

When problems are identified by the therapist and client working in co-operation, some modification procedures are often thought to help gain better control. Wallace recommends that clients visualize a square or rectangle. Each side has a time value allocated to it and the client works around the four sides, paying attention to the instructions and time values given, as in Figure 12.1. According to Burnard (1991), this type of exercise prevents a tendency towards overbreathing, regulates the pace of breathing and distracts the mind from other thoughts.

Another 'convenient' way of teaching clients controlled breathing is to use 'pacing tapes' (Clark *et al.*, 1985). The pacing on these tapes consists of a voice say 'In' for two or three seconds and then 'Out' for the same time period. By prolonging the words, gentle and extended inspirations and expirations are achieved. This limits clients taking sharp gasps characteristic of hyperventilation syndrome during instruction. The client uses the pacing tape until confident that they can maintain the set pace independently.

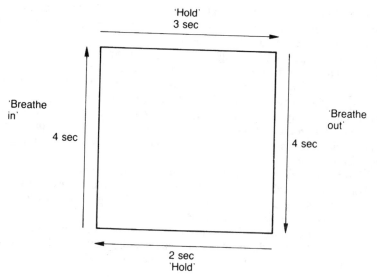

Figure 12.1. Wallace's breathing square

An example of a breathing awareness exercise

1. Lie down on your back, with spine straight, knees slightly bent and feet flat on the floor.
2. Focus upon your breathing. Help yourself to do this by placing your hands on the chest. Notice the movement which takes place there, its rate and rhythm. Is it hurried and shallow, or steady and deep?
3. Move one hand down over the abdomen. Again, notice the movement which takes place there. Does your abdomen move in harmony with your chest as it should?
4. Notice whether there are any areas of tension around your throat, chest or abdomen. Does your clothing restrict your breathing in any way?
5. Now, attempt to focus upon your heart beat in the middle of your chest. Is it affected by your breathing in any way – its speed or intensity?
6. Lift up one arm so it points towards the ceiling. Notice whether your breathing changes during this movement, or as a result of this new position. Repeat this exercise, lifting one foot approximately 1 cm from the floor.
7. Using these exercises, you can learn to appreciate how you breathe and what factors affect it. This is important when using breath control to aid relaxation.

Specific relaxation techniques

Beech *et al.* (1982) outline some important points to consider when teaching relaxation techniques:

1. Relaxation is essentially a self-control method. Evidence suggests that substantial improvement only occurs if the client realizes that relaxation is a

coping skill to be practised and applied to daily life. In addition to the increased feeling of control which is gained, the client also develops some self-responsibility for actions and health.

2. Paradoxically, perhaps, although relaxation is an active process, individuals gains control over themselves by 'letting go' – a passive attention.
3. If it is accepted that learning to relax involves learning a skill, like learning a new sport, then it follows that disciplined, regular practice is essential.
4. Relaxation is only one method among many which is used to help control tension. Thus relaxation may be seen as part of a therapeutic programme, rather than existing alone, used alongside cognitive restructuring, desensitization, etc.
5. Due to the lowering of tension levels and slowing of body processes, there is sometimes a tendency to drift to sleep. This should be resisted unless a technique is being used to overcome insomnia. The goal of most training is to be deeply relaxed while remaining wide awake.
6. In everyday life, most tension builds up by an insidious process over a period of time, and the individual may not recognize this build up of tension as a result. Relaxation training should increase the client's self-awareness of body tension.

Progressive muscular relaxation techniques

Edmund Jacobsen, who was a Chicago physician, is seen as a pioneer of progressive muscle relaxation, publicizing this type of training over 50 years ago (Jacobsen, 1938). He asserted that his form of muscle relaxation requires no imagination, will-power or suggestion, which makes it an easy technique to learn. He based his work on the premise that the body responds to anxiety-provoking thoughts and events with muscle tension. This in turn increases an individual's subjective experience of anxiety and a vicious cycle develops. He argues that progressive muscle relaxation reduces both physiological and psychological tension as a consequence.

This technique provides a way of identifying particular muscle groups which are tight due to stress and distinguishing between feelings of tension and relaxation. This is done by teaching the client systematically to contract and relax groups of muscles, and pay attention to the sensations that this action evokes, see Script 1, below.

Classically, Jacobsen's subjects were trained to relax 44 different muscles in turn, taking up to an hour to practice each one. Fortunately, shorter versions of this technique have been developed since, by such influential figures as Joseph Wolpe, who used tense–relax techniques as the introductory part for his successful phobia desensitization programme.

Research has shown progressive muscle relaxation to be effective in the treatment of a number of stress-related conditions. These include bruxism (teeth grinding), where special attention is paid to the relaxation of the masseter muscle; essential hypertension; gastrointestinal disorders; headaches and phobias.

Another type of progressive muscular relaxation is that developed by Laura Mitchell in the 1950s. This method differs from that of Jacobsen's in so far as it involves contracting muscles acting as antagonists to muscles held tense by stress. Mitchell (1977) argues that this action brings about reciprocal inhibition and therefore decreases tension in tight muscle groups.

Mitchell's method also uses changes in resting postures to bring more neutrality and balance to the muscles (see Script 2 below). Scarrot (1993) argues that this technique is easier to apply and is less obtrusive than the Jacobsen method.

Another conceptually sound alternative to Jacobsonian 'tense–relax' exercises is muscle stretching (Carlson *et al.*, 1987). They point to evidence which suggests that tensing muscles may actually inhibit relaxation of the skeletal musculature, especially in those with chronic muscle tension.

Valbo (1973) argues that this form of exercise stimulates motor neurons which elevates muscle tension. Rather, muscle stretching should be incorporated into a programme aimed at increased relaxation of the body.

Carlson *et al.* (1990) highlight the benefits of muscle stretching:

- More length receptors in the muscle fibres are activated while stretching muscles rather than tensing them. Stretching therefore has a stronger contrast effect than tightening muscles, helping to foster client learning to discriminate tense muscle groups.
- Muscle stretching produces muscle relaxation as long as the action is slow and does not cause microscopic tearing of the connective tissue.
- Muscle stretching is also said to reduce excitability of the motor neurone pool which may lead to decreased levels of muscle tone, ischaemia and pain.

According to Anderson (1983), muscular relaxation training based on stretching incorporates the beneficial effects of muscle sensation contrasts typically associated with muscle-tensing exercises, with reduction in muscle activity from the stretching procedure itself.

Carlson *et al.* (1987) argue that muscle stretching is more effective at lowering both subjective and objective states of arousal than 'tense–relax' techniques.

Differential relaxation training

This technique was developed by Jacobsen (1964) as his 'self-operations control' methodology. It involves applying the concepts of his 'tense–relax' techniques to everyday activities. The client learns to recognize and relax non-essential muscles during activities and to reduce the tension level in the working muscle to a necesssary level only.

Training may progress in stages, from sitting activities in a quiet environment to standing and walking in noisy surroundings.

The theoretical basis involves that of straightforward muscle relaxation training taken further to include learning to distinguish between 'primary tensions' (those needed to perform an act) and 'secondary tensions' (which are superfluous to the task). The client observes this distinction in daily tasks and learns to reduce secondary tensions, thus achieving 'self-operations control'.

Mitchell (1977) also describes a similar development in her 'simple relaxation technique'.

Relaxation 'in action' is also the basis of the Alexander technique, which describes the 'use' and misuse of the body while performing an action or posture. Accordingly, misuse is acquired through inappropriate learning of excess tension habits which lead to inco-ordination between the mind and the body.

Script 1: A Jacobsonian self-help technique

You should get into a comfortable position, e..g. lying or sitting reclined. The technique should preferably be done with the eyes closed.

Whole muscle groups will be contracted; these should be held for approximately 10 seconds and then released for 15 seconds. This is repeated three times before moving to the next muscle group. You should attempt to discriminate between feelings of tension and release throughout. During untensing, try to think relaxing expressions to accompany this action, e...g...

- 'My tension is evaporating/draining/dissolving away.'
- 'My muscles are untying and becoming longer – they are relaxing.'
- 'My body is becoming more calm and rested.'

Step 1. Get in a comfortable position with eyes closed. Free from interruption.

Step 2. Scan your body and notice where any areas of tension lie. Take some time to appreciate how that tension feels, e..g. aching, tightness, pain.

Step 3. Notice your breathing – how it feels to breathe in and out. Use your hands on your chest to appreciate how your ribs move. If your breathing is fast/hesitant and/or shallow, attempt to slow it down by taking slightly deeper, more rhythmic breaths, allowing the air further into the lungs. Again, feel the difference this modification makes and now notice whether your heart rate slows at all because of it. Most importantly of all, your breathing should feel comfortable.

Step 4. Clench both hands tight.

Step 5. Hunch both shoulders as high as possible.

Step 6. Return to your breathing for approximately 1 minute.

Step 7. Push your head back into its support. Be careful here not to exert too much force that might cause injury to your neck.

Step 8. Screw your eyes up tight.

Step 9. Clench your jaw. Again, make sure you do not exert too much force that could damage your teeth. You may also find it uncomfortable to hold longer than 4 seconds.

Step 10. Return to your breathing for approximately 1 minute.

Step 11. Concentrate on any other areas in which you noticed tension during step 2. Tighten and release these areas as directed.

Step 12. Return to your breathing for approximately 1 minute.

Step 13. Scan your body again and decide whether the overall tension is any less.

Step 14. Ending – move fingers first, then roll shoulders, roll head from side to side, deep breathe in–out, open eyes and stretch slowly.

Practice this technique daily. It should take approximately 20 minutes to begin with. As you become familiar with the technique and find it more effective, you can shorten the time of its application. This can be done by reducing the number of repetitions or just focusing upon the areas which feel tense to you.

Script 2: A short stretch relaxation technique

Step 1. Push up your eyebrows with your fingers and at the same time push down both cheeks with your thumbs, slowly. Hold for 10 seconds and notice the feeling of stretch, then release quickly. Notice now the feeling of letting go and of the muscles relaxing – wait approximately 30 seconds.

Step 2. Let your head sag over to your left shoulder slowly. Hold for 10 seconds and notice the tension on the right side of your neck. Return your head back up to the neutral position quickly and enjoy the release which accompanies it on the right. Wait 30 seconds. Repeat this sequence with the head on the right side.

Step 3. Interlock your fingers and raise your hands above your head, straightening the elbows and rotating the palms outwards. Let your arms fall back over the head until resistance is felt at the shoulders – hold for 10 seconds – notice the tightness under the shoulders and across the chest. Release quickly, returning your arms to your side. Notice the release of tension in the tight muscles. Wait 30 seconds.

Step 4. Slowly side-bend over to your left, tracing your left hand down the outside of your left thigh. Take it as far as is comfortable and then hold this position for 10 seconds. Realize the tightness on the right side of your middle. Straighten back up quickly and feel the tension disappear from this area. Wait 30 seconds and then repeat the movement over to the right side.

Step 5. Place your hands together at chest height, palms touching. Keeping your palms together, slowly move your hands downwards along your body until you feel resistance to further movement. Notice where the muscles are tense and hold for 10 seconds. Quickly release, and appreciate the change of sensation which accompanies it in the lower arms and wrist.

Step 6. Focus your attention on all the muscle groups stretched, one after the other for 30 seconds. Evaluate in your mind whether tension has been decreased in any or all of them. Repeat any of the exercises once again if tension remains.

Script 3: The Mitchell method of relaxation

ARMS

Shoulders

Order: Pull your shoulders towards your feet. *Stop!*

Result: Feel that your shoulders are further away from your ears. Your neck may feel longer.

Elbows

Order: Elbows out and open. *Stop!*

Result: Feel your upper arms away from your body and the wide angle at your elbows. The weight of both arms should be resting on floor, chair arms, or pillow.

Hands

Order: Fingers and thumbs long and supported. *Stop!*

Result: Feel your fingers and thumbs stretched out, separated, and touching support, nails on top. Especially feel your heavy thumbs.

LEGS
Hips
Order: Turn your hips outwards. *Stop*!
Result: Feel your thighs rolled outwards. Kneecaps face outwards.

Knees
Order: Move slightly until comfortable if you wish. *Stop*!
Result: Feel the resulting comfort in your knees.

Feet
Order: Push your feet away from your face, bending at the ankle. *Stop*!
Result: Feel your dangling heavy feet.

BODY
Order: Push your body into the support. *Stop*!
Result: Feel the contact of your body on the support.

HEAD
Order: Push your head into the support. *Stop*!
Result: Feel the contact of your head on the support of pressure on the pillow.

BREATHING
Choose your own rate, but try to keep it slow. Breathe in gently. Expand the area in front above the waist, and between the angles of the rib cage, and raise your lower ribs upwards and outwards like the wings of a bird. Then breathe out gently. Feel your ribs fall downwards and inwards. Repeat once or at most twice.

FACE
Jaw
Order: Drag your jaw downwards. *Stop*!
Result: Feel your separated teeth, heavy jaw, and soft lips gently touching each other.

Tongue
Order: Press your tongue downwards in your mouth.*Stop*!
Result: Feel your loose tongue and slack gullet.

Eyes
Order: Close your eyes. *Stop*!
Result: Feel your upper lids resting gently over your eyes, without any screwing up around the eyes. Enjoy the darkness.

Forehead
Order: Begin above eyebrows and think of smoothing gently up into your hair, over the top of your head and down the back of your neck. *Stop*!
Result: Feel your hair move in the same direction.

Mind
Order: Repeat the above sequence around the body, possibly more quickly.
RETURN TO FULL ACTIVITY
Always stretch limbs and body in all directions and yawn. Do not hurry. Sit up slowly and wait for a minute or two before standing up.

'Hands-on' techniques

The Jacobsen, Mitchell and stretching techniques all have scientifically based research which supports their effectiveness, despite their own disagreements. Although these physiologically based techniques rely on verbal command and demonstration as a means of instruction, this should not discourage a 'hands-on' approach to help the client gain relaxation. For those clients who are not uncomfortable being touched (something the physiotherapist should assess carefully before attempting to handle anyone) there are a number of techniques which may prove beneficial:

1. The physiotherapist can invite the client to see and palpate a muscle in contraction and at rest for themselves, so helping the client recognize and appreciate how/what a tight muscle looks/feels like. They can then be encouraged to explore their own bodies, searching out areas where tension exists in muscle groups with their hands.
2. During contraction of muscles using a Jacobsen technique, the physiotherapist can offer resistance to those muscles, increasing the client's awareness of tension.
3. Passively moving the client's limbs can help them more accurately assess what level of muscular relaxation they have gained – the less their resistance to the physiotherapist's handling, the more physically relaxed they are said to be. This is also a simple, but useful, evaluation technique for the therapist to use.
4. Passive stretches performed by the physiotherapist on the client can also prove beneficial. This technique is particularly useful for releasing tension in muscle groups which are difficult to stretch independently.
5. Auto-assisted active movements done with the therapist, and/or sling support, using such techniques as proprioceptive neuromuscular fascilitation (PNF), not only helps reco-ordinate and balance movements, but brings fluency to muscle group action that might be compromised because of tension. This can help release muscle tightness and again initiate physical relaxation.
6. Massage is an effective way of releasing muscle tension and also helps the client recognize where tightness exists in their body. This is discussed further in Chapter 11.

All these techniques can help heighten a client's awareness of their state of physical arousal and promote some self-control in its reduction.

Cognitive techniques

Guided imagery, visualization and enhanced relaxation
Coue insisted that the power of the imagination far exceeds that of the will. He asserts that it is hard to will yourself into a relaxed state, but you can imagine your body becoming relaxed. He also argues that 'we are what we think we are', and therefore a person who has anxious thoughts will become physically tense.

Both guided imagery and visualization are techniques that incorporate the use of mental images to promote psychological and physical relaxation.

With guided imagery, clients are encouraged to conjure up mental pictures which will act as a distraction from their source of stress. The assumption here is that an individual cannot concentrate on more than one thing at a time. The images used are usually of a calming, peaceful nature, e.g. a walk on a deserted beach, sitting on a hill in the countryside. However, more powerful scenes are sometimes used to divert attention away from a particularly painful stressor.

Another variation is to ask the client to concentrate on real-life situations. Patients draw upon past experiences that have contributed to feelings of pride, self-assertion or self-esteem. In this way they gain confidence in dealing with present stressors, e.g. preoperative anxiety. This technique is known as 'in-vivo' imagery (Horan, 1973). In many ways it resembles the reminiscence therapy used with the elderly.

'Visualization' is yet another variation on an imagery theme. It differs from guided imagery in so far as the client is encouraged to imagine actions and/or scenes they would like to occur in 'the future', e.g. that they do not get tense at work, that they will win at squash, that they will survive cancer. The client repeats the desired image over and over again in their mind, increasing their confidence with every thought and will to be successful. According to Davies *et al.* (1988), this also acts as a way of bridging the conscious and unconscious mind, allowing the latter to make the wish come true.

This technique has proved popular with cancer patients, agoraphobics and athletes wishing to improve their performance.

The power of visual imagery, however, varies widely between individuals. Some clients are unable clearly to visualize themselves in a relaxing or successful scene despite repeated practice. To help the subject imagine the scene more clearly, the therapist may also be tempted to paint in the details too closely, causing anxiety in the client if it does not correspond with their own imaging. In an attempt to minimize these problems, King (1983) added several sense modalities to imagery techniques, which he called enhanced relaxation. These include:

- *Stereophonic sound effects.* The client listens to the whole relaxation programme on an audio tape. Headphones are used to obtain full stereophonic quality and to block off extraneous noise. The first half of the tape is instruction in progressive muscular relaxation, with low-level background music. The second is then guided imagery where a pleasant scene is introduced, accompanied by appropriate sound effects, e.g. in the case of a seaside scene, the sound of the waves breaking on the shore, seabirds calling, etc. The narrative is kept to a minimum to allow the client to fill in details from their own experiences.
- *Use of heat and light.* Gentle warmth, conducive to relaxation, is provided by an infrared lamp.
- *Use of fragrance.* King asserts that odour contributes most powerfully to the overall experience and effectiveness of this particular technique. Again, using a seaside scene, a smelling strip is dipped into Indian ink and intermittently held under the client's nose. Alternatively it is put in front of a fan directed towards them. According to King, the latter is a good mimic of a sea breeze. One of the advantages of using fragrances is that over time it can be used as a cue-controlling medium to promote immediate relaxation responses. Just smelling the chosen odour can begin to have a calming effect on an individual.

Autogenic training

Autogenic training (see Script 4, below) was developed in the early part of this century by the German hypnotherapists Vogt and Schultz (Massey, 1990). Born out of traditional hypnosis procedures, this technique utilizes their recuperative effects without the need of a hypnotist.

Autogenic training recreates the psychophysical effects of a hypnotic state by concentrating the client's mind upon trigger phrases or formulae, which are repeated over and over again. Through suggestions, these phrases help diminish the client's consciousness of the external environment and focus instead upon inner physical and emotional awareness. This is said to calm thought processes, reverse physiological effects of arousal and increase a client's confidence, esteem and control.

Shultz divided autogenic training into three categories of exercises:

- standard exercises, which concentrate upon the body, encouraging physical wellbeing, e.g. 'My heart beat is strong and regular'.
- meditative exercises, which focus upon the mind and thought processes, e.g. 'I am calm and free of worry'.
- special exercises, designed to normalize specific problems, such as phobia and panic attacks, e.g. 'I can get on the bus'.

Script 4: An autogenic standard exercise technique

Position, sitting; 3 times daily.

EXERCISES

Formulae/phrase	Repetition	Time span
I am completely calm	Once	1st and 2nd Week
My right arm is heavy	Six times	
I am completely calm	Once	
My left arm is heavy	Six times	
I am completely calm	Once	
My right arm is warm	Six times	
I am completely calm	Once	
My left arm is warm	Six times	
I am completely calm	Once	
My right arm is heavy and warm	Six times	
I am completely calm	Once	
My left arm is heavy and warm	Six times	
I am completely calm	Once	
My heart beats calmly and strongly (or regularly)	Six times	3rd and 4th Week
I am completely calm	Once	
My breathing is calm and regular	Six times	
I am completely calm	Once	
My abdomen is flowing and warm	Six times	5th and 6th Week
I am completely calm	Once	
My forehead is pleasantly cool	Six times	
I am completely calm	Once	

Ending with every session: arms firm – breathe deeply – open eyes.

Meditative relaxation

Meditative relaxation was developed by Herbert Benson and colleagues in America during the 1970s, becoming very popular in the USA over the past decade. It derives from various religious meditative practices, although it has no religious connotations itself.

Meditation involves a conscious effort to focus attention on a single thought or image, along with an effort not to be distracted by other thoughts away from it. Bensonian relaxation combines this with muscular relaxation in a 'no-nonsense' approach (see Script 5, below). He neither tries to mystify the process nor insist that the client must relax. He argues that it is impossible to implore a person to do so and it therefore should not be attempted (Burnard, 1991).

Using this technique, participants have reported feelings quite similar to those generated by other meditative practices – peace of mind, a feeling of being at peace with the world, and a sense of well-being (Atkinson *et al.*, 1983).

Script 5: Bensonian relaxation

Step 1. Sit quietly in a comfortable position and close your eyes.

Step 2. Deeply relax all your muscles, beginning at your feet and progressing to your face. Keep them deeply relaxed.

Step 3. Breathe through your nose. Become aware of your breathing. As you breathe out, say the word 'one' silently to yourself. Continue for 20 minutes. You may open your eyes to check the time, but do not use an alarm.

Step 4. When you finish, sit quietly for several minutes, at first with eyes closed and later with eyes opened.

Step 5. Do not worry if you do not achieve a deep level of relaxation. Maintain a passive attitude and permit relaxation to occur at its own pace. Expect other thoughts. When these distracting thoughts occur, ignore them by thinking 'oh well' and continue repeating 'one'. With practice, the response will come much quicker with less effort.

Step 6. Practice the technique once or twice daily, but not within 2 hours after any meal.

Progressive and applied relaxation regimens

Many therapists use the relaxation techniques outlined in the framework of wider progressive regimens. These aim to decrease the time span necessary to gain relaxation and make the techniques more practical in everyday situations.

One such regimen, supported by research as to its effectiveness, is the applied relaxation (AR) regimen (Ost, 1987). The application of this regimen is as follows – the full programme runs 10–12 sessions over a duration of 10–12 weeks:

Session 1–rationale
The rationale of treatment is explained, which is to:

- teach the patient to recognize early signals of anxiety
- learn to cope with anxiety.

Homework assignments are then given to self-observe and record any reactions tabulated as follows:

Date	Situation	Reaction – focus on early signals	Intensity (0–100)	What action did you take?

Session 2 – progressive muscular relaxation
A Jacobsonian technique is taught lasting 15–20 minutes. The client is asked to practice twice daily in a place they find comfortable and relatively free of interruption.

Sessions 3–4 – release-only relaxation
The therapist deletes instructions concerning the contracting of muscle groups. Instead the patient is instructed in 'release-only' techniques of 5–7 minutes' instruction.

Sessions 5–6 – cue-controlled relaxation
The patient is taught a 'cue-controlled' relaxation technique over a 2-minute time span. The purpose of cue-controlled relaxation is to create a conditioning between the self-instruction 'relax' and the state of being relaxed. Here the focus is upon breathing.

The client first relaxes using release-only and signals to the therapist when relaxed. The therapist then directs the pattern of breathing with instructions; just before inhalation the therapist says 'inhale' and just before exhalation the therapist says 'exhale'. This is repeated a number of times and then the client is encouraged to keep the sequence going silently. The aim is eventually to be able to bring about a state of relaxation by focusing upon breathing only, and therefore, speed up this process.

Sessions 6–8 – differential relaxation
In order for autogenic relaxation to be an efficient coping skill, the patient should be able to use it practically in any situation and not be confined to a comfortable chair or 20 minutes of their time. This is why at this stage differential relaxation is taught, usually of 60–90 seconds' duration. The primary purpose of this technique is to teach the client to be able to relax in situations other than in an armchair. The second purpose is to teach them not to tense muscles that are not being used for the particular body activity they are engaged in at that moment.

First the client is asked to relax using cue-controlled relaxation in an armchair. They are asked to move various body parts while maintaining this relaxed state. This is progressed to various starting positions, including standing and eventually walking.

Sessions 8–10 – rapid relaxation
'Rapid relaxation' is now taught. The aim is to reduce further the time it takes to relax to between 20–30 seconds. Also, to give clients extensive practice in relaxing in natural, non-stressful situations.

The therapist and client identify a series of cues which can help remind the client to relax, e.g. looking at one's watch, making a telephone call. The client should aim to relax 15–20 times daily following this routine:

- take 1–3 deep breaths, slowly exhaling after each breath
- think 'relax' before each exhalation

- scan the body for tension and try to mentally unwind any which exists.

Sessions 10–12 – application training
Here the client is introduced to 'application training'. This involves exposing the client briefly to an array of anxiety-arousing situations. The purpose of this phase is to build the client's confidence that they can cope with the anxiety experienced and eventually abort it altogether.

Maintenance programme
For AR to be effective, it is important to keep practising the techniques after the end of the treatment sessions in order not to 'forget the skill' or become 'rusty'. The client is encouraged to develop a habit of scanning the body at least once a day and use rapid relaxation if any tension exists. He/she should also practice differential or rapid relaxation twice a week.

Other physiotherapy-based regimens which have enjoyed attention include the Whitchurch method of relaxation (Ricketts and Cross, 1985) and multi convergent technique (MCT) (Sadlier and Heptinstall, 1991).

All these regimens are used alongside other coping strategies or stress management interventions, e.g. coping skills training or counselling.

Use of voice

There is no definitive way in which one should use their voice during relaxation training, apart from to communicate information. Some argue that the voice can be a very effective tool in helping to evoke a state of decreased arousal. If it is soft and quiet, with words spoken slowly in low tones, it is argued this will help calm a client and induce a relaxation response.

Similarly, if the content of a techniques narrative is detailed with many adjectives describing release of tension, increasing sense of relaxation, etc., then this too is reasoned to be supportive of effect, and therefore should be used.

However, others such as Mitchell feel that therapists should not attempt to exert their influence upon the effectiveness of a technique. Rather the action of that technique alone should reduce tension levels. This lessens the chance of clients becoming therapist dependent for relaxation.

Cue-controlled techniques, such as meditation and autogenic training, use directive narratives which are kept to a minimum and said only by the client. In the former, repeated pairings of a sub-vocalized word such as 'calm' or 'relax' is used simultaneously with expiration. This word becomes synonymous with relaxation over time. Eventually only that one word is needed to control anxiety by producing an opposite response. With autogenics, whole phrases are used, but again these are kept to a minimum.

One way around this dilemma is to help the client initiate relaxation responses at the early stage of therapy by using the voice, but steadily withdraw this support as they progress. This is, of course, somewhat dependent upon which techniques you are attempting to teach, and also the client's initial presentation and needs.

Use of audio tapes

As with any coping skill, the emphasis of relaxation training should be on self-mastery of techniques and independent, effective use. At the early stages of intervention, a recording of the relaxation techniques can be given, which the client takes home and which may be useful in aiding self-sufficiency.

However, the author advises care that the use of a tape is not excessive and continues to the end of therapy. If possible, the client should be encouraged not to use it very often once they have learnt the technique, as this lessens the possibility of dependency for relaxation upon the tape.

Occasional use is permitted, or even the making of their own relaxation tape by putting other techniques, music, etc., on it. The passivity of being told what to do can be a healthy alternative and, as mentioned earlier, music, sound effects, etc., can actually enhance the effectiveness of self-help techniques. Many advertisers now postulate on the effectiveness of subliminal tapes to aid relaxation. However, the client's focus should remain on self-application for the most part.

Measurement techniques

Many methods and implementation have been employed in an attempt to gain some objective measure of the effectiveness of relaxation training. One of the most popular and revolutionary contributors to this is biofeedback.

In biofeedback, biological responses are measured by instruments which can display the status of those responses immediately to the person being tested. This is most commonly done by auditory, tactile or visual signals. In this way a person is able to monitor any changes in these responses and/or attempt to alter them if required, using the information supplied as a gauge.

Although first clinically used in the 1950s by Jacobsen, biofeedback machines only really appeared on the market in the early 1970s, measuring brainwaves, gastric motility and skin conductance, as well as many other physiological processes.

The two most common types of biofeedback used in relaxation training are electromyographical (EMG) and temperature biofeedback. EMG is the most popular type of biofeedbvack in clinical use. It shows the activity of skeletal muscle by measuring the electrical discharges in muscle fibres. The level of activity reflects the degree of tension of the muscles. The measurement is taken by attaching electrodes to the surface of the skin over the muscles to be monitored. The electrodes can be placed anywhere, but are commonly positioned on the forehead during relaxation training.

High stress tends to constrict superficial blood vessels and cool the skin, whereas relaxation opens blood vessels and warms the skin. Therefore, a cool surface skin temperature may indicate a person is under stress. Temperature biofeedback measures this by placing a thermistor (a temperature-sensitive resistor), which signals changes, on the skin surface, usually the fingers or toes.

Stoyva and Anderson (1982) argue that biofeedback techniques, as contrasted with verbal induction of relaxation, do offer certain practical advantages in the operation of stress management programmes.

- it helps measure objectively whether desired physiological changes due to relaxation are being achieved
- clients are more likely to be aware that they are beginning to master an anti-stress response, or at least make some progress towards this goal, a realization that can act as a potent source of motivation

- if there is any difficulty learning how to relax using only verbal induction, biofeedback can be offered as an alternative strategy or a variant of the old one.

Beech *et al.* (1982) also highlight its advantages when dealing with hard-headed, executive, goal-oriented individuals who may refute relaxation training, seeing the whole proposition as being far too nebulous and 'wishy-washy'. Biofeedback, with its emphasis on instrumentation and the display of precise accurate information, can be more appealing to this sort of person, who is hungry for tangible figures and results.

However, Brannon and Feist (1992) claim that early enthusiasm over biofeedback has waned in recent years. This is due to the fact that research has failed to demonstrate an advantage of biofeedback over much less expensive relaxation training. It can be argued further, however, that even where there is no cear-cut evidence for the superiority of biofeedback over cheaper techniques, there is still a case to be made for the provision of biofeedback equipment.

Other simple short- and long-term measures that the therapist may wish to use to demonstrate the effectiveness of their relaxation training include:

- blood pressure measurement
- pulse rate
- respiration rate
- validated subjective psychological measures
- validated objective psychological measures
- subjective visual analogue scales measuring anxiety, pain, etc.
- changes in medication intake
- subjective and objective changes in behaviour – cigarette smoking, caffeine, alcohol intake, illness behaviour, aggressiveness
- observation – of posture, function, movement, co-ordination, balance
- palpation – of muscle tone, fluency of movement.

References

Anderson, B. (1983) Stretching and sports. In *Sports Medicine*, 2nd edn (eds Appenzeller, O. and Atkinson, R.), Urban and Schwarzenberg, Baltimore

Atkinson, R.L., Atkinson, R.C. and Hilgard, E.R. (1983) *Introduction to Psychology*, Harcourt, Brace, Jovanovich, London

Beech, H.R., Burns, L.E. and Sheffield, B.F. (1982) *A Behavioural Approach to the Management of Stress – A Practical Guide of Techniques*, John Wiley, Chichester

Beitman, B.D., Basha, I.M. and Trombka, L.H. (1987) Panic attacks and their treatment: an introduction. *Journal of Integrative and Electic Psychotherapy*, 6(4), 412–420

Bird, J. and Wilson, A. (1991) In *The Runners Handbook* (eds Gower, B. and Shepherd, J.), Penguin Books, London

Blanchard, E.B. and Andrasis, F. (1985) *Management of Chronic Headaches: A Psychological Approach*, Pergamon Press, New York

Blanchard, E.B., Schwarz, S.P. and Radnitz, C.R. (1987) Psychological assessment and treatment of irritable bowel syndrome. *Journal of Behaviour Modification*, 11(3), 348–372

Brannon, L. and Feist, J. (1992) *Health Psychology: An Introduction to Behaviour and Health*, 2nd edn, Wadsworth

Burnard, P. (1991) *Coping with Stress in the Health Professions – A Practical Guide. Therapy in Practice 21*, Chapman and Hall, London

Burns, L.E. (1981) Relaxation in the management of stress. In *Coping with Stress* (Marshall, J. and Cooper C.L., eds), Gower, London

Carlson, C.R., Collins, F.L. Jr., Nitz, A.J., Sturgis, E.T. and Rogers, J.L. (1990) Muscle stretching as an alternative relaxation training procedure. *Journal of Behaviour Therapy and Experimental Psychiatry*, **21**(1), 29–38

Carlson, C.R., Ventrella, M.A. and Sturgis, E.T. (1987) Relaxation training through muscle stretching proceedures – a pilot case. *Journal of Behaviour Therapy and Experimental Psychiatry*, **18**(2), 121–126

Clark, D.M. (1989) Anxiety states – panic and generalised anxiety. In *Cognitive Behaviour Therapy for Psychiatric Problems – A Practical Guide* (eds Hawton, K., Salkovskis, P.M., Kirk, J. and Clark, E.M.), Oxford Medical Publications, Oxford

Clark, D.M., Salkovski, P.M. and Chalkley, A.J. (1985) Respiratory control as a treatment for panic attacks. *Journal of Behaviour Therapy and Experimental Psychiatry*, **16**, 23–30

Davies, M., Eshellman, E.R. and McKay, M. (1988) *The Relaxation and Stress Reduction Workbook*, 3rd edn, New Harbinger Publications, Oakland, NJ

Dodge, V.H. (1991) Relaxation training: a nursing intervention for substance abusers. *Archives of Psychiatric Nursing*, **5**(2), 99–104

Eppley, K.R., Abrams, A.I. and Shear, J. (1989) Differential effects of relaxation techniques on trait anxiety: a meta-analysis. *Journal of Clinical Psychology*, **45**(6), 957–974

Glantz, K. and Himber, J. (1992) Sex therapy with associated disorders – a protocol *Journal of Sex and Marital Therapy*, **18**(2), 147–153

Horan, J.J. (1973) 'In-vivo' emotive imagery: a technique for reducing childbirth, anxiety and discomfort. *Psychological Reports*, **32**, 1328

Jacobson, E. (1938) *Progressive Relaxation: A Physiological and Clinical Investigation of Muscle States and their Significance in Psychology and Medical Practise*, 2nd edn, University of Chicago Press, Chicago

Keable, D. (1985a) Relaxation training techniques – a review – Part 1: What is Relaxation? *British Journal of Occupational Therapy*, April, 99–102

Keable, D. (1985b) Relaxation training techniques – a review – Part 2: How effective is relaxation? *British Journal of Occupational Therapy*, 201–204

King, J.R. (1983) Anxiety reduction using fragrances. In *The Psychology and Biology of fragrance*, (eds Van Toller, S. and Dodd, G.H.), Chapman and Hall, Oxford

Kirsh, C.A., Blanchard, E.B. and Parnes, S.M. (1987) A multiple baseline evaluation of the treatment of subjective tinnitus with relaxation training and biofeedback. Biofeedback and Self Regulation, 12(4), 295–312

Lammers, C.A., Naliboff, B.D. and Straetmeyer, A.J. (1984) The effects of progressive relaxation on stress and diabetic control. *Journal of Behavioural Research and Therapy*, **22**(6), 641–650

Massey, P. (1990) Autogenesis – the way forward. *Journal of Chartered Physiotherapists in Psychiatry*, **2**, 3–11

Meichenbaum, D. (1985) *Stress Inoculation Training*, Pergamon Press, London

Miller, T.W. and Kraus, R.F. (1990) An overview of chronic pain. *Hospital and Community Psychiatry*, **41**(4), 433–440

Millis, J.E. and Schonell, M. (1981) Relaxation therapy in asthma: a critical review. *Journal of Psychosomatic Medicine*, **43**, 365–372

Mitchell, L. (1977) *Simple Relaxation*, John Murray, London

Nicassio, P.M. and Buchanan, D.C. (1981) Clinical Application of Behaviour Therapy for Insomnia. *Comprehensive Psychiatry*, **22**(5), 512–521

Ost, L.G. (1987) Applied relaxation: description of a coping technique and review of controlled studies. *Journal of Behaviour Research and Therapy*, **25**, 297–410

Patel, C. and Marmot, M.G. (1988) Efficacy versus effectiveness of relaxation therapy in hypertension. *Stress Medicine*, **4**(4), 433–440

Prima, A., Agnoli, A. and Tambruell, A. (1979) A review of the application of biofeedback to migraine and tension headaches. *Acta Neurologica*, **34**(6), 510–521

Ricketts, E. and Cross, E. (1985) The Whitchurch method of stress management by relaxation exercises. *Journal of Chartered Society of Physiotherapy*, **71**(6), 262–264

Ritson, B. (1992) Treatment of alcohol related disorders and alcohol abuse. *International Journal of Mental Health*, **21**, 43–67

Rosa, K.R. (1976) *Autogenic Training*, Victor Gollancz, London

Sadlier, M. and Heptinstall, S.T. (1991) Overcoming stress. *Therapy Weekly*, 31 Oct., 1991

Scarrot, J. (1993) A comparison of the effects of the Whitchurch method of stress management with relaxation and group exercise therapy in the management of psychiatric patients (unpublished)

Stoyva, J.M. and Anderson, C.D. (1982) A coping–rest model of relaxation and stress management. In *Handbook of Stress – Theoretical and Clinical Aspects* (eds Goldberger, L. and Breznitz, S.), Free Press, New York

Surwit, R.S. (1981) Behavioural approaches to Raynaud's disease. *Journal of Psychotherapy and Psychosomatics*, **36**(3–4), 224–245

Tomes, H. (1990) Cardiac rehabilitation: an occupational therapist's perspective. *British Journal of Occupational Therapy*, **53**(7), 285–287

Valbo, A.B. (1973) Muscle spindle afferent discharge from resting and contrasting muscles in normal human subjects. In *New Developments in Electrotherapy and Clinical Neurophysiology*, Vol. 3 (ed. J.E. Desmedt), Karger, Basel

Wilson, D. (1985) *Occupational Therapy in Long Term Psychiatry*, Churchill Livingstone, Edinburgh

13

Exercise and mental health

John Smeaton

Introduction

Let us remind ourselves of two contemporary stereotypes. The sporty couple running along the beach – fit, perfect and happy. The thirty-something squash player, so tanned positive and successful. The belief that exercise is good for the body and the mind, the 'whole person', is flourishing, and not just in the advertising community. A survey of 1750 American 'primary-care physicians' (Ryan, 1983) revealed that 85% regularly prescribed exercise as a treatment for depression and a few psychiatric clinicians are starting to supplement their treatment protocols with exercise prescription (Morgan and Goldston, 1987; Chastain and Shapiro, 1987). There now appears to be a consensus among exercise psychologists that physical fitness is associated with psychological well-being (Morgan and Goldston, 1987).

Physiotherapists working in the mental health field are in a position to contrast the 'healthy lifestyle' image with the reality of many psychiatric wards. Here the picture is one of low energy, poor body image and inactivity. The same physiotherapists quickly realize that trying to motivate and energize patients whose psychiatric disorders affect their energy levels, mood and motivation demands an approach grounded in the psychology of exercise.

Largely due to the efforts of exercise psychologists, an increasingly convincing body of research has built up over the past 20 years, suggesting that exercise has preventative and therapeutic benefits for individuals with psychiatric disorders. Despite this research and considering the costs of pharmacological and psychological treatment approaches, it is surprising that the systematic prescription of therapeutic exercise has not been more widely reported.

One of the barriers to a more widespread use of exercise in mental health may be that professionals are unaware of the research base; another may be patient compliance, a problem common to all interventions; a third, the influence of the 'medical model' and the consequent pharmacological bias.

Thus the first step in extending the role of exercise in psychiatry may be the need to convince clients and professionals of the value (and limitations) of exercise for those with mental health problems. Designing programmes of physical activities that meet the needs of specific groups of patients may be the next problem, closely followed by the biggest challenges of all – trying to get patients active and then to 'stick with it'.

This chapter is intended to be as practical as possible, while also being an overview of the value of exercise as a therapeutic approach to mental health problems. It looks first at exercise in mental health from a broad perspective and then focuses on specific psychiatric conditions, before considering the problems of exercise adherence and motivation and strategies to overcome them.

Rationale for the role of exercise in mental health

Theories and mechanisms

Psychiatry is concerned with both mental and physical processes. The relationship between these two processes is addressed by the 'biopsychosocial model' (Engel, 1980). This views nature as an interconnected hierarchy; a change in one level will effect changes in the others. At the 'top' of the personal hierarchy, mental phenomena 'emerge', generated by biochemical and physiological events. Thus physical changes could effect mental ones. The recently proposed 'organic unity theory' views the distinction between the mental and the physical as a semantic one (Goodman, 1991) and would see no contradiction in exercise being described as a psychological treatment.

A theoretical framework may be in place, but our knowledge of exactly *how* exercise affects mental states is a little more shaky. However, we can make a start by looking at the reasons *why* people exercise. They can be grouped under the following headings: to increase health and fitness; to improve appearance; enjoyment; social and psychological benefits (Johnsgard, 1985). Ideas about why exercise might cause mental health improvements can be similarly subdivided. The physiological view is that aerobic exercise causes biochemical changes that affect the mental state. One psychological stance is that group cohesiveness and social support are responsible for changes in mood and emotion, while the more 'cognitive' opinion is that fitness training is a coping behaviour; by reducing 'somatic turmoil' we can improve our relations with our environment (Folkins and Sime, 1981). Another variation, proposed by Davidson and Schwartz (1976), is that physical activity such as running demands the total response of mind and body so that previous inputs, such as the somatic tension and cognitive 'noise' of anxiety, are overwhelmed by the signals of aerobic activity. The feeling of relaxation after exercise, they suggest, is the result of cleared cognitive and somatic channels.

Perhaps exercise merely distracts people from their problems. The 'distraction hypothesis' may underlie other stress-reducing activities such as watching fish (Katcher *et al.*, 1983) or eating lunch (Wilson *et al.*, 1981). Getting 'nice and warm' is associated with a feeling of well-being whether after a sauna (deVries, 1968) or after exercise. To confuse the picture even further there is a correlation between *perceived* fitness and well-being. A feeling that one should be doing more exercise (sound familiar?) and should be fitter, is negatively correlated with well-being. Whereas, exercise may lead to feelings of mastery and increased self-esteem.

Providing support for the physiological view are studies that have paid attention to effective placebo groups. For example, Mutrie (1988) provides evidence that it is not participants' expectations or the attention that they get that are responsible for beneficial effects. Indeed the above study demonstrated a strong positive correlation between exercise intensity and an antidepressive effect.

If aerobic exercise itself is the active ingredient, what biological mechanisms might be responsible? Changes in people's behaviour are associated with variations in the levels of psychoactive substances. Catecholamines are probably involved in the regulation of effect. Fit people can be distinguished from the less fit by a combination of catecholamine and psychological variables (Ismail and Sothmann, 1983). Antidepressant drug therapy raises the brain levels of norepinephrine (noradrenaline) and serotonin, as does exercise (Morgan, 1985).

Raised plasma endorphin levels are part of the body's response to physical stress. Endorphins ('natural opiates') have analgesic and euphoric effects, but a relationship between raised levels and elevated mood has not been established.

Clearly, biochemical changes are associated with mental variation, and exercise produces biochemical changes. However, the gap in our knowledge – how does body chemistry affect psychology? – may take some time to fill.

Biological influences may be crucial, but the behavioural effects of the interaction between the client and the exercise situation cannot be discounted. Which of these factors is responsible for specific mental health improvements is still unclear. It is imperative for physiotherapists working in psychiatry that these questions are answered. If, for example, mood elevation is our goal, should our activity sessions be pleasant and distracting or should we be 'pushing hard' for biochemical changes?

The psychological effects of exercise

Before we summarize the beneficial effects of exercise it is well to remember that exercise has, as the Americans say, a down-side (as anyone who has worked in a sports injury clinic will testify). Injuries, obsession, pain and strained relationships are among the negative outcomes that occur in 7–20% of marathon runners (Morgan, 1979; Robbins and Joseph, 1985). Although largescale surveys in the US and Canada (Brown, 1990) reveal a direct relationship between positive mental health and exercise, it is not clear whether people are able to endure the rigours of running, etc., because they are happy and well adjusted or if it is exercise that produces this euphoria. This 'chicken and egg' problem has still to be resolved.

Table 13.1 lists some of the psychological effects of exercise programmes mentioned in the literature, while Table 13.2 summarizes the therapeutic effects.

Table 13.1 Psychological effects of exercise programmes

Accepted	Tentative
Mood elevation	Improved sense of body image
Improved self-concept	Reduced aggression
Improved work behaviour	Improved cognition
Reductions in some indicators of stress	Greater emotional stability
	Increased assertiveness
	Greater sexual satisfaction
	Memory improvements
	Greater confidence

Table 13.2 Therapeutic effects of exercise programmes

Accepted	Tentative
Reduced state anxiety	Reduced trait anxiety
Reduced mild/moderate depression	Adjunct to the treatment of
Enhanced ability to resist stress	severe depression

In both cases an important distinction is made between findings that are widely accepted and those that are more tentative.

Exercise and stress, anxiety and depression

Stress

Stress is associated with depression and anxiety, but what exactly is 'stress'? It can be seen as a process. If an external or internal stimulus ('stressor') is perceived as threatening, an unpleasant emotional reaction may be the result, accompanied by activation of the autonomic nervous system. Reactions to stress vary; some people have effective 'coping strategies', others have high trait anxiety and are more vulnerable, especially when being evaluated by others, as they may lack self-confidence and self-esteem.

Personal resources that are thought to increase resistance to stress include self-esteem, confidence and 'wellness'. 'Wellness' encompasses physical fitness, controlled weight and high energy (Matheny *et al.*, 1986).

A meta-analysis of 34 studies by Crews and Landers (1987) demonstrated that irrespective of the sorts of measures used, aerobically fit individuals have a reduced psychosocial stress response. Fitter people have lower baseline levels of cardiovascular activity and their blood pressure and heart rate response to stress are less dramatic (McGilley and Holmes, 1988).

Exercise may be a cheap and 'natural' coping strategy for dealing with acute stress and there is also evidence that it has a protective role against long-term exposure to stress (Tucker *et al.*, 1986; Brown and Siegel, 1988). These studies suggest that physical fitness along with social support and 'hardiness' (a sense of control and purpose, a perception of problems as opportunities of personal growth) provide a buttress against the impact of life's stress on health. Exercise can maintain or increase fitness, whereas other components of the triad may not be so easily manipulated. Exercise has played a limited overt role in stress management so far, but surely this must increase.

Anxiety

Let us just remind ourselves that anxiety is linked to stress, commonly involves challenges to self-esteem and self-worth that the individual feels powerless against, and is associated with high levels of sympathetic nervous system activity. 'State anxiety' is a temporary emotional reaction to an identifiable trigger and may result in elevated heart rate and muscle tension. Individuals with high 'trait anxiety' react to stressors, especially perceived threats to self-esteem, with high levels of state anxiety.

Relaxation has physiological components; neuromuscular tension correlates positively with anxiety. A convincing study by deVries and Adams (1972) compared the effect of four interventions: meprobamate, an anxiolytic drug; walking at a heart rate of 100 beats per minute (bpm); walking at 120 bpm; and a lactose placebo – against a control. Muscle tension was significantly reduced after 100 bpm walking compared to the control and slightly but not significantly reduced after more energetic walking, the other conditions did not differ significantly from the control.

This study raises two interesting points. Could exercise replace minor tranquillizers for some patients? What is the optimum exercise dosage for anxiety reduction? Although neither question is resolved, Sime (in Morgan and Goldston, 1987) reports the case of a client with a two-year history of severe anxiety and depression. Tranquillizing and antidepressant medication provided only minimal symptom relief; eventually exercise was tried and proved to be a potent acute antidepressant agent. Interestingly the researcher complains about having to supervise the client's exercise himself as nobody else was willing.

Bahrke and Morgan (1978) measured the state anxiety of 75 men who were randomly assigned to one of three interventions – walking, meditation or quiet rest. Each treatment lasted 20 minutes. All three groups demonstrated significantly reduced levels of anxiety, leading the researchers to wonder whether distraction or 'time-out' was the common mechanism.

Studies support the prescription of exercise as a treatment for anxiety, but they also highlight the role of a client's personality or history in mediating the magnitude of its effects. Exercise is not for everyone; some people derive more benefit from less strenuous strategies like meditation, relaxation or, indeed, watching fish. But for clients who are normally involved in a strenuous occupation and who are deprived, by illness, of exercise and the structure of the working day, a programme that is physically demanding may be especially beneficial.

Although the evidence for exercise-related reductions in state anxiety is considerable, fewer studies have looked at changes in trait anxiety. Lion (1978) randomly assigned volunteers ($n = 6$) residing at a home for discharged psychiatric patients to either an exercise group or a control group. Following 1 mile (1.5 km) of running–walking three times per week, for 2 months, the exercisers showed significant drops in trait anxiety scores. Other studies show support for an exercise effect (e.g. Sexton *et al.*, 1989) and chronic exercise is usually associated with reductions in trait anxiety, but more evidence is required before definite conclusions can be reached.

Finally, it is worth mentioning that exercise has been successfully used as an anxiety inhibitor in phobic states (Orwin, 1973, 1974).

Depression

Depressive illness and anxiety are clinically distinct, but the two syndromes are very commonly found in combination. They are our most prevalent mental health problems.

In the majority of studies that look at the effects of exercise on moderately depressed non-elderly patients, the findings are that sustained aerobic exercise reduces depression (e.g. Greist *et al.*, 1979; Martinsen *et al.*, 1985). There is no convincing body of evidence that exercise has beneficial effects for people suffering from depressive psychosis.

Martinsen *et al.* (1985) randomly assigned 49 inpatients, who satisfied DSM-III criteria for major depression, to an exercise and a control group. The 9-week exercise programme consisted of walking, jogging, cycling, skiing and swimming at 50–70% of predicted aerobic capacity. There were three one-hour sessions each week. The control intervention was occupation therapy. The mean reduction in depression scores was significantly larger ($p < 0.05$) in the exercise group who also demonstrated improved fitness. The age range for these patients was 17–60 years (mean = 40) and the mean number of years since the first depressive episode was 11.

Greist *et al.* (1979) randomly assigned young adults, who were moderately depressed, to one of three 10-week regimens: behavioural therapy; cognitive therapy; walking and running (for 30–65 minutes three times a week). The exercisers had at least as much improvement in their depression as the other groups.

Doyne *et al.* (1983) demonstrated significant improvements in the affective states of women with major depressive disorder following the introduction of an aerobic exercise programme. This study controlled for patient expectancies and contact time with therapists. Despite the association of a fitness effect with relief of depression, recent studies have found non-aerobic exercise to be as effective an antidepressant as aerobic exercise (Martinsen *et al.*, 1989; Doyne *et al.*, 1987). Perhaps a programme of *regular* exercise is the key, rather than a specific type. As the effects of exercise on depression are comparable with those of psychological therapy and given the undesirable side effects of antidepressant medication and ECT, the emergence of exercise, cheap and relatively side effect free, as a potential treatment for depression is an exciting prospect.

Alcohol dependency

Among problem drinkers there is a high incidence of depression and state anxiety and, as we have seen above, exercise has been shown to be effective in dealing with these problems.

Part of the growing evidence that exercise can be an effective adjunct to treatment for this client group is the well-designed study by Donaghy *et al.* (1991). Forty-five male problem drinkers were randomly assigned to one of three groups: aerobic exercise, weight training and relaxation. Each group met three times a week for 30–40 min. After eight weeks the two exercise groups had lower scores on measures of depression and anxiety compared with pre-exercise. No such differences were demonstrated by the relaxation group. As with other client groups, exercise adherence is a problem once regular contact with the therapist is tailed off (Sell and Christensen, 1989).

While there is no indication, as yet, that exercise leads to improved function or abstinence, physical activity seems to merit a place in a multidisciplinary approach to what is a many-sided and intractable problem.

Severe psychiatric disorders

People with severe mental illness commonly present with multiple problems, many of which may be physical. Psychiatric inpatients, particularly those with schizophrenia, score very badly on most measures of fitness (Lindquist, 1981). The side effects of medication, altered body image and low self-esteem further complicate the picture. In many instances a client's physical problems form the major barrier to independent living or employment (Gordon *et al.*, 1966). Physiotherapists are already hard at work with many of these patients, but nevertheless hospitalized patients lose their fitness (Morgan, 1974).

Research into the effects of exercise on the mental health of clients with problems such as schizophrenia and major affective disorder is not plentiful but is encouraging. Pelham *et al.* (1993) describe three interesting studies involving patients with these diagnoses. In the first experiment, 5 patients undertook 8 weeks of aerobic exercise while 6 clients followed an anaerobic programme. A post-programme interview revealed that 9 of the 11 clients reported either moderate or very significant benefits from the programmes. The clients also remarked that exercise helped them become more motivated towards other components of their rehabilitation programme.

In the second study, 10 clients were randomly assigned to either an aerobic or anaerobic exercise group. A time series analysis (measurements at 3, 6, 9 and 12 weeks) showed that the aerobic exercisers had significant fitness and mood improvements, whereas the anaerobic group had neither.

Chastain and Shapiro (1987) describe a collaborative pilot project involving a physical therapist, a psychiatric nurse and an occupational therapist. Twenty-four inpatients with various psychiatric conditions attended aerobic exercise sessions three times per week for 6 weeks. The psychological goals of the programme were to promote a more positive body image and raise self-esteem. The majority of the patients, including sufferers from Huntingdon's chorea and schizophrenia, were able to fulfil their commitment to see out the programme. Several participants stated that it was the most useful experience of their hospitalization. Similar client praise is reported by Karen Unger and her team (Unger *et al.*, 1992) in an evaluation of an exercise programme for students with severe psychiatric disabilities. The high exercise compliance rate in this study may have been helped by goal-setting and client self-selection of exercises. However, the other researchers quoted above, working with older clients, seem to think a highly structured exercise regimen is more likely to succeed.

Chamove (1988) used the Nurses' Observation Scale for Inpatient Evaluation to rate the behaviour of 38 patients with chronic schizophrenia on active and less active days. Participants had a mean age of 50 years and had been hospitalized for an average of 14 years. On active days the patients showed less psychotic symptoms, less movement disorder, less depression and more social competence. The encouraging results of the above interventions, plus the evidence that patients with schizophrenia who are involved in active leisure pursuits are more likely to find employment (Gordon *et al.*, 1966) and the finding that schizophrenia sufferers use exercise as a strategy for coping with auditory hallucinations (Falloon and Talbot, 1981), all point to the usefulness of exercise in an area where fruitful interventions are not commonplace.

Exercise in the community

Increasingly, physiotherapists working in mental health will be working in the community and our collective attentions should be focusing more and more on collaboration with GPs, early intervention in acute mental health problems and even prevention (the only strategies to have had a big impact on major health problems have been preventative ones).

A large-scale survey and 8-year follow-up by Farmer *et al.* (1988) found that inactive women without baseline depression were twice as likely to develop depression compared to active women. Men with depressive symptoms at baseline were 12 times more likely to report similar symptoms at follow-up than active men depressed at baseline. The possibility that exercise is a protective factor in women without depression is extremely interesting.

Mutrie (1988), extending the external validity of North American studies, looked at the effects of exercise on depressed sedentary adults referred by Glasgow GPs. The referrals (30 women, 6 men) exercised on an individual basis, guided by fortnightly visits from a physical education specialist. Her study indicated that depression does not remit spontaneously in 4 weeks, but aerobic exercise does reduce depression over the same period. Two-thirds of her exercising group maintained their regimens and reduced depression scores up to a 20-week follow-up. Interestingly, some clients reported that aerobic exercises were more enjoyable and easier to maintain than anaerobic exercises.

Another study (King *et al.*, 1989) looked at the psychological effects of a home exercise programme in a group of inactive middle-aged men and women. Participants were randomly allocated to either the exercise or an assessment-only control group. Perceived physical fitness, satisfaction with physical shape and weight were all significantly greater in the exercise group than for the controls. There were no corresponding fitness changes. The average adherence rate during this study was at least 75%.

As Nanette Mutrie states: 'These results have important implications for GPs and the NHS....It would therefore seem cost-effective for the NHS to employ an exercise specialist who could be used by GPs on a referral basis' (Mutrie, 1988).

What kind of exercise?

Although the balance of research opinion seemed to favour aerobic exercise rather than non-aerobic as a relaxant and antidepressant, more recent work supports the efficacy of the latter (e.g. Doyne *et al.*, 1989). In addition, the usefulness of the numerous lower intensity exercise possibilities has not been sufficiently explored. The cautionary note by Berger and Owen (1988) that 'the research focus on jogging seems to reflect a large number of researchers who jog' should be borne in mind. These same researchers found that hatha yoga was associated with mood benefits similar to those reported by swimmers and runners (this finding made them wonder whether deep abdominal breathing might be the secret of stress reduction rather than any aerobic component!).

Nevertheless, if the objective is to enhance mood or reduce anxiety, then there is some evidence that exercise should be regular, non-competitive, predictable and rhythmical (Berger, 1987). Repetitive rhythmical movement requires a minimal amount of attention; the mind is free to wander. Predictability may have similar advantages. 'Certain' activities, like jogging, allow you to pay a minimum amount of attention to the environment and 'think pleasant thoughts'.

Activities that fit the bill include walking, swimming, aerobics, step aerobics, running, cycling, weight training and, of course, jogging. Clients can easily continue with these activities independently. Interpersonal competition can be stressful and allows the possibility of losing. perhaps competitive activities should be avoided if relaxation is a main goal (Glasser, 1976). Interactive sports (e.g. tennis, squash) seem to be, as one might expect, invigorating rather than relaxing (Berger and Owen, 1988), although research in this area is sparse.

For some people, improvements in self-confidence and image may be produced by changes in physique. For them progressive resisted exercise may be especially useful. Most importantly, if people are going to persist with it, exercise has to be enjoyable. One kind of activity cannot be 'all things to all men'; a range of activities should be available.

Exercise dosage

A lot is known about the amount of exercise required for physical improvements, but very little about the dosages needed for psychological benefits, although the following comments on frequency, intensity and duration may prove useful. Before going on, however, it is worth noting, especially for those of us who work with more disabled clients, that persuading people who are doing nothing to do a little, but often, results in tangible mental and physical benefits (Collingwood and Willett, 1971; King *et al.*, 1989). Many people will need to start exercising very gently and may eventually progress to the levels recommended below.

Frequency

Whilst opinion is divided on the questions of exercise intensity and 'aerobic versus non-aerobic', researchers do agree that the reported benefits of exercise tend to be short term and therefore frequent exercise is necessary if improvements are to be maintained. Exercising every 2–3 days is recommended (Morgan, 1979).

Intensity

There is some indication that high-intensity aerobic exercise is stress-inducing (Morgan and Horstman, 1976). Conversely, there is not enough support for the beneficial effects of low-intensity exercise. For the moment, moderate intensity is recommended: 60–85% of maximum age-adjusted heart rate. The formula, maximum exercise heart rate = 220 minus age in years, can be used, but see 'Measuring exercise intensity' below.

As regards non-aerobic exercise, a standard approach based on the principle of progressive resisted exercise seems to be acceptable.

Duration

It is a struggle to find guidelines for duration; however, it seems that 20–30 minutes might be enough time for clients to become involved in an activity, but up to 60 minutes may result in even more psychological benefits (Berger, 1984). Energy expenditure of 4 kilocalories per kilogram of body weight is seen as adequate to induce the biological benefits of exercise. Healthy adults expending 400–700 kcal per hour doing moderate aerobic exercise like cycling or jogging reach the 4 kcal goal in 25–45 minutes. However, gentler activities such as gardening or walking, if performed frequently and for longer periods, also seem to result in physical benefits, so may have the potential to produce psychological changes.

Exercise adherence

'This year I am going to get fit' is a familiar cry. Getting started may be difficult, but sticking to an exercise programme is even more tricky. Commonly, half those who start a supervised exercise regimen, even if recommended to do so by their doctor, drop out (Dishman, 1982). 'Blue collar workers', smokers (Oldridge and Jones, 1983) and those who are overweight are more likely to relapse, as are people who are hostile or depressed. Low self-motivation (Dishman, 1983) and lack of support from family or friends (Andrew *et al.*, 1981) are associated with non-adherence, whereas a good credit rating (linked to socioeconomic status) is associated with better adherence.

The above information will be of no consolation to therapists working in psychiatry who also have to contend with the side effects of medication and the problems of institutionalization. As one might expect, people are more likely to start and persist with exercise programmes that are at convenient times and locations (Gettman *et al.*, 1983). Some people prefer to set their own exercise targets, others like more structure (Tu and Rothstein, 1979). Physiotherapists are aware that some people set themselves unattainable exercise goals and so set themselves up for failure; those reporting greatest discomfort from exercising are likely to discontinue (Ingjer and Dahl, 1979).

Practical implications

Strategies to improve adherence and increase motivation

Exercise, whether in a mental health setting or not, will only produce lasting physical or psychological change if people adhere to an appropriate programme of physical activity and exercise at an optimal level. Below are some ideas, drawn from the literature and personal experience, that should help clients commit themselves enthusiastically to an exercise programme.

- *Enjoyment.* Exercise can be demanding but it should also be *fun*. Music, jokes, tea and biscuits are all grist for the mill. People do not enjoy cramped airless rooms, broken equipment, tatty decor or cold grimy showers.
- *Variety.* If clients are to become habitual exercisers they need to find an activity that suits them. Making full use of community facilities will increase exercise options, but carefully 'managed' the combined staff and client population of typical psychiatric units should be able to sustain a wide range of exercise options (e.g. aerobic classes open to all – clients, staff and public).
- *Clear overall objectives.* It would be hard to exaggerate the usefulness of goal-setting. Written, explicit short- and long-term goals should be agreed. Hard to quantify objectives such as 'feeling better' should be avoided. Instead, process (attend aerobics 3 times a week) or outcome (able to jog twice round the grounds within 30 minutes) goals can be used. For promoting adherence,

'time' goals have been found superior to 'distance' goals and 'five-week goals' better than weekly goals (Martin *et al.*, 1984).

- *Client participation.* Involving patients in selecting activities and goal-setting will give them a sense of ownership of their programme. Self-motivation, essential if they are going to continue with exercise in the long term, will also be enhanced by participation (Martin *et al.*, 1984).
- *Monitoring realistic goals.* Having attained at least a few goals, an individual is more likely to persevere with an exercise regimen (Danielson and Wanzel, 1977). It is important that participants set realistic but *challenging* goals and monitor their progress in reaching these objectives. Achieving realistic goals may mean that day-to-day goals need to be flexible. Visual records, such as graphs or bar charts, can be displayed in the gym and are instant indicators of progress and keep clients interested (even if it involves a sneaky look at someone else's chart).
- *Positive self-monitoring.* Encouraging people new to physical activity to record their successes rather than their failures (Kirschenbaum and Flanery, 1983) increases their persistence.
- *Contracting* provides a framework for self-monitoring and goal-setting and should be part of the agreed treatment plan. Contracting has included the client leaving something of value as a deposit, retrievable only if agreed goals are reached (Gettman *et al.*, 1982).
- *'Decision balance sheets'.* Asking clients about to start an exercise programme to list the positive outcomes ('able to eat more') and the negative outcomes ('less time to watch television') that might result from attaining *specific exercise goals* increases their commitment and the likelihood they will 'stick with it' (Janis and Mann, 1977).
- *Group activity.* For most people, exercising with others rather than alone will encourage adherence. Friendship, mutual support and comparing progress are all possible in group approaches.
- *Positive feedback.* Common sense and research evidence (Smith *et al.*, 1979) support the crucial role of plenty of support and encouragement. Recognizing client's achievements increases their self-esteem. Support can be gradually phased out if a client's self-motivation improves.
- *Music. Suitable* background music, either by distracting or energizing exercisers, makes exercise seem easier but increases actual effort (Franklin, 1978). Music is a very important component of indoor exercise, but beware of copyright implications!
- *Exercise partners.* Patients can be paired off, each member of the duo being responsible for encouraging the other to exercise. An alternative is to make use of volunteers. making friends in an exercise group will encourage participants to continue.
- *Relapse prevention training.* If you think someone may well lapse and that feelings of loss of control or guilt may lead to a total relapse, then it is worth preparing for such an eventuality. Exercisers can be warned that they may well lapse, that everybody slips now and again, that exercise is not an all-or-nothing process. It should be stressed that they should not feel guilty, and a definite strategy for returning to exercise should be worked out.
- *Preventing over-exercising.* As we know, clients who exercise too hard may experience pain, injury and anxiety. Physiotherapists can educate and advise (see 'Monitoring realistic goals', above).

- *Easy access.* Obviously, to maximize adherence, exercise facilities should be local, cheap (or free).

In general, research demonstrates that the use of behavioural management techniques (goal-setting, contracting, etc.) increases adherence by roughly 20% and that if clients can persevere with a programme of physical activity for 3–6 months then they may be more likely to become long-term exercisers (Dishman, 1982). If help is needed with psychological strategies then your local psychology department is obviously the first choice.

Keeping a group going can be difficult and requires effective interdisciplinary communication and collaboration. Regular meetings for all staff concerned with the group should help boost morale and ensure continued good intercommunication (Chastain and Shapiro, 1987). Rotating staff through a demanding programme is a good idea if you have the option.

As a final word on adherence, the following quote from Professor R.S. Brown, an American psychiatrist, will suffice: 'The prescription of exercise for mental disorders, like anxiety and depression, fell on deaf ears except when phrased in special terms, incorporated in the treatment plan, and added to traditionally accepted psychiatric treatment' (Morgan and Goldston, 1987).

Evaluation

Measuring exercise intensity

The criterion exercise intensity measure is the percentage of maximal oxygen uptake (VO_2 max). Heart rate has a linear relationship to VO_2 max and is easier to measure; percentage maximum age-adjusted heart rate (220 minus age) is commonly used. However, this dosage indicator does not allow for factors like fitness, smoking, respiratory disease, etc. A method that avoids this problem is *rating perceived exertion* (RPE). Table 13.3 illustrates one version of the scale. The scale numbering approximates to one-tenth of the corresponding heart rate. The range 12–15 corresponds to 50–85% VO_2 max.

RPE can be used for exercise prescription and may be preferable to pulse

Table 13.3 Perceived exertion rating scale

6	
7	Very very light
8	
9	Very light
10	
11	Fairly light
12	
13	Somewhat hard
14	
15	Hard
16	
17	Very hard
18	
19	Very very hard
20	

counting for some clients. At lower exercise intensities, RPE correlates less well with heart rate, so care should be taken with cardiac patients. Interested readers are referred to Borg (1970) and Birk and Birk (1987).

Measuring fitness improvements

RPE could also be used as a rough guide to fitness improvements (e.g. RPE of a task). Other practical methods to quantify cardiovascular fitness improvements include measuring resting heart rate and heart recovery rates. A patient performs, say, 3 minutes' worth of stationary cycling at a given resistance and RPM. Pulse rate is measured before the test, immediately after and 3 minutes after. The test can be repeated.

The views of the client

At the moment there is no standardized measure for assessing clients' views of exercise programmes. Pelham *et al.* (1993) used a structured interview combined with a key word 'content analysis' to obtain the views of participants as to the efficacy of their programme. The Group Environment Questionnaire (Carron *et al.*, 1985) might be useful as it assesses group cohesion and considers group goals and objectives.

Psychological outcomes

Psychometric tests (Table 13.4) have been widely used by exercise psychologists. Advice on use, applicability and availability should be obtained from a clinical psychologist.

Safe exercising

Physiotherapists should already be aware of the potential hazards of exercise. However, it might be useful to look at the potential problems that could arise from the interaction between exercise and psychotropic medication. Very large doses of chlorpromazine (1.5–3.6 g/day – the average dose in our unit is 50–100 mg) tend to reduce stroke volume and increase plasma noradrenaline levels, limiting exercise performance. Within the normal dosage range, occasional postural hypotension is likely to be the only problem, along with

Table 13.4 Some psychological outcome measures

Measure	What it measures	Reference
Depression inventory	Depression	Beck *et al.* (1961)
State–trait anxiety inventory	State anxiety Trait anxiety	Spielberger *et al.* (1970)
Rosenberg self-esteem inventory	Self-esteem	Rosenberg (1965)
Profile of mood states	Affective states, including anger, vigour, inertia, etc.	McNair *et al.* (1971)
Nurses' Observation Scale for Inpatients Evaluation	Behaviour change	Walls *et al.* (1977)

drowsiness and Parkinsonism. Exercise is indicated for patients on these drugs to increase their fitness and reduce the level of circulating noradrenaline (Martinsen, 1987).

Large doses of beta-blockers will impair exercise performance by reducing cardiac output and cause a sensation of muscle fatigue while exercising. Beta-blockers also inhibit the response of blood glucose to exercise so hypoglycaemia is a potential problem, but again only with large doses. However, exercisers taking beta-blockers should be on a sensible diet (i.e. plenty of carbohydrates). It is prudent to be cautious with patients taking tricyclic antidepressants, while their dosage is being increased. Once their circulation has adjusted to the medication and provided that there are no other contraindications, more intensive exercise can start (Martinsen *et al.*, 1985). Patients with a history of heart problems would normally be prescribed an alternative drug.

Conclusion

Research in the field of exercise and mental health has come a long way in the past 10 years. There is now a considerable knowledge base indicating that exercise has the potential to become the treatment of choice for clients suffering from anxiety and moderate depression. What is needed now, to establish exercise as a 'psychological treatment' (and to persuade those of a determined pharmacological stance), is clinical replication.

Physiotherapists in psychiatry are ideally placed to initiate exercise programmes or evaluate existing projects. We need to know more about mechanisms of effect, optimal dosages, the role of exercise in prevention, etc.; the scope for research is vast.

Exercise in mental health provides a fascinating opportunity for collaborative work between physiotherapists, other mental health disciplines and primary care workers.

References

Andrew, G.M., Oldridge, N.B., Parker, J.O. *et al.* (1981) Reasons for dropout from exercise programs in post-coronary patients. *Medicine and Science in Sports and Exercise*, **13**(3), 164–168

Bahrke, M.S. and Morgan, W.P. (1978) Anxiety reduction following exercise and meditation. *Cognitive Therapy and Research*, **2**(4), 323–333

Beck, A.T., Ward, C.H., Mendelson, M., Mock, J. and Erbaugh, H. (1961) An inventory for measuring depression. *Archives of General Psychiatry*, **4**, 561–571

Berger, B.G. (1984) Running away from anxiety and depression: a female as well as a male race. In *Running as a Therapy: An Integrated Approach* (eds Sachs, M.L. and Buffone, G.W.), University of Nebraska Press, Lincoln

Berger, B.G. (1987) Stress reduction following swimming. In *Exercise and Mental Health* (eds Morgan, W.P. and Goldston, S.E.), Hemisphere, Washington

Berger, B.G. and Owen, D.R. (1988) Stress reduction and mood enhancement in four modes: swimming, body conditioning, hatha yoga, and fencing. *Research Quarterly for Exercise and Sport*, **59**(2), 148–159

Birk, T.J. and Birk, C.A. (1987) Use of ratings of perceived exertion for exercise prescription. *Sports Medicine*, **4**, 1–8

Borg, G.A.V. (1970) Perceived exertion as an indicator of somatic stress. *Scandinavian Journal of Rehabilitation Medicine*, **2**, 92–98

Brown, D.R. (1990) Exercise fitness and mental health. In *Exercise Fitness and Health* (ed. Bouchard, C.), Human Kinetics, Champaign, Illinois

Brown, J.D. and Siegel, J.M. (1988) Exercise as a buffer of life stress. a prospective study of adolescent health. *Health Psychology*, **7**(4), 341–353

Carron, A.V., Widmeyer, W.N. and Brawley, L.R. (1985) The development of an instrument to assess cohesion in sport teams: the Group Environment Questionnaire. *Journal of Sport Psychology*, **7**(3), 244–266

Chamove, A.S. (1988) Exercise improves behaviour: a rationale for occupational therapy. *British Journal of Occupational Therapy*, **49**, 83–86

Chastain, P.B. and Shapiro, G.E. (1987) Physical fitness program for patients with psychiatric disorders. *Physical Therapy*, **67**(4), 545–548

Collingwood, T.R. and Willett, L. (1971) The effects of physical training upon self-concept and body attitudes. *Journal of Clinical Psychology*, **27**, 411–412

Crews, D.J. and Landers, D.M. (1987) A meta-analytic review of aerobic fitness and reactivity to psychosocial stressors. *Medicine and Science in Sports and Exercise*, **19**(5), S114–120

Danielson, R.R. and Wanzel, R.S. (1977) Exercise objectives of fitness program dropouts. In *Psychology of Motor behaviour and Sports* (eds Landers, D.M. and Christina, R.W.), Human Kinetics, Champaign, Illinois

Davidson, R.J. and Schwartz, G.E. (1976) The psychobiology of relaxation and related states: a mutli-process theory. In *Behavior Control and Modification of Physiological Activity* (ed. Mostofsky, D.I.), Prentice-Hall, Englewood Cliffs, New Jersey

DeVries, H.A. (1968) Immediate and long term effects of exercise upon resting muscle action potential level. *Journal of Sports Medicine and Physical Fitness*, **8**, 1–11

DeVries, H.A. and Adams, G.M. (1972) Comparison of exercise response in old and young men: 1. The cardiac effort/total body effort relationship. *Journal of Gerontology*, **27**(3), 344–348

Dishman, R.K. (1982) Compliance/adherence in health-related exercise. *Health Psychology*, **1**(3), 237–267

Dishman, R.K. (1983) Predicting exercise compliance using psychometric and behavioural measures of commitment (Abstract). *Medicine in Science and Sports and Exercise*, **15**(2), 118

Donaghy, M., Ralston, G. and Mutrie, N. (1991) Exercise as a therapeutic adjunct for problem drinkers. *Journal of Sports Sciences*, **9**(4), 440

Doyne, E.J., Chambliss, D.L. and Beutler, L.E. (1983) Aerobic exercise as a treatment for depression in women. *Behaviour Therapy*, **14**, 434–440

Doyne, E.J., Ossip-Klier, D.J., Bowman, E.D. *et al.* (1987) Running versus weight-lifting in the treatment of depression. *Journal of Consulting and Clinical Psychology*, **55**, 748–754

Engel, G.L. (1980) The clinical application of the biopsychosocial model. *American Journal of Psychiatry*, **137**, 535–544

Falloon, I.R.H. and Talbot, R.E. (1981) Persistent auditory hallucinations: Coping mechanisms and implications for management. *Psychological Medicine*, **11**, 329–339

Farmer, M.E., Locke, B.Z. and Moscickic, E.K. (1988) Physical activity and depressive symptoms: the NHANES I epidemiologic follow-up study. *American Journal of Epidemiology*, **128**, 1340–1351

Folkins, C.H. and Sime, W.E. (1981) Physical fitness training and mental health. *American Psychologist*, **36**(4), 373–389

Franklin, B.A. (1978) Motivating and educating adults to exercise. *Journal of Physical Education and Recreation*, **49**(6), 13–17

Gettman, L.R., Pollock, M.L. and Ward, A. (1983) Adherence to unsupervised exercise. *The Physician and Sportsmedicine*, **11**(10), 56–66

Gettman, L.R., Ward, P. and Hagan, R.D. (1982) A comparison of combined running and weight training. *Medicine and Science in Sports and Exercise*, **14**, 229–234

Glasser, W. (1976) *Positive Addiction*, Harper and Row, New York

Goodman, A. (1991) Organic unity theory: the mind–body problem revisited. *American Journal of Psychiatry*, **148**(5), 553–563

Gordon, H.L., Rosenberg, D. and Morris, E.E. (1966) Leisure activities of schizophrenic patients after return to the community. *Mental Hygiene*, **50**, 452–459

Greist, J.H., Klein, M.H., Eischens, R.R. *et al.* (1979) Running as treatment for depression. *Comprehensive Psychiatry*, **20**, 41–54

Ingjer, F. and Dahl, H.A. (1979) Dropouts from an endurance training program. *Scandinavian Journal of Sports Sciences*, **1**, 20–22

Ismail, A.H. and Sothmann, M.S. (1983) Discrimination power and catecholamine-related variables to differentiate between high and low fit adults. In *Health Estimation, Risk Reduction and Health Promotion* (eds Landry, F. *et al.*), Proceedings of the Society of Prospective Medicine,

Janis, I.L. and Mann, L. (1977) *Decision Making*, Free Press, New York

Johnsgard, K. (1985) The motivation of the long distance runner: I. *Journal of Sports Medicine*, **25**, 135–139

Katcher, A.H., Friedmann, E., Beck, A.M. and Lynch, J.J. (1983) Talking, looking, and blood pressure: physiological consequences of interaction with the living environment. In *New Perspectives on Our Lives with Animal Companions* (eds Katcher, A.H. and Beck, A.M.), University of Pennsylvania Press, Philadelphia

King, A.C., Taylor, C.B., Haskell, W.L. and Debusk, R.F. (1989) Influence of regular aerobic exercise on psychological health: a randomized controlled trial of healthy middle-aged adults. *Health Psychology*, **8**, 305–324

Kirschenbaum, D.S. and Flanery, R.C. (1983) Behavioral contracting: outcomes and elements. In *Progress in Behaviour Modification*, Vol. 15 (eds Hersen, M., Eisler, R.M. and Miller, P.M.), Academic Press, New York

Lindquist, J.E. (1981) Activity and vestibular function in chronic schizophrenics. *Occupational Therapy Journal of Research*, **1**, 56–78

Lion, L.S. (1978) Psychological effects of jogging: a preliminary study. *Perceptual and Motor Skills*, **47**, 1215–1218

McGilley, B.M. and Holmes, D.S. (1988) Aerobic fitness and response to psychological stress. *Journal of Research in Personality*, **22**, 129–139

McNair, D.M., Lorr, M. and Droppleman, L.F. (1971) *Manual for the Profile of Mood States*, Educational and Industrial Testing Service, San Diego

Martin, J.E., Dubbert, P.M., Kattell, A.D. *et al.* (1984) The behavioral control of exercise in sedentary adults: studies 1 through 6. *Journal of Consulting and Clinical Psychology*, **52**, 795–811

Martinsen, E.W. (1987) Exercise and medication in the psychiatric patient. In *Exercise and Mental Health* (eds Morgan, W.P. and Goldston, S.E.), Hemisphere, Washington

Martinsen, E.W., Hoffart, A. and Solberg, O. (1989) Comparing aerobic and non-aerobic forms of exercise in the treatment of clinical depression: a randomised trial. *Comprehensive psychiatry*, **30**(4), 324–331

Martinsen, E.W., Medhus, A. and Sandvik, L. (1985) Effects of aerobic exercise on depression: a controlled study. *British Medical Journal*, **291**, 109

Matheny, K.B., Aycock, D.W., Pugh, J.L. *et al.* (1986) Stress coping: a qualitative and quantitative synthesis with implications for treatment. *The Counseling Psychologist*, **14**(4), 499–549

Morgan, W.P. (1974) Exercise and mental disorders. In *Sports Medicine* (eds Ryan, A.J. and Allman, P.L. Jr.), Academic Press, London

Morgan, W.P. (1979) Negative addiction in runners. *The Physician and Sportsmedicine*, **7**(2), 57–70

Morgan, W.P. (1985) Affective beneficence of vigorous physical activity. *Medicine and Science in Sports and Exercise*, **17**, 94–100

Morgan, W.P. and Goldston, S.E. (eds) (1987) *Exercise and Mental Health*, Hemisphere, Washington

Morgan, W.P. and Horstman, D.H. (1976) Anxiety reduction following acute physical activity. *Medicine and Science in Sports and Exercise*, **8**, 62

Mutrie, N. (1988) Exercise as a treatment for moderate depression in the UK Health Service. In *Sport, Health, Psychology and Exercise Symposium*, Sports Council, London

Oldridge, N.B. and Jones, N.L. (1983) Improving patient compliance in cardiac exercise rehabilitation: effects of written agreement and self monitoring. *Journal of Cardiac Rehabilitation*, **3**, 257–262

Orwin, A. (1973) 'The running treatment': a preliminary communication on a new use for an old therapy (physical activity) in the agoraphobic syndrome. *British Journal of Psychiatry*, **122**, 175–179

Orwin, A. (1974) Treatment of a situational phobia – a case for running. *British Journal of Psychiatry*, **125**, 95–98

Pelham, T.W., Campagna, P.D., Ritvo, P.G. and Birnie, W.A. (1993) The effects of exercise therapy on clients in a psychiatric rehabilitation program. *Psychosocial Rehabilitation Journal*, **16**(4), 75–84

Robbins, J.M. and Joseph, P. (1985) Experiencing exercise withdrawal: possible consequences of therapeutic and mastery running. *Journal of Sport Psychology*, **7**, 23–39

Rosenberg, M. (1965) *Society and the Adolescent Self-Image*. Princeton University Press, Princeton, New Jersey

Ryan, A.J. (1983) Exercise is medicine. *The Physician and Sportsmedicine*, **11**, 10

Sell, E.H. and Christensen, N.J. (1989) The effect of physical training on physical, mental and social conditions in drug and/or alcohol addicts. *Ugeskr-Laeger*, **151**(33), 2064–2067

Sexton, H., Maere, A. and Dahl, N.H. (1989) Exercise intensity and reduction in neurotic symptoms. *Acta Psychiatrica Scandinavica*, **80**, 231–235

Smith, R.E., Smoll, F.L. and Curtis, B. (1979) Coach effectiveness training: a cognitive-behavioural approach to enhancing relationship skills in youth sport coaches. *Journal of Sport Psychology*, **1**, 59–75

Sonstroem, R.J. (1984) Exercise and self-esteem. *Exercise and Sports Science Reviews*, **12**, 123–155

Spielberger, C.D., Gorsuch, R.L. and Lushene, R.E. (1970) *Manual for the State–Trait Anxiety Inventory*, Consulting Psychologists Press, Palo Alto, California

Tu, J. and Rothstein, A.L. (1979) Improvement of jogging performance through application of personality specific motivational techniques. *Research Quarterly*, **50**(1), 97–103

Tucker, L.A., Cole, G.E. and Friedman, G.M. (1986) Physical fitness: a buffer against stress. *Perceptual and Motor Skills*, **63**, 955–961

Unger, K.V., Skrinar, G.S., Hutchinson, D.S. and Yelmokas, A.M. (1992) Fitness: a viable adjunct to treatment for young adults with psychiatric disabilities. *Psychosocial Rehabilitation Journal*, **15**(3), 21–28

Walls, R.T., Werner, T.J., Bacon, A. and Zane, T. (1977) Behaviour check-lists. In *Behavioral Assessment* (eds Cone, J.D. and Hawkins, R.P.), Brunner/Mazel, New York

Wilson, V.E., Berger, B.G. and Bird, E.I. (1981) Effects of running and of an exercise class on anxiety. *Perceptual and Motor Skills*, **53**, 472–474

Agoraphobia and panic attacks: a physical cause for a psychiatric problem

A discussion of the work of the Institute for Neuro-Physiological Psychology*

Peter Blythe

Introduction

Doctors and psychologists at the University of Pittsburg Medical School (1985) conducted a battery of vestibular and audiological tests on 8 patients with panic attacks and 13 patients with agoraphobia and panic attacks. The results were that 75% of those with panic disorder, and 60% of the agoraphobes, had abnormal vestibular responses. The researchers, Jacob, Moller, Turner and Wall, commented: 'In this preliminary study, we found that a surprisingly high proportion of patients suffering from panic attacks with dizzying, had abnormal vestibular and audiological function according to a standard criteria of the University laboratory.' They went on to say: 'Physical causes probably account for about a quarter of the phobias. ...It has been found, for instance, that *some phobics have a very minor impairment of the parts of the brain which affect balance, co-ordination and vision. The fact is sudden, inexplicable attacks of dizziness and instability which a person may wrongly associate with surroundings and come to anticipate and fear*' (emphasis added).

Levinson (1986) has claimed that his research has shown that over 90% of all phobics had 'an underlying dysfunction of the inner-ear system' and 'when I say inner-ear system, I am really referring to the cerebellar-vestibular system'.

More recently, Yardley *et al.* (1991) published a study of 23 people suffering from various types of vertigo, an acknowledged vestibular–oculomotor reflex (VOR) arc disorder, and showed how the vestibular problems led to individuals imposing the same restrictions upon themselves as those found in the agoraphobic population.

However, despite all the evidence, of which only a small part has been outlined above, either it has been ignored, or those researching into the role played by the vestibular and cerebellum have failed to follow up their research

* The INPP, 4 Stanley Place, Chester, England was established in 1975 to research into the effects of central nervous system dysfunctions on children with specific learning difficulties. The work also includes help for those adults suffering from agoraphobia and panic attacks which may have a neurological impairment as a basis of their problem. Appropriate CNS remediation programmes are built on the basis of eliminating retained primitive reflex patterns.

to try to ascertain exactly what is causing the underlying vestibular–oculomotor dysfunction.

It is the latter area of trying to isolate 'why' agoraphobics and panic sufferers have an impaired balance and oculomotor functioning which has occupied the writer for many years.

As from the mid-1970s the writer and others at the Institute for Neuro-Physiological Psychology (INPP) began to examine the central nervous system of patients suffering from agoraphobia and panic attacks. This involved, in addition to the normal 'soft signs', such tests as getting a patient to complete the tandem walk (placing one foot in front of the other, with heel touching the toes), the 'fog walk' (walking on the outsides of the feet), etc., but also examining for the continued presence of the primitive reflexes and the absence of the postural reflexes.

It is an accepted neurological fact that if there is a continued presence of a cluster of primitive reflexes, which should have been inhibited within the first year of life, there is a definite neurological dysfunction which is measurable (Fiorentino, 1981; Capute and Accardo, 1991).

The primitive reflexes

Among the many primitive reflexes which are tested for within the INPP's 'Neuro-Developmental Diagnostic Assessment' are the following.

Asymmetrical tonic neck reflex (ATNR)

This reflex emerges at approximately 20 weeks *in utero*; it is present at birth and should be inhibited by the developing CNS by, at the latest while awake, 8 months.

This particular reflex is activated by slowly turning the infant's head to one side, causing marked extension of the jaw-arm and to a lesser degree the jaw-leg, and flexion of the occipital arm and leg.

If the ATNR remains uninhibited into adulthood it affects the patient's balance and adversely affects oculomotor functioning (Holt, 1993; Goddard, 1994).

Tonic labyrinthine reflex (TLR) (in flexion and extension)

The TLR in flexion emerges *in utero* and the crude aspects of the reflexive response should be inhibited at about 16 weeks of life, whereas the TLR in extension emerges at birth and is slowly inhibited from 6 weeks up to $3\frac{1}{2}$ years of age. As it is inhibited, it precipitates the simultaneous development of certain of the postural reflexes, the symmetrical tonic neck reflex (STNR) and the Landau reflex, etc. (Goddard, 1994).

When the TLR fails to be inhibited, it not only affects the emergence of the head-righting reflexes, but it affects the development of the balance mechanism and significantly affects oculomotor functioning and visual-perceptual performance.

Oculo-head-righting reflex (OHRR) and labyrinthine head-righting reflex (LHRR)

As mentioned above, as the crude response of the TLR is controlled between the second and fourth month of life this enables the HRRs to emerge. The former, the OHRR, is elicited by slowly moving the patient's torso over to one side, then the other, and finally backwards and forwards.

Because the patient can see their position in space, this should facilitate the function of the semicircular canals, the labyrinth, which in turn activates the neck muscles so that the head adjusts to being in the midline position. In the case of the latter, if the eyes are closed, then the semicircular canals should 'sense' where the body is in space and reflexively brings the head to midline.

If the OHRR fails to emerge, eye functioning and visual perception is impaired, and the eyes cannot assist the patient in maintaining a stable position in space. When this aberrant reflex is found in conjunction with a retained or strongly residual ATNR, and a TLR, there is no gravitational security and the patient exists in a state of continual anxiety. Should the LHRR fail to emerge, and there is the cluster of other aberrant reflexes, the eyes have to take over and they require fixed reference points at all times to compensate for the labyrinthine–vestibular dysfunction. If there are no fixed reference points available, even for a very short period of time, the person experiences sudden and severe insecurity. Of course, if oculomotor functioning is dramatically impaired, the eyes cannot even attempt to compensate and the feelings of near panic are virtually always present.

The Moro reflex

This reflex emerges *in utero* and should be fully developed immediately after birth, and its function is to act as a 'danger alarm'. This is necessary because the cortex, the decision, logical and sensory interpreting part of the brain, is not operative, and the neonate is solely dependent upon reflexive responses which even it does not understand. Therefore, if there is, for example, a sudden loud noise or the position of the head or trunk is altered quickly, the baby cannot determine whether that stimulus is threatening or not, and the Moro 'panic alarm' response is triggered as a means of summoning help.

The physical movements involved in the Moro reflex are that the arms, and to a lesser degree the legs, abduct, and there is a rapid intake of breath. At the point of extension there is a momentary freeze, and then a return of the arms across the body. As the arms, and to a lesser degree the legs, return across the body, the earlier deep breath is released together with a loud cry.

Although the Moro reflex in its crude form should be inhibited between the second and fourth months, and slowly transformed into the adult startle or Strauss reflex, it can still be activated in later life by a major life-threatening situation. However, it should not be triggered off by minor stimuli.

According to Goddard (1994), if the Moro reflex remains strongly residually present or fully retained, the following symptoms may be observed:

'(a) Vestibular related problems such as motion sickness. Poor balance and co-ordination. ...
'(b) Physical timidity.

'(c) Oculo-Motor and Visual-perceptual problems, e.g. Stimulus Bound effect (cannot ignore irrelevant visual material within a given visual field, so that the eyes tend to be drawn to the perimeter of a shape, to the detriment of perception of internal features.
'(d) Poor pupillary reaction to light, photo-sensitivity, difficulty with black print on white paper. Tires easily under fluorescent lighting.
'(e) Possible auditory confusion – cannot discriminate between sounds easily, or occlude miscellaneous sound.
'(f) Allergies and lowered immunity, e.g. Asthma, Eczema, history of frequent E.N.T. infections.
'(g) Adverse drug reactions. Tires easily. Dislikes change or surprise.'

Oculomotor functioning

In addition to checking the above-mentioned reflexes, and many others, the INPP's diagnostic assessment also investigates oculomotor functioning, with particular attention being paid to the patient's ability, or lack of it, to get the eyes to fixate upon a stimulus – to determine whether the eyes can track a moving object or along a straight line without the balance being markedly affected. Also, to determine whether the patient is stimulus bound, particularly being unable to ignore irrelevant movement within a given visual field.

As a result of having examined approximately 2000 agoraphobes and panic victims over many years, the INPP has discovered that most of these have failed to respond to the various therapies of choice or been recidivists, and the INPP's 'Screening Questionnaire' has provided sufficient indication of an underlying CNS dysfunction. Subsequent examination of these patients revealed that they have a strongly residual or retained ATNR bilaterally or unilaterally, a strong TLR, lack of the appropriate HRRs, a Moro reflex, and are stimulus bound, together with oculo-tracking problems.

To illustrate how this combination of dysfunctions may well affect an agoraphobe–panic victim would be useful at this stage. One may imagine the agoraphobe and a companion going into a large, fluorescently-lit department store on a very warm and busy afternoon. The companion could well find the store oppressive, and through the various senses detect the heat, the masses of moving people and make a conscious decision: 'I do not like all this, and the quicker we get out of here the happier I shall be.' That would be a normal response, but the agoraphobe who is stimulus bound, has a Moro reflex, etc., does not have the time to come to that conscious decision. Instead all the varied stimuli overload the sensory system and activate the brainstem Moro reflex. The agoraphobe immediately goes into a panic state, with the cortex being temporarily bypassed. Only when the agoraphobe gets out of the store, the panic subsides and the sensory system is no longer overloaded by stimuli, can he or she utilize the cortex to try to sort out why the panic ocurred.

Blythe and McGlown (1982) published the results of a pilot study of 23 agoraphobes who had been examined for aberrant reflexes and oculomotor dysfunction. They wanted to test the hypothesis that if a cluster of aberrant reflexes did emerge in this group, it pointed towards the presence of an underlying organic dysfunction. The question had to be faced: 'In certain agoraphobes, is the presence of CNS deficits the primary factor in their condition, with the neurotic symptoms being of a secondary nature?'

The findings of the study were that 19 (82%) of the subjects studied had a sufficiently large cluster of dysfunctions to warrant the diagnosis of 'secondary agoraphobia'.

Later that same year a Swedish psychologist (Ljunggren, 1982), at the University of Gothenburg, chose for her MSc thesis to do a replica study of Blythe–McGlown, and '...using the identical test procedure as in the Blythe and McGlown study, to examine a group of agoraphobes, and make a descriptive presentation of the results'.

Although her sample consisted of only 8 patients, Ljunggren found that:

'...all subjects failed to perform adequately on the majority of the tests. Six subjects can be said to have severe gross-muscle coordination and balance problems, manifesting difficulties with 5 or all 6 tests administered.

'All subjects showed some degree of ocular-motor weakness. ...Four or more abnormal signs out of a total of 7 functions examined were found in as many as six subjects, including major impairment of their oculo-motor functioning.

'Only one subject had less than 5 aberrant reflex responses, and as many as five subjects manifested a cluster of uninhibited or untransformed primitive and postural reflexes, showing some abnormality in 6 out of the 9 reflexes examined. ...'

In the discussion section of her thesis she wrote: 'The claim made by Blythe and McGlown (1982), that there is an organic basis – dysfunction of the central nervous system with accompanying balance and motor-system disturbances and oculo-motor problems – underlying the presenting symptoms in certain cases of agoraphobia, is undoubtedly a controversial one. It is, to some degree, running against the currently accepted theories of the origins and nature of agoraphobia. However, it is a neurologically accepted fact that the continued presence of primitive reflexes in older children and adults is indicative of either a pathology or marked central nervous system dysfunction (Capute *et al.*, 1978; Bobath, 1979), and that patients, who have been suffering from a variety of psycho-pathological disorders, have been subsequently found to have detectable CNS dysfunctions (Hartocollis, 1968; Bellak, 1979).'

Retief (1990) completed a study entitled 'A psychophysiological approach to panic disorder'. Taking 10 patients suffering from agoraphobia and panic disorder, and 10 controls who had never suffered from any emotional, balance or oculo disorder, she examined them for the continued presence of (a) primitive reflexes, (b) gross-muscle co-ordination, (c) oculomotor functioning, and visual perception when measured broadly, and (d) neurological function.

Her study found that statistical analyses, 'supported the Blythe/McGlown hypothesis of CNS dysfunction as a prime aetiological factor'.

The examination for the continued presence of primitive reflexes, and using a scoring method that '0' meant no abnormality detected, '1' a residual presence of a reflex to 25%, '2' present to 50%, '3' present to 75% and '4' to be fully retained as a neonate, she found that the subjects scored 215, while the control group scored 85. This Retief demonstrated as statistically significant and supported the hypothesis that 'Subjects would exhibit more CNS dysfunction than would be shown by controls. ...'

As Ljunggren pointed out, the work at INPP does appear on the surface to fly in the face of current psychiatric thought, which gives grounds for further research and discussion.

Testing for CNS dysfunction

It is proposed that all diagnosed agoraphobes and those who are victims of recurrent panic attacks should be tested to ascertain if there might be an underlying CNS dysfunction which is the primary factor in their presenting problem. This could easily be done by using the INPP's 'Neuro-Developmental Screening Questionnaire'. Then, if there was sufficient evidence as a result of completing the questionnaire, which takes about 20–30 minutes, the patient could subsequently have a full neurodevelopmental assessment.

Opposition to the above suggestion could be that, even if a CNS dysfunction is found to be present, there is nothing that can be done to correct the abnormal reflex responses. Equally it could be argued that if a patient is told there is an underlying physical basis, this could have a detrimental psychological affect on the patient and compound the already severe symptoms. Concerning this, Hartocollis (1968) wrote: 'A patient who presumably has an organic deficit should be helped to recognise and accept his limitations so that he may behave and plan accordingly.' And Wender (1971) stated: 'The evidence for the usefulness of drug therapy is sometimes less than perfect, but that supporting the usefulness of psychological intervention is far from convincing.'

This particular argument or objection is contested here. Many year's experience by the writer and his colleagues, in the UK, Sweden, the Netherlands and the USA, have shown that when patients are told that there is an underlying physical basis for their presenting symptom or syndrome they experience a marked uplift in emotional functioning and adopt a new attitude towards themselves, their problem and their future. Of course, the patients have to be told exactly what the underlying factors are and have fully explained to them exactly how these play a part in their illness.

The INPP remedial programme

The claim made by the INPP that for the majority of agoraphobes and panic victims there is a cluster of aberrant reflexes can easily be verified by anyone familiar with the diagnostic methodology. However, it is when the INPP asserts that the aberrant primitive reflexes can successfully be inhibited in later life, either in childhood or during adulthood, that the work becomes controversial.

The INPP's remedial programme is based on the concept that all normally developing babies make the same repetitive stereotyped movements, among a number of apparently random movements, at approximately the same age. This fact was noted by Thelan (1979). Furthermore, INPP claims that if the therapist knows the age at which the primitive reflexes are normally inhibited, and knows what reflexive movements are involved in each of the primitive reflexes, then it can easily be seen and understood that the repetitive stereotyped movements directly assist the developing brain in the reflex inhibitory process. This concept can be summarized by stating that, in exactly the same way that the primitive, survival reflexes are programmed into the brainstem, so a physical-movement antidote to these reflexes is available at a higher brain developmental level to be activated at the appropriate stage and thereby inhibit the earlier reflexes. There is evidence to support this fact.

In normal development, after a baby has crawled on its stomach for a period of time, a synchronized movement which can only be accomplished after certain of the primitive reflexes have been inhibited, the baby at approximately 9 months is developmentally ready to defy gravity. To assist that major leap forwards, the developing brain releases the symmetrical tonic neck reflex (see Appendix to this chapter) which permits the baby to raise the trunk from the floor and go onto hands and knees. However, although the baby can now begin to defy gravity due to the STNR, the reflex does impose certain movement limitations on the infant. When the baby is on hands and knees and lifts the head to look straight in front, the arms reflexively straighten, the knees bend, and the infant's bottom sinks back onto the ankles. Still on hands and knees, if the infant looks down, the elbows bend until the head touches the floor.

Until the STNR is inhibited, the voluntary locomotion of creeping on all fours is impossible. Accordingly, all normal developing infants at about 10–11 months will reflexively rock backwards and forwards, thus directly inhibiting the STNR. Only after the rocking has successfully inhibited the reflex can the infant proceed to creep.

In exactly the same way that the reflex was there in the lower part of the brain, so the movement antidote was reflexively available to the infant to inhibit it.

By assessing what primitive reflexes are uninhibited, and knowing what repetitive stereotyped movements the neonate and infant would have made to inhibit them, a specific programme is given to each adult patient. Initially, this remedial programme aims to inhibit the earliest primitive reflex and then work developmentally upwards through the reflex hierarchy. The only difference between the baby's or infant's inhibitory movements and those used by the INPP is that the latter are completed daily in a slow, deliberate stylized sequence. The reflex-inhibition programme takes approximately 4–14 minutes per day, and is done in the patient's own home.

Each patient is seen at regular intervals for a 'review', when the reflexes and the earlier effect of the aberrant reflexes are retested. As one primitive reflex is inhibited, another reflex-inhibition movement is introduced to inhibit the next reflex in the hierarcy.

As the aberrant reflexes are corrected, the brain 'releases' the appropriate postural reflexes, both groups of reflexes being testable and measurable, and as that happens the majority of agoraphobes find their earlier presenting symptoms abate.

Finally, although this chapter has focused primarily on the possibility of re-educating aberrant reflexes found in panic disorder victims and agoraphobes, this could and should also be extended to patients suffering from balance problems and vertigo, as the same fundamental principles apply. There is also evidence available to suggest that those patients who do not respond to the therapies of choice may also have underlying CNS dysfunctions which prevent the various therapies, be they drugs, psychotherapy or behaviour modification, etc., from being effective (Hartocollis, 1968; Gustafson, 1970; Blythe and McGlown, 1978, 1980; Bellak, 1979; Levinson, 1986). This is yet a further avenue to be explored in an interesting new area of mental health care.

Appendix: Example of a reflex examination: the symmetrical tonic neck reflex (Field and Blythe, 1988)

Emergence: c. 6–8 months neonatal. Inhibition: c. 9–11 months.

STANDARD TEST
Subject position: 'Table', without glasses or contact lenses.

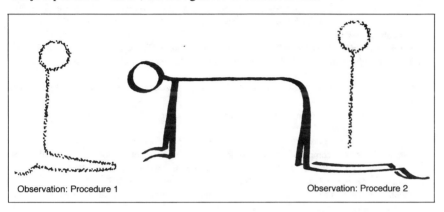

Observation: Procedure 1   Observation: Procedure 2

TEST PROCEDURE 1. Subject instructed to:
  1. Maintain body position and look down *very slowly*, as if looking behind him/her between the thighs.
  2. Hold this position for 2–3 seconds. See Observations.

TEST PROCEDURE 2. Subject instructed to:
  1. Maintain body position and look up *very slowly* to ceiling.
  2. Hold maximum lift for 2–3 seconds. See Observations.

REPEAT PROCEDURES 1 and 2 twice.

OBSERVATIONS
  Procedure 1. As subject looks down, does one/both arm(s) bend?
  Procedure 2. As subject looks up, does bottom move back and/or down towards the feet, or one or both feet lift?

SCORING Procedure 1
  0. No arm movement.
  1. Tremor in one or both arms.
  2. Slight but definite elbow bending in one or both arms.
  3. One or both arms bend and/or elevation of one or both feet.
  4. One or both arms bend to the floor.

SCORING Procedure 2
  0. No backward movement of bottom.
  1. Slight movement backwards, or slight arm extension.
  2. Definite movement backwards.
  3. Backward movement 3 cm, or one/both feet raised from floor.
  4. Complete backward movement, or one/both feet lifted at an acute angle.

References

Bellak, L. (1979) (Ed.) *Psychiatric Aspects of Minimal Brain Dysfunction in Adults*, Grune and Stratton, New York

Benedikt, M. (1870) Uber platschwindel. *Allgemeiner Wierner Medizinische Zeitung*, **15**, 488

Blythe, P. and McGlown, D.J. (1979) *An Organic Basis for Neuroses and Educational Difficulties*, Insight Publications, Chester

Blythe, P. and McGlown, D.J. (1980) *An Organic Basis for Neuroses and the Existence, Detection and Treatment of Secondary Neuroses*, The Swedish Institute for Neuro-Physiological Psychology, Gothenburg,, Sweden

Blythe, P. and McGlown, D.J. (1982) *Agoraphobia: is it organic?* World Medicine, London, July 10

Capute, A.J. and Accardo, P.J. (1991) *Developmental Disabilities in Infancy and Childhood*, Paul H. Brookes, Baltimore

Field, J. and Blythe, P. (1988) *Towards Developmental Re-education*, Field Publication, Wichenford, Worcester

Fiorentino, M.R. (1981) *Reflex Testing Methods for Evaluating CNS Development*, Charles C. Thomas, Springfield, USA

Goddard, S. (1994) *Reflexes – the basis of education.* INPP Monograph No. 1, Chester

Gustafson, F. (1970) A comparison of basic reflexes with the subtests of the purdue perceptual-motor survey. Unpublished thesis. Quoted in Rider, B.A., Relationship of postural reflexes to learning disabilities. *American Journal of Occupational Therapy*, July/August, 1972

Hartocollis, P. (1968) The syndrome of minimal brain dysfunction in young adult patients. Bulletin of the Menninger Clinic, **32**, No. 2. March 1968

Holt, K.S. (1991) *Child Development, Diagnosis and Assessment.* Butterworth-Heinemann, Oxford

Jacob, R.G., Moller, M.B., Turner, S.M. and Wall, C. (1985) Otoneurological examination in panic disorder and agoraphobia with panic attacks: a pilot study. *American Journal of Psychiatry*, **142**(6)

Levinson, H.N. (1986) *Phobia Free*, Evans, New York

Ljunggren, M. (1982) Agoraphobia: an organic basis? An exploratory neuropsychological approach. M.Sc. thesis, Gothenburg University, Sweden

Marks, I. (1981) Space 'phobia': a pseudo-agoraphobic syndrome. *Journal of Neurology, Neurosurgery, Psychiatry*, **44/5**, 387–391

Retief, L. (1990) A psychophysiological approach to panic disorder. Doctoral thesis

Sauvages, E.B. de, (1770) *Nosologie Methodique*. Vol. 2, pp. 606–617, Translated by J. Nicolas, Herissant, Paris

Schilder, P. (1933) The vestibular apparatus in neurosis and psychosis. *Journal of Nervous and Mental Disease*, **78**, 1–23, 137–164

Thelan, E. (1979) Rhythmical stereotypes in normal infants. *Animal Behaviour*, **27**, 699–715

Wender, P.H. (1971) *Minimal Brain Dysfunction in Children.* Wiley-International, New York

Westphal, C. (1871–72) Die agoraphobie: ein neuropathische erscheinung. *Archiv fur Pscyiatrie und nervenkrankheiten*, **3**, 138–71, 219–21

Yardley, L., Todd, A.M., Lacoudraye-Harter, M.M. and Ingham, R. (1991) *Psychosocial Consequences of Recurrent Vertigo*. Psychology and Health

15

Movement therapy:
old roots, new profession

Terri Fresko

Introduction

Movement and dance can be a healing creative process that many people in psychic distress often find helpful. The intimate link between psyche and soma, together with the power of play, means that movement and rhythm has a capacity to reach the non-verbal parts of ourselves. Dance movement therapists, who carry this deep conviction, can be found working with families, children and adults, individually or in groups, to help them find a healthier and more satisfying 'dance of life'. They work in educational institutions, mental health day centres, psychiatric hospitals, in private practice and in the community. Due to the pioneering nature of this profession in the UK, other professionals and clients are often unaware of the rationale and working methods of this therapy. This chapter therefore defines dance movement therapy, outlining the historical background to its emergence, the basic principles in practice, and provides examples to illustrate some of the pertinent clinical issues when working in this modality. The focus will be mainly on work with psychiatric populations, as this is the brief of the present publication.

The terms dance movement therapy, DMT, dance therapy, movement psychotherapy and movement therapy are used interchangeably by therapists, sometimes depending on the emphasis they wish to put on the guiding principles of their practice. This text will use the term movement therapy for simplicity and it is hoped that this choice of words does not detract from an acknowledgment that the roots of this form of therapy lie firmly in the universal human experience of dance.

Definition

Movement therapy is often confused with other disciplines such as physiotherapy and occupational therapy or thought of as a preconceived set of dance exercises. In fact, it is more accurately described as a form of psychotherapy, but one that can be applicable to those who are either non-verbal or those who find words hinder getting in touch with feelings that may have their roots in pre-verbal experiences. Movement therapy groups are more than simply 'activity' groups; they combine activity with a psychodynamic point of view. Stanton-Jones (1992) suggests movement therapy has the potential to fill the gap between occupational therapy and psychotherapy. As in all psychotherapies, the main principle is that the client and therapist enter a therapeutic relationship based on trust, in which problems and conflicts can be examined and integrated into the personality. The process of integration will enable the individual to cope with the residues of the past and with present difficulties in a manner that cause them the least distress.

Depending on the client's or group's level of functioning, it may be possible to work in an 'insight-orientated' way. Those who are less able to recognize the connections between their own movements and their emotional states can use the artistic medium to discover for themselves other ways of being in the world. What distinguishes movement therapy is its use of expressive movement and dance, often initiated by the client, and its focus on the individual meaning, feelings and images that these movements might evoke in the mover. The associations and reactions of the client are then used within the therapeutic relationship to help the client to move to a more appropriate level of functioning – physically, emotionally and mentally.

There is widespread acknowledgement that dance and exercise leads to effective stress reduction. The release of endorphins in the brain during physical activity leads to a sense of well-being and relaxation. However the use of movement therapy is not solely for cathartic and relaxation purposes. Movement therapists work from the assumption that this technique can be used for change both on body-movement and psychological levels. One of the pioneers of movement therapy in the USA has put it thus:

'If psychoanalysis brings about a change in mental attitude, there should be a corresponding physical change. If dance therapy brings about a change in the body's behaviour, there should be a corresponding change in the mind. Both methods aim to change the total human, mind and body' (Schoop, 1974)

Movement therapists' conviction about the close link between motion and emotion, between body and soul, is derived on one hand from our personal experiences and, on the other, from a great body of knowledge that probably reaches back to our ancestors.

The origins of movement therapy

Dance in society

People have used dance and movement for expression, communication and healing purposes since the dawn of history. Harvest time, wars, rites of passage have all been accompanied by dances to unite people in a common rhythm. In religious contexts, dance can at times lead to altered states of consciousness, as is the case with the dervishes who express their link with divine energy through their whirling. Across the ages, one of the crucial functions of dance may be the 'prevention of depression and accumulation of other psychic stresses' (Lamba, 1965). Today, across the globe, in flamenco, tap dancing, rock and roll or African rhythms, the joy and vitality that dance can bring is unmistakable. The joy is perhaps especially poignant as adults in Western cultures often lose their basic capacity to dance spontaneously. It is as if large numbers of us have somehow internalized the cultural inability to nurture both body and mind:

'Dance may ... function like play, exploratory behaviour, rituals of rebellion' or cathartic outlets for deviance, in which a segment of the psyche or world is represented in a non-threatening manner in order to understand or cope with it' (Hanna, 1967).

Exploring the psychobiological bases of dance in different societies, Hanna suggests that the power of dance in social situations may be due to its encompassing all the senses, i.e. auditory, tactile, visual, kinaesthetic, smell. Movement therapists also recognize the value of using the senses and attempting to integrate them with verbal and symbolic material that emerges within sessions. Ayres (1991) has written about the role of sensory integration for the development of body image, cognitive learning and motor skills, with implications not just for children but throughout adult life.

Modern dance as a catalyst

The advent of modern dance since the turn of the century has perhaps been the great impetus that gave birth to the practice of movement therapy as we know it today. The early modern dancer valued spontaneity, authenticity of expression, awareness of the body and was propelled by 'the desire to express the totality of the human experience without limitations'. In Martha Graham's words, one can clearly sense her appreciation of movement as a gateway to one's personal history. 'It [dance] comes from the depths of man's inner nature, the unconscious, where memory dwells.... It goes into the experience of man, the spectator, awakening similar memories' (Morrison Brown, 1980).

It was a dancer, Marian Chace, who, in the 1940s, introduced rhythmic group movement and dance into the wards of St. Elizabeth's Hospital in Washington, DC, before the widespread practice of drug therapy. Psychiatric staff at the hospital recognized how dance-movement techniques could help reach many disturbed and withdrawn patients. Other dancer/teachers working in private and public mental health settings gradually emerged, and in 1966 a group of such pioneers came together to form the American Dance Therapy Association (ADTA).

These pioneers and their students have developed different approaches to movement therapy, ranging from the psychoanalytical (Siegel, 1984) to Jungian (Chodorow, 1991), While deriving inspiration from theorists such as Winnicott, Stern, Foulkes and Bion. However, the basic principle that binds all movement therapists is the understanding that body-movement reflects unconscious processes, personality characteristics and feeling states and that it can be used for the integration of the ignored, split-off parts of the individual. Let us first look at what is communicated in movement, before we consider how movement can be healing.

Movement and child development

From conception to death, movement is ever present; even during sleep, the rhythm of the breath, the subtle growing and shrinking movements in the chest are observable. Observers of human development have consistently theorized that the mastery of motor skills is critical to a young child's ability to develop a sense of itself as separate from its surroundings, to learn certain cognitive concepts and to gain a sense of control in relation to its environment (Erikson, 1950; Piaget. 1952; Gessell and Amatruda, 1952). It was Freud who pointed out that 'the ego is first and foremost a body ego' (Freud, 1923). The early physical experiences of internal sensations (hunger, pain) and external stimuli (visual, tactile, auditory, etc.) combine to help the infant develop a sense of itself as distinct and separate from the world around.

Similarly, Mahler and her colleagues (Mahler *et al.*, 1975) regard bodily experiences to be at the crux of the psychological birth of the individual, in so far as separation and individuation processes which render it possible are 'dependent upon and coincide with the acquisition of the autonomous locomotor function of the ego'. The achievement of standing and finding stability in the upright posture go hand in hand with a sense of emerging from infancy to join the ranks of the adult. Often in therapy, it is our task to help clients retrace certain crucial developmental experiences and enable them to make a transition from a dependent position that signals their dependency, to an upright, grounded, well-balanced posture that coincides with greater self-esteem and autonomy.

Researchers who have studied the communications of infants with their care-takers have concluded that, through the interpersonal relationship, the infant learns to regulate his state of arousal and to control motor impulses (Brazelton, *et al.*, 1974; Stern, 1974). Interactional synchrony is to do with our unconscious movement reactions to others' speech rhythms or movements. Condon's research has found interactional synchrony to be present in neonate movements in relation to human speech, indicating that human infants are born neurologically equipped with responsiveness on a kinaesthetic level. It is one aspect of communication that has been seen to be deficient in psychotic patients.

Contributions of a psychoanalyst

For the movement therapist, perhaps one of the most important contributions to the greater understanding of body-movement behaviours of children has been made by Dr Kestenberg who, starting with a psychoanalytic framework, researched into the movement patterns in infancy and childhood, analysing them in Laban's Effort–Shape terms. She has found that movement patterns and body attitudes progress through specific stages, correlating with psychosexual developmental stages outlined by Anna Freud (1965). Kestenberg explains this by suggesting that 'motor apparatus are put into the service of developing mental structures' (Kestenberg, 1975). Moreover, she regards observable rhythms of tension flow and shape flow to be manifestations of personality that is constitutional to a certain extent and that is shaped and reshaped in coping with psychological needs and environmental influences.

For example, during the first year of life, when the infant is learning about its environment mainly through the erogenous zone of the mouth, rhythms of sucking and later biting become the means of tension discharge and of expressing needs and feelings. On the other hand, modes of relatedness to the environment are expressed in the infant's shaping of his body. Through narrowing or widening, the infant either shrinks away from its surroundings or reaches out to it. Using different terminology, Stern (1974) also has identified the approach and withdrawal patterns that infants engage in, in relation to their care-givers.

Perhaps the more significant aspect of these patterns experienced in infancy and childhood is that the movement experiences remain somehow ingrained within the individual's neurological pathways. The characteristic quality of our earliest relationships are 'imprinted' into our muscle memory. In later life, it is likely that the unique, repetitive 'missteps' of approach and withdrawal will be re-enacted, often within other intimate and significant relationships. These are precisely the sorts of difficulties that impel people to seek therapy, to begin the process of changing long-established patterns.

Movement and non-verbal communication

Detailed research into non-verbal communication during the 1960s and 1970s has contributed to the development of a coherent rationale for the use of movement in psychotherapy (Condon, 1967; Birdwhistell, 1970; Kendon, 1979). Through microanalysis of sound films it has been shown that units of observable body movement tend to change patterns and direction simultaneously with units of speech. This was observed to be true both for the speaker (self-synchrony) and for the listener (interactional synchrony). These findings seem to be strong indicators of the unity of our verbal and non-verbal behaviours.

There are other studies that suggest movement and personality are inter-related, North (1990), also using Effort–Shape analysis, has found that her movement assessments of school-age children were compatible with assessments from educational psychologists and teachers in making inferences about personality traits. Another colleague of Rudolf Laban, Warren Lamb, devised the 'action profiling' technique. In this method, by noting the effort and shape qualities present in one's movement repertoire and by noting whether these occur as total body movements or only gesturally, it is possible to discover the person's managerial qualities, such as communication with others, decision-making and anticipating. It is also claimed that in reassessments over long term, the action profile is constant, despite the fact that different situations bring out different aspects of our movement patterns.

Movement and psychopathology

In psychoanalytical thinking, the work of Reich represents a major development in that it focused specifically on the body as revealing character structure. He recognized chronic muscular tensions as representing 'defensive armouring' that individuals have developed in the process of protecting themselves from painful experiences. As defensive posturing becomes habitual it ceases to fulfil its original adaptive function and instead prevents a healthy expression of emotions through the medium of energy discharge, the body. The creator of bioenergetics, Lowen, similarly stresses that emotion means 'motion outward' and outward is synonymous with discharge: 'A therapy which encourages expressive movement increases the motility of the organism, improves its aggression and creates a feeling of strength on both the physical and psychic levels' (Lowen, 1971).

Deutsch (1962) has worked in the psychoanalytic process to reach unconscious memories and feelings through the body's sensations. Similarly, Mahl (1979) has noted that certain body movements precede what he calls 'primitive ideation' such as dreams, images and perceptions which in turn precede verbalization of wishes or memories that have gained access to consciousness.

Clinical experience leads us to suspect that psychiatric breakdowns often correlate with changes in movement patterns. Dulicai (1980) suggests that a drastic change in a person's usual repertoire is a strong indicator of increased suicidal risk. Bartenieff recounts an incident where, observing a group therapy session through a one-way screen, she correctly identifies a patient as suicidal, when the movement phrasing of the patient ends with an abrupt cutting off of the action (Bartenieff and Lewis, 1980).

By applying the Effort–Shape system of analysis, Davis and Bartenieff systematically analysed the movement patterns of psychiatric patients (Davis, 1970). The diagnostic scale consisted of pathological movement characteristics that Davis had observed in hospitalized patients. Results indicated that there was an important correlation between the clinical features of depression and the movement characteristics of diffusion (unclear spatial patterns, diffuse over-lapping of actions, unclear effort patterns) and flaccid and limp features. Moreover, certain forms of disorganization were found to correlate significantly with the diagnosis of chronic schizophrenia.

A common vocabulary

The movement therapists' search for a universal language of movement has been greatly aided by the efforts of Rudolf Laban, who was an architect and painter before taking up choreography and dance. He worked in Paris and Germany where he founded dance and movement schools, and developed a dance notation system call Labanotation. The variables in this system describe the structural aspects of movement – where, what, when – which make it valuable for record-ing and reproducing dance sequences. Just before World War II, Laban moved to England, where he collaborated with, among others, Marion North, Warren Lamb and Valerie Preston-Dunlop. The latter has been influential in introducing educational dance to Britain's schools.

Laban also became involved in efficiency studies in British factories during World War II. In this context, he analysed individual movement styles to deter-mine whether a particular worker would be suitable for a specific job and made recommendations to minimise fatigue and maximise efficiency. From this grew Effort analysis, which describes the qualitative and expressive aspect of movement: how, and with what intensity. Movement therapists are most interested in this aspect of movement.

Effort and shape theory

Each of the four factors of motion – space, weight, time, flow – occur on a continuum, the extremes of which are in either indulging in or fighting against the use of that factor. In view of the fact that Freud in his psychoanalytical frame-work believed in the existence of two drives – aggression and libido – it is interesting to note here that Laban (1960) regarded fighting and indulging attitudes to motion factors as forming the basic aspects of the emotions of hatred and love. In the middle of the range for each motion factor, there is not an active attitude or intention towards the factor; this neutral state does not constitute a predominant quality of the movement.

The proportion of the various combinations of two Effort factors and three Effort factors any person uses will vary according to the task at hand. Similarly, this proportion will vary between different individuals, depending on their characteristic coping styles. For a detailed description of Effort combinations, their variations and behavioural correlations, the reader is referred to North (1990) and Dell (1977).

The theory of Shape, on the other hand, was developed by Warren Lamb, a colleague and collaborator of Laban. The concept of Shape involves three kinds of movement in increasing complexity: Shape flow involves growing and shrinking movements, gathering towards and scattering away from the body centre. This is the kind of movement seen in young infants. Directional movement is linear action through space, e.g. forward, backward, downward, upward. Shaping involves three-dimensional use of space and enables one to accommodate one's body shape to the environment.

Together, Effort–Shape analysis provide a comprehensive system of movement observation that yields information about the individual's coping mechanisms and his relationship to the environment. North (1990) stresses the importance of movement phrases, i.e. the sequences of different elements and their combinations, in 'revealing a person's characteristic routes of mental and emotional activities'.

Movement observation and assessment of an individual's level of functioning is perhaps one of the most essential aspects of the therapist's tasks. It is important to stress here that this observation, whilst being objective, is at the same time informed by the movement therapist's own training and experience in various movement forms, whether they be yoga, the Alexander technique, tai-chi, contemporary or improvised dance. These and other methods in different ways support and expand our knowledge of the body–mind.

While none of the British training programmes requires prospective therapists to be skilled ballerinas or dancers, there is nevertheless a strong expectation that students will be conversant in the use of their bodies, This knowledge of our own bodies and movement patterns enables us to use our kinaesthetic responses within the therapy sessions.

The movement data that observation will yield can be categorized under the four broad headings shown below.

Body attitude

This relates to the characteristic shape that the body takes on in stillness, whether standing or sitting. It involves such questions as: does the person stress their verticality, how wide is the base of support, are there any tension areas such as the neck or pelvis, do any parts appear to be split off from the others, is there an overwhelming preference for one sitting position?

One woman with unexpressed and unmet dependency needs who attended groups in a psychiatric day hospital habitually sat collapsed to her right side, so that she almost appeared to be reclining like a baby at the breast. A torso that is sunken and concave signals weak back muscles and may well be correlated with a depressed state, as if the person literally cannot hold themselves up.

Dynamic range

This category will yield information about the individual's use of Effort elements as outlined above. Can the person be direct in their actions as well as multi-focused? What is the relationship to the floor: does the person appear to be firmly grounded or to be walking as if on clouds? Is there a preference for slow movements to the exclusion of quick ones? Does the person show extremes of tension, perhaps in constantly wringing the hands? Do two or more different rhythms appear simultaneously in different parts of the body? Does the person actively use all body parts or are there some that are held still for long periods? Is there evidence that the client can use the whole range of developmental movement rhythms, or only the early rhythms characteristic of the oral phase of development? What are the preferred types of phrasing movement: are they impulsive phrases with the emphasis at the beginning, is there a clear beginning, middle and end to actions or do they run-on?

One long-term psychiatric patient had minimum use of strength that was outwardly directed; instead she coped by adjusting muscle tension, that is by continual changes between high muscle tension (bound flow) and low muscle tension (free flow). Another patient frequently swings his leg in a steady smooth rhythm, while a more uneven staccato action can be observed in the hands and arms.

Use of space

This relates to how a person relates to the space around them. Do they take up a lot of space, with an unawareness of boundaries (their own and other people's)? Do they seem to shrink away, can they extend forward and upwards as well as backward and downward? Are the movements primarily on the horizontal plane of action? Is it possible to rise or advance with full postural support for the action? Most schizophrenic patients have some deficit in the way they relate to their environment. They may have limited use of personal space with perhaps little or no awareness of their back-space. Not surprisingly, these physical difficulties correlate with cognitive difficulties as well as emotional ones.

Interactional

Here we focus on interpersonal aspects of non-verbal behaviour: the extent and quality of eye contact in different contexts; the extent that the person is willing and able to stay in synchrony with others' movements with a group context as well as on a one-to-one level; the clients' movements towards and away from people; any blocking movements. All provide valuable information regarding a person's range and quality of interaction with others. Unusual fear of touch or physical proximity, or disregard for other people's personal space. e.g. inappropriate touching, are all common disturbances that one might encounter within a psychiatric setting. To the movement therapist, these difficulties communicate corresponding problems in the area of relationships.

Some useful concepts

Mirroring

Having gathered information about the client's use of the body, the movement therapist will attempt to establish rapport non-verbally. This is done by attuning to the non-verbal style of the client, whether by reflecting the intensity of the movement, spatially taking on a similar position or 'mirroring' their rhythms in a way that is supportive and communicates an understanding. Winnicott (1967) writes about mirroring in the context of the mother–infant relationship, wherein the infant sees itself reflected in the mother's face. Through this process the infant learns eventually to distinguish between itself and the outside world. Winnicott draws a close parallel with psychotherapy, which he sees as as 'long-term giving back what the patient brings', that will enable the patient to find their own real self.

One new group member, after experiencing the non-verbal attuning of the therapist, said 'it was like finding a kindred spirit'. Occasionally, a client will resist the therapist mirroring and may feel 'engulfed'. This communicates to the therapist the extreme pain of seeing oneself, as is sometimes the case with anorexics, both literally in front of the mirror and through the therapist.

Play as problem-solving

Another concept relevant to movement therapy is that of play as specified by Winnicott (1988), who theorized that 'psychotherapy takes place in the overlap of two areas of playing, that of the patient and that of the therapist'. According to him, if a client is unable to play, then the work of the therapy involves moving the client to a stage where he can play. This concept is especially helpful when working with chronic patients who, through years of psychic distress and dependency on carers, appear to have lost all sense of mastery and control over their lives, as well as having diminished access to a range of spontaneous emotional responses. Movement-play, word-play, the symbolization of internal conflicts in any modality helps us to gain a handle on life again (Erikson, 1965). The emphasis of such play is on the active manipulation of the environment, on changing the passive experiencing of life to the active, through the movement process (Dosamantes-Alperson, 1981).

Healing factors

Schmais (1985) outlines eight healing processes in group therapy, as a preliminary attempt to categorize the ways in which non-verbal groups support change. These factors are: synchrony, expression, rhythm, vitalization, integration, cohesion, education and symbolism. Through synchrony, a 'group achievesa sense of solidarity' and cohesion as people moving together identify withone another. Expression relates to the way in which 'internal states are made conscious through external expression'; frightening feelings become less dangerous as they are shared with others symbolically in the movement.

In breathing in and out, in resting and working, in giving and taking, in moving towards and moving away, rhythms of life have a regulating and healing influence. Movement therapy focuses on rhythm as the major organizer of our actions and feelings. Vitalization is another function of movement and dance in helping people to regain an enjoyment in activity; Schmais suggests that 'the inability of patients to function can be linked to their misdirected use of energy', resulting in powerlessness.

Integration relates to the way in which body actions, sounds, words, images and feelings are connected in movement therapy. Past experiences are understood and linked with present patterns. Cohesiveness results from people actively participating in each other's symbolic expression; 'finding a commonality of experience' through sharing similar feelings as reflected in movement.

When patients try out new patterns and understand old ones, by leading and following, by learning to trust others as well as support them, movement therapy provides an avenue for education. Movement therapy is also an excellent platform for symbolism, which according to Schmais 'allows for psychic distance from private preoccupations' (Schmais, 1985).

Therapy in action

The group now considered has been running for two years and is open to patients within the rehabilitation services of a large mental hospital. The group members are long-stay patients suffering from schizophrenia. They come to the group from hospital wards or from supported housing in the community. Some patients use the group as a place to support them through their move into progressively more independent lodgings. For others who will always need high levels of support, the group can help to improve the quality of life in hospital.

The group meets weekly for 1 hour in the movement therapy room within the hospital. A therapist is also an administrator who ensures that the time and space boundaries of sessions are maintained and unnecessary changes are kept to a minimum. Regularity of attendance is also advisable for a group that aims to work psychodynamically. However, regularity and commitment is universally problematic for these long-term hospitalized clients who may be influenced by a multiplicity of factors such as lack of motivation, memory deficits and difficulty in establishing and maintaining meaningful relationships. Moreover, these disabled clients also have difficulties 'maintaining an internal representation of the group' (Sandel and Johnson, 1983); the notion of a group identity is out of reach for those whose self-identity is so fragile.

The present author attempted to deal with this issue by establishing a group culture among group members, by pointing out absences, explicitly acknowledging attendances and even remembering absent members through their preferred movement suggestions. In addition to this, contacting carers and nursing staff before and after sessions, written reports and, where possible, attendance at reviews, became an important part of communicating the emphasis on regular attendance. The issue of therapist and staff relations and their ramifications for the therapy process are dealt with at greater length elsewhere (Liebowitz, 1992; Stanton-Jones, 1992).

Regarding the structure of therapy sessions, we generally start in a circle, a democratic formation where each member can easily see and hear others. This formation may remain throughout the hour depending upon the needs of the group. Various balls, pieces of stretchy cloth or stretch bands can be used to facilitate movement and connection between group members. Objects used in this way are frequently imbued with symbolic meaning, with personal and group significance. A stretchy piece of cloth can represent the sea, a universal metaphor for feelings. A journey taken together can symbolize the solidarity which group members feel with each other. For some in the group, it can bring back memories of journeys from the past.

Music is often a good organizer of bodily rhythms and therefore an essential part of most sessions with clients coping with long-term mental illness. Care has to be taken that the choice of music reflects and supports the emotional state of the group, i.e. an animated group will not react favourably to a meditative slow piece of music. Often the group itself chooses the extent to which they will make physical contact; negotiating how much contact occurs, with what body parts, and perhaps even how to refuse it, are all parts of the work of the group in relearning social rules and asserting personal needs and boundaries. Sometimes the therapist can suggest hand-holding in a circle, as a way of starting or concluding a session. It is generally advisable to conclude sessions with some verbal sharing, partly to aid retention of session events and partly as a transition to the everyday mode of talking that we willall return to.

Some specific group members

Rose

Rose is a 48-year-old patient with a 10-year history of psychiatric illness. She is tall, thin, and holds extreme amounts of tension all over her body. This leads to her head being perpetually bowed, while her torso takes on an exaggerated S-shape, with a retreating chest and a lower torso advancing before her. Her arms are always held close to her, with elbows nearly resting on her stomach, her hands always closed, fingers appearing as claws in their frozen position. Her walk is slowed down, probably due to the effects of medication. Every move she makes looks as if a great deal of effort is spent to keep it under control. One can only imagine the distress and discomfort of being in Rose's body.

Rose joined the group when it was first established 2 years ago. At the time she was extremely irregular in her attendance, perhaps not confident that she could bring her difficult feelings. Rose challenges her carers to be able to 'hold' her despair, rage and terror. This is expressed in her absolute conviction that she is in the grip of some deadly disease, such as cancer or diabetes, in spite of repeated reassurances and test results proving negative. This conviction in Rose may be seen as a metaphoric expression of the terrible feelings that she is carrying inside, that 'attack' her in a very devastating way.

The movement process gave Rose an opportunity to externalize and symbolize the fury in her stamping that is reminiscent of a 2-year-old's temper tantrum, and in her beating a huge ball, while being supported and understood by other group members. During the past year, Roses's attendance became more regular but her tolerance of the group was still limited. She would either arrive furious and walk out again or she would stay for 15-20 minutes and then storm out after a huge outburst. In both eventualities, Rose was acting out a process of dumping all her unbearable feelings, without giving herself the chance to re-own them.

Rose then went through a phase of being able to verbalize her envy of those who she perceived as healthy. She simply could not accept help or caring or affection; in Melanie Klein's terms the 'good breast' could not be there for her. Though still convinced she was carrying all the 'badness', and others had the 'goodness', this represented a progression for Rose, who could now remain in the same room with others.

More recently, Rose has come to the session with greater composure, this time complaining about not being able to eat and feeling weak. This made sense, one could see that Rose was also unable to 'eat' within the sessions, more and more taking on a passive role, which one can speculate as conveying her internal spiritual deadness. A turning point came when the writer reflected to Rose that she was not 'feeding' in the session that day. Rose then came out of her passive reclining sitting position and actively started pulling at the piece of stretch cloth she and the group had been holding. This is an example of how the verbal metaphors can be used in movement therapy to bring about changes in behaviour (Cox, 1987).

Jane

Jane is a 40-year-old single person who had recently moved to supported housing before joining the group two years ago. She maintained a one-piece torso, with little mobility through the waist. Her stance was more like a toddler, but without the strong relation to the ground and gravity. When Jane walked, she waddled from side to side. There was a sense of her being quite floppy and loose in the periphery of the body. Pointing at her solar plexus, she complained of a 'trapped nerve' in the chest, which she felt was the cause of the tension in that area.

When she initially joined the group, Jane found it difficult to remain within the boundaries of the circle and would regularly 'break away', flitting around the room like a practising bird in flight. She liked free-flowing swinging movements of the arms, as she saw these as helping her tension.

Jane gradually became more attached to the group, as evidenced in more regular attendance to group sessions. Around this time, she was more able to associate feelings and images in relation to the movement process. As the huge ball was beaten wildly, she was able to share her fury and frustration at the psychiatric services which she accused of not knowing what they were doing. In a way, they became substitutes for her parents who had not known what to do with her. She carried around a continual sense of guilt for causing everyone problems. Later, it became clear that beyond the guilt was intense anger, directed mainly at her parents.

When the ball was rocked gently, Jane thought of the ball as a huge pregnant tummy or her dead boyfriend's head. These experiences became avenues for Jane to integrate some of her unresolved feelings of loss to do with the recent death of her boyfriend and her abortions. Related to these losses was a sense of hopelessness that she would never lead an independent, fulfilled life.

After 2 years of group membership, she decided she wanted to leave the group. One sensed it was important for Jane not to feel stuck, to feel that she had achieved certain things in the therapy and that she could 'graduate'. It was also becoming clearer that the group, due to its composition, could not challenge Jane to work at a deeper level. She left, still quite disabled from her illness but somehow with an experience of being held as well as being in charge.

Maggie

Maggie is a 24-year-old black patient with a recent history of violent attacks on staff and fire-setting. When the author met her within the rehabilitation services, she was spending most of her time sleeping in the day room of the ward. She was initially reticent to join the group as she felt uneasy about her weight and her body. Once engaged, she immediately became a very keen participant, with a strong sense of rhythm, carrying on the movement when others had stopped.

It seemed as if her need to move was like an unstoppable impulse, the movement enjoyed for the body sensations that it evoked.

Maggie speaks softly with a child-like voice and comes across as a very sweet 3-year-old in an adult body. In fact her sweetness is rather one-dimensional as she often denies angry, destructive feelings. For her, the group and what goes on in it are always positive. However, her strength of feeling does surface when she is banging a drum, pulling a stretch-band or tapping her feet on the floor.

Initially, one felt that Maggie's identification with the therapist was so strong that there might be a confusion about our psychic boundaries. She would, for example, say: 'you feel like a small baby'. When asked if she feels like a small baby, she would be surprised that this was known, but confirm that it was the case. I also wondered if Maggie actually wanted to be me; being slim, I probably came close to the 'ideal image' that she had portrayed in her art therapy sessions while in a different ward.

In the first 9 months of her group membership, Maggie brought her pre-occupation with food into the sessions. One could also say that she was a hungry baby in the group, taking in what was on offer with a huge appetite. For example, the stretch cloth, a regular prop in the group, is most often held with a minimum of emotional investment by other members. Maggie, on the other hand, derives great pleasure from pulling it, gathering it to herself, grabbing it with enthusiasm and joy. It is as if Maggie is trying to incorporate everything in an attempt to drown the inner void. For the time being, she cannot face the monsters within her; instead she probably feels safer projecting them onto the creations in her mind.

Robert

Robert is a 67-year-old patient with a 35-year history of hospitalization. He has moved to supported housing in the community, while being supported by attendance in OT, music therapy and movement therapy. After 18 months, he still continues his membership of the two arts therapies groups.

Robert is bony and highly tense; he demonstrates a degree of energy unusual for his fellow patients. Characteristically, he holds himself in a hunched posture with his head forward of the rest of the body and arms held close to the torso. At certain times, this posture becomes exaggerated and he sits in an almost fetal position, holding his hand against his forehead. On these occasions, he appears anxious and preoccupied. He denies that this may reflect any change in his feelings, but describes it as 'habit'. He has acknowledged now that this habit is not particularly comfortable.

In the movement, Robert initially chose to initiate strong, clear rhythms as in clapping. This structure seemed to provide him with the predictability and reliability of a strong rhythm without the need to change his body shape or posture. When standing around in a circle for a specific movement activity, he would be the first to sit down again, preferring the safety of his chair, even though he is strong enough to walk briskly and for considerable distances.

For some months now, Robert is initiating movements that involve stretching and extending beyond his limited personal space. He does this with a big smile, as if he has discovered something new for himself. It is as if he is slowly extending his repertoire of possibilities; although a limited change, it represents an increased capacity to reach out, both physically and psychologically.

Sean

Sean is 30 years old and has been involved in psychiatry for 8 years. There are plans for him to move to a hostel when a suitable placement is found. Sean's major behavioural problem now is his periodic loss of temper, which involves physical aggression towards objects. These episodes are then followed by strong feelings of guilt.

Sean is overweight, wears thick glasses and walks with a downward emphasis throughout his body. After any extended exercise he gets easily out of breath and usually sweats profusely. His shoulders appear almost non-existent as his neck and arms are connected by a continuous curved line. His hands are child-like and lack tonus. He has a degree of body awareness and has talked about how, in the past, he would carry his head bowed when he was 'drugged up', but that now he can carry his head straight, though he does revert when particularly stressed. He is also observant on a body-movement level, both about his own and others' movements.

On the whole, Sean prefers to initiate movements that he perceives will strengthen his arm muscles. He also seems to seek out group activities that involve a common rhythm, free-flowing movements such as swinging or those that involve a strong emphasis or impact. In a recent session when he had talked about times when he had lost his temper, the group movement evolved into working with the stretch cloth, and members talked about imagining that it was like the sea. Sean derived a certain pleasure from shaking the cloth vigorously to make the sea rough. This then became a metaphor for turbulent feelings, which both the group and Sean could use creatively.

Sean joined the group 2 months ago, when he approached the therapist with questions about the way the movement therapy group worked. Initially, he was probably attracted to the idea of movement as a means of feeling stronger, more energetic and active; movement as an antidote to the lethargy that strikes most hospitalized patients. The group is already a place for Sean to deal symbolically with outbursts of feelings that seem uncontrollable, inexplicable and potentially destructive.

Fred

Fred is another relatively new member, having joined at the same time as Sean. He has spent more than 20 years in hospitals, initially in locked wards because he would hit children. Now, there is little outward aggression in him, except that his hands are often locked into fists and he sometimes gestures semi-threateningly with them. He is thin, holds his torso in a concave shape, with tremendous amounts of tension in his muscles, but he belies the tension by slouching casually into his chair.

Fred can only attend to one stimulus at a time; this can be seen in the inflexibility of his torso, which only faces forward. His gaze is intense, sometimes sideways, perhaps because he dare not turn his head. Fred's clearest verbal communications consist of slight lip movements to indicate his wants.

In the group, Fred's involvement is very variable. At times he will slouch, almost unaware of anyone else. At other times he will sit up straight, make eye contact with group members but remain largely unresponsive to the group activity, with perhaps brief tokens of involvement and then a quick retreat back. In a session where his fist movement was expanded on by the therapist and used as part of the group work, Fred transformed into a highly involved member.

For now, Fred's repertoire is very limited. One sometimes gets the sense that conscious initiation of a movement or an action for him is somehow not an option, and that his movement behaviour is made up of habitual residues from his past life. Therapeutic goals for Fred would include encouraging him to feel part of the group by sharing symbolic experiences and expanding his repertoire of relating to others. When assessing and treating severely socially and emotionally disabled people like Fred, therapists have to be aware of setting themselves realistic goals.

Conclusion

This chapter has attempted to introduce some of the theoretical underpinnings of movement therapy and highlighted these with practical examples of the way it can be used within psychiatric rehabilitation services. The focus on concrete actions means that those clients whose hold on reality is tenuous can literally 'get a grip on life' again. Working with symbolic associations, on the other hand, enables the therapist to enter the world of dreams, fantasies, psychotic phenomena and artistic creations and to ease the patient back to the world of reality.

The rationale for movement therapy is evident; it is developmentally based and therefore provides the therapist with a diagnostic and treatment tool that allows us to make contact with regressed patients to whom the medium of verbal language does not always reach. Thus, as with other arts therapies, non-verbal clients can make use of the communicative, creative, playful and ultimately healing aspects of the artistic medium. Higher-functioning clients appreciate the opportunity to express themselves in a different way, as words can often be experienced as an inadequate medium to communicate extremely frightening, dangerous and apparently illogical feelings.

The process of therapy is more like a journey of discovery for all those involved. In movement therapy, it is often the case that a new language of movement is discovered and this discovery becomes a metaphor for the possibility of being understood in a very fundamental way, much more like a mother will understand the wordless communications of her infant.

Appendix: Useful addresses

Association for Dance Movement Therapy UK
c/o Arts Therapies Dept.
Springfield Hospital
61 Glenburnie Road
London SW17 7DJ

Laban centre for Movement and Dance
Laurie Grove
London SE14 6NH

Roehampton Institute
Digby Stuart College
Roehampton Lane
London SW15 5PJ

University of Hertfordshire
7 Hatfield Road
St. Albans
Herts. AL1 3RS

References

Ayres, A.J. (1991) *Sensory Integration and the Child*, Western Psychological Services, California
Bartenieff, I. and Lewis, D. (1980) *Body and Movement: Coping with the Environment*, Gordon and Breach, London
Birdwhistell, R. (1970) *Kinesics and Context*, University of Pennsylvania Press, Philadelphia
Brazelton, T.B., Koslowski, B. and Main, M. (1974) The origins of reciprocity: the early mother–infant interaction. In *The Origins of Behavior* (eds Lewis, M. and Rosenblum, L.), Wiley, New York
Chodorow, J. (1991) *Dance Therapy and Depth Psychology*, Routledge, London
Condon, W. (1967) Linguistic-kinesic research and dance therapy. Proceedings, 3rd Annual Conference, American Dance Therapy Association 1968, ADTA, Baltimore
Condon, W. and Sander, L.W. (1974) Neonate movement is synchronized with adult speech: interactional participation and language acquisition. *Science*, **83**, 99–101
Cox, M. (1987) *Mutative Metaphors in Psychotherapy*, Tavistock, London
Davis, M. (1970) Movement characteristics of hospitalized psychiatric patients. In *Therapy in Motion* (ed. Costonis, M.N.) University of Illinois Press, Illinois
Dell, C. (1970) *A Primer for Movement Description Using Effort–Shape and Supplementary Concepts*, Dance Notation Bureau, New York
Deutsch, F. (1962) *Body. Mind and the Sensory Gateways,* Karger, New York
Dosamantes-Alperson, E. (1981) Experiencing in movement psychotherapy. *American Journal of Dance Therapy*, **4**, 33–44
Dulicai, D. (1980) Personal Communications, quoted in Flint, L. (1981) A pilot study exploring the relationships between body movement parameters and suicidal risk in suicidal and non-suicidal psychiatric patients. *Unpublished Master's thesis*, Hahnemann Medical College and Hospital, Philadelphia
Erikson, E. (1965) *Childhood and Society*, Penguin, Harmondsworth, Middlesex, UK
Freud, A. (1965) *Normality and Pathology in Childhood*, International University Press, New York
Freud, S. (1923) The Ego and the Id, Hogarth Press, London
Gesell, A. and Amatruda, C. (1975) *Developmental Diagnosis*, Harper and Row, New York
Hanna, J.L. (1987) *To Dance is Human*, University of Chicago Press, Illinois
Kendon, A. (1979) Movement coordination in social interaction: some examples described. In *Nonverbal Communications: Reading with Commentary* (ed Weitz, S.), Oxford University Press, London
Kastenberg, J.S. (1975) *Children and Parents: Psychoanalytic Studies in Development*, Jason Aronson, New York
Laban, R. (1960) *The Mastery of Movement* (ed Ullman. L.), Macdonald and Evans, London
Lambo, T.A. (1965) The place of the arts in the emotional life of the African. *AMSAC Newsletter*, **7**, 1–6
Leibowitz, G. (1992) Individual dance movement therapy in an in-patient psychiatric setting. In *Dance Movement Therapy: Theory and Practice* (ed. Payne, H.), Routledge, London
Lowen, A. (1975) *The Language of the Body*, Collier Macmillan, London

Mahl, G.F. (1979) Body movement, ideation and verbalization during psychoanalysis. In *Nonverbal Communication: Reading with Commentary* (ed. Weitz, S.), Oxford University Press, London

Mahler, M. Pine, F. and Bergman, A. (1975) *The psychological Birth of the Infant: Symbiosis and Individuation,* Basic Books, New York

Morrison Brown, J. (1980) *The Vision of Modern Dance,* Dance Books, London

North, M. (1990) *Personality Assesment Through Movement,* Northcote House, Plymouth, UK

Piaget, J. (1952) *The Origins of Intelligence in Children,* International Universities Press, New York

Sandel, S. and Johnson, D.R. (1983) Structure and process of the nascent group: dance therapy with chronic patients. *The Arts in Psychotherapy,* **10,** 131–140

Schmais, C. (1985) Healing processes in group dance therapy. *American Journal of Dance Therapy,* **8,** 17–36

Schoop, T. (1974) *Won't You Join the Dance? A Dancer's Essay into the Treatment of Psychosis,* Mayfield Publishing, California

Siegel, E. (1984) *Dance-Movement Therapy: Mirror of Our Selves,* Human Sciences Press, New York

Stanton-Jones, K. (1992) *An Introduction To Dance-Movement Therapy in Psychiatry,* Routledge, London

Stern, D.N. (1974) Mother and infant at play: the Dyadic interaction involving facial, vocal and gaze behaviors. In *The Origins of Behavior* (eds Lewis, M. and Rosenblum, L.), Wiley, New York

Winnicott D.W. (1967) Mirror-role of mother and family in child development, In *Playing and Reality,* Penguin, Harmondsworth, Middlesex, UK

Winnicott, D.W. (1988) *Playing and Reality,* Penguin, Harmondsworth, Middlesex, UK

16

Complementary medicine

A. An introduction to the subject

Maureen Dennis

'He's a devout believer in the department of witchcraft called medical science.' (G.B. Shaw)

Scepticism of medical science is nothing new. The reductionist model, dealing with symptoms rather than a person and using surgery and medication as methods of treating illness, reduces the patient to the role of passive victim. By assuming authority as professionals, doctors can exclude by licence others whose skills could perhaps benefit the sick. There is always conflict between the need for professional standardization and space for innovation and diversification. Doctors however, by their trade union, the British Medical Association (BMA), maintain the exclusive right to prescribe drugs, handle X-rays and operate surgically.

Physiotherapists were and still are, but to a much lesser extent, subservient to that authority and dependent on doctors for diagnosis and treatment recommendation. The Welfare State, by creating a National Health Service, reinforced this hierarchy and monopoly in its institutions.

Physical and mental symptoms were divided and treated by specialists. Mental illness was reduced to a physical or genetic cause to be treated by medication, shock therapy, social restraint, or even lobotomy. Individual psychotherapy or family therapy was given to very few patients after hospitalization. Segregation was preferable to integration.

The mass of population suffer at one time or another from stress-related disorders which do not cause them to cease functioning but which considerably impair their efficiency, reasoning and happiness of their lives. Prolonged anxiety does cause physical changes, fatigue and eventual breakdown. In most pre-industrial cultures there exists local healers who have gained a reputation for their knowledge of herbal remedies, massage, midwifery or even bone-setting skills. This, combined with a certain insight into parapsychological phenomena and a shrewd knowledge of human nature, gave them within the community something of the enhanced status of the contemporary doctor. Consultation with such a healer would involve some payment for the advice given which, if heeded, no doubt did something to allay the fears of the afflicted and may even have relieved symptoms.

The unassailable prestige of the post-industrial medical profession was considerably shaken by many major pharmaceutical disasters, the most famous and tragic of which was the birth of 'thalidomide babies' with limb abnormalities in the 1960s. The public became fearful of the side effects of prescriptions, not least because they were rarely if ever indicated to the patient as a pre-prescription advice. The power and pressure of major pharmaceutical companies to market their drugs had placed too much emphasis on chemical therapy as a means of treating a crisis. Too few trials took place before commercial sales commenced, and very rarely was an alternative approach considered. Lifestyle, nutrition, social and economic circumstances and philosophical attitude were all given scant attention as causative factors. Indeed no emphasis was placed, except perhaps in primary care, in Western medical training, on prevention, education and developing the body's resources to heal itself.

In 1972 President Nixon signed a treaty with the Communist leaders of China, which permitted cultural and economic exchange. Western doctors were able to observe the traditional Chinese medical practices of acupuncture, moxibustion, herbal prescription and exercise. Chinese medicine is based on a philosophy which is radically different from Western Cartesian thought. Modern Cartesian thought, which splits mind from body, has permeated our culture, and as we think ourselves the centre of our universe. It dominated medical dogma and practice.

Throughout the 1970s and 80s there permeated a gradual awareness among those interested in 'alternative therapies' that, within Chinese medicine, there existed a school of philosophy uncorrupted by eighteenth century reductionist thinking. In addition, osteopathic and chiropractic principles though not indebted to Chinese medicine, have as their foundation a belief in homeostasis or a well-balanced fluid medium through the body's tissues. This is dependent on a unified and well-balanced relationship between body structure and function. Pathology is provoked by displacement or distortion of joint tissue which if prolonged for long enough can impair organ function, hormonal balance and immune strength.

Herbal remedies are particular to local cultures and ecology and the British School of Homeopathy, founded in 1844, and the National Institute of Medical Herbalists are also exceptions to this Oriental revolution.

Acupuncture, reflexology, shiatsu (a Japanese method of acupressure based on using the hands on acupuncture points instead of needles) and aromatherapy are all Oriental healing skills which are based less on crisis intervention and more on earlier prevention by reharmonizing the organs of a system or personality which may be going out of balance.

Chinese medical practice, however, has not transferred wholesale to the West because of the basic premise within the Chinese practice that medication and therapy is created specifically for each patient and there are no universal prescriptions for specific diseases. This has made it a poor commercial proposition in the eyes of large pharmaceutical companies in the West. Here, the pharmaceutical industry dictates a universal prescription for a similar pattern of symptoms.

The Western public, however, had made that important psychological leap that the role as patient did not require passivity in the face of authority and that the process of caring is just as important as prescriptive treatment. The contract of care created between therapist and patient requires confidentiality, agreement and sharing and not impersonality, fragmentation, nor distant authority assumed on specialization as role-played by the majority of Western medical experts.

The opportunities for complementary practitioners expanded enormously in the 1970s, but there were few regulatory bodies to monitor standards of training and practice. the Council for Complementary and Alternative Medicine (CGAM) was founded in February 1985, among whose members were practitioners of Chinese medicine, chiropractitioners, osteopaths and medical herbalists. All these had well-established standards of training, but peripheral to these were practitioners of complementary skills who put less emphasis on diagnosis and more on therapeutic technique, e.g. aromatherapists and reflexologists. The various specialities decided individually to put their training schemes and professional qualifications in order, and are gradually being integrated within the tertiary levels of mainstream educational institutions. (*Complementary Therapies in Medicine*, 1993)

The role of all complementary therapies has expanded enormously. In 1983, the BMA journal surveyed and found that 80% of trainee doctors wished to train in some form of complementary therapy. (Reilly, 1983). A modest percentage were already referring patients to complementary therapies.

Where lies the profession of physiotherapy in relation to complementary therapies? It has a highly regulated standard of formal education, well integrated in mainstream educational understanding of human physiology and utilizing exercise, electrotherapy, massage and, to a lesser extent, mobilization and manipulation with the hands. It has obtained the right, within the boundaries of these skills, to recommend treatment without being dependent on medical advice. It remains, however, 'supplementary' to medicine and not independent from the profession. Meanwhile, greater numbers of the general public are consulting complementary therapists. These are not gullible ill-informed people, but articulate citizens capable of making informed choices.

Is there an innate criticism of the inadequacy of the deductive medical model which attacks specific symptoms but may ignore the person experiencing those symptoms? By reflection, is there a criticism of the physiotherapeutic approach which is also based on the deductive medical model. Complementary therapies are gaining ground because they are holistic, often treating highly successfully minor symptomatic conditions which threaten to become more chronic, but which are averted because of good advice and intervention from the therapist. This is not to say that physiotherapists do not do the same, but often the advice they offer is not integral to the whole person but a specific remedy for a specific condition.

In the field of mental health, it may be said that the crisis of comprehension due to the mind/body specialization of orthodox medicine does not arise in complementary therapies. They work through the body, so that the patient is not instructed how to feel better – they experience feeling better. Time is given to the patient; the average length of consultation with a complementary therapist is 36 minutes as opposed to 6 minutes with the general practitioner (BMA, 1986). Touch is given to the patient, and therapeutic touch has remained central to the complementary professions rather than pushed to the periphery by technology such as electrotherapy machines. Touch as a diagnostic and therapeutic tool has fallen by the wayside of orthodox medical practice in the rush for placebo prescription. Technique, though idiosyncratic to each complementary therapy, is on a simple humanistic level and not complicated by expensive technology. Though seen by some as fad and fashion, and not examined by a good foundation of research, it has survived for hundreds of years and at its heart deals with the very essence of what is human.

The public, in a sense, has already chosen. To ignore the need for a simple humane treatment of public malaise and anxiety will impoverish the physiotherapy profession. Most physiotherapy practices are enriched by the additional acquisition of a complementary skill which marries well with the physical skills of the established profession. In the grey area, where spiritual malaise and physical imbalance can conspire to make very sick human beings, the physiotherapist has the advantage of a sound analytical knowledge with the freedom and capacity to study and utilize the wider understanding of holistic healing.

References

Complementary Therapies in Medicine (1993), Vol. 1, Longman, London

Reilly, D.T. (1983) Young doctor's views on alternative medicine. *British Medical Journal,* **287**, 337–339

BMA (1986) *Report of the Board of Science and Education on Alternative Therapy,* British Medical Association, London

B. Aromatherapy in the mental health setting

Lynne Dunham

Introduction

Aromatherapy has an advantage as a form of stimulus because we respond emotionally and not intellectually to the sense of smell. A high proportion of what we respond to as taste is actually smell and many have strong associations related to experiences of our personal life. Can this strong association be used to influence mood and behaviour?

Physiologically the olfactory nerve endings are in direct contact with both the external environment and the limbic system of our brain which is important in the control of emotions. This limbic system is part of the primitive brain concerned with survival and is the source of very basic emotional responses such as anger, aggression, sexual arousal, and tears.

The close association of the olfactory nerves to that part of the limbic system known as the hippocampus, which is associated with long-term memory, explains why smells can arouse very deep and long-forgotten memories and their emotional associations in adult life. (Figure 16.1).

Animals respond at a very basic level to the hostile smells emitted by fellow and predatory species. We too may experience arousal of the sympathetic nervous system when faced with unpleasant threatening smells. Correspondingly, enjoyable smells with their pleasant associations can be said to have a calming effect on both memory and emotion. Smells associated with sexual arousal can be said to fall somewhere between the two processes and create a vast endocrine and behavioural response.

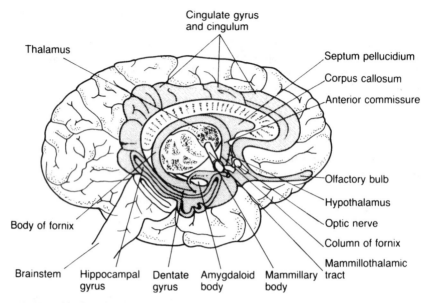

Figure 16.1 The limbic system in the mid-portion of the cerebrum (From Warwick and Williams, 1973, by permission)

Van Toller (1988) has demonstrated that when we smell something pleasant the whole of the cortex is stimulated, whereas when we smell something equally unpleasant we attempt to block it off. The right side of the brain responds more to the euphoric effect and this in turn has a beneficial effect on the intuitive side of brain functioning.

Aromatherapy creates a response by oily infiltration through the skin, increased by massage and by the direct process of smelling. Our response to and need for touch is as primal as our sense of smell. It is hard to censure our spontaneous response to comforting or hostile touch intellectually.

Essential oil therapy is therefore useful in altering mood without becoming addictive. We are unable intellectually to block the process of response to smell, but we may also respond positively to the empathetic touch of a good therapist. The interaction between patient and therapist is as important to the success of the process as is the process itself.

Aromatherapy is a skill which is therefore useful to assist the relaxation process in common stress-related illnesses (e.g. mild to moderate depression, agitated depression. lethargy, postnatal depression, insomnia, fatigue, post-bereavement, low mood/changes or loss of motivation) rather than as an intervention in major illnesses. The oils can also be used to uplift and stimulate, to aid fitness and well-being.

Is a qualification in aromatherapy necessary?

At present (1995) the professional indemnity cover provided by the UK Chartered Society does not include the practice of aromatherapy. Therefore, any physiotherapist who is also trained as an aromatherapist will need to obtain secondary cover, either on a personal basis or through their health authority or Trust. It is essential to obtain high-quality training and some useful addresses for this are given in Appendix II of this chapter. There is also a cost implication as regards purchasing the oils and maintaining good supplies of stock, which will be depleted by use on clients, especially if the oils are blended to be used in between sessions.

An aromatherapist has to ask detailed questions concerning physiological and psychological symptoms and creates a particular mixture of oils to suit the requirements of a particular patient. There also has to be an awareness not only of the needs of the patient but of the medication which they are taking. There may be an incompatibility between the prescription consumed and the oils, however blended and diluted, to the skin. Some medications suppress the immune system, whereas aromatherapy attempts to boost the same system. It is important to check with the person who prescribed before any interventions take place.It is also important to be aware of those essences which are contra-indicated for pregnancy, respiratory conditions and epilepsy.

Helpful hints for the non-qualified

The physiotherapist may wish to utilize simple aromatherapy techniques to reduce anxiety and depression, but sensibly they may be hesitant to use oils for skin contact when they are not trained as aromatherapists. However, essences can safely be used to create aromas within the room which can create calm and relaxing atmospheres for those experiencing mental stress. Aromas can be created by placing six drops of the essential essence in a vaporizer or on a burner, or one or two drops can be placed on a tissue for inhalation. Indeed, a few drops of oil added to a ball of cotton wool and placed on a radiator can be sufficient to influence the atmosphere and the minds within it. No techniques, however, should take place without the agreement of ward management and staff. Mentally ill patients tend to smoke heavily and essential oils are inflammable. The fire risk with six drops of essence is practically negligible, but it would be against Health and Safety rules to use it without permission. On the positive side, nursing staff would probably be pleased to have such a positive innovation.

What essences to use

The Institute of Classical Aromatherapy (1 Belvedere Trading Estate, Taunton, Somerset TA1 1BH) publishes a booklet entitled *Aromatherapy for the Family* edited by Jan Kusmirek, which gives a useful list of mental and emotional symptoms and the oils which will help. For example, specific oils which have an effect on mood are:

Chamomile, Clary, Sage, Frankincense, Geranium, Lavender, Orange, Sandalwood, Tangerine and Ylang Ylang can help diminish the symptoms of depression.

Cedarwood and Sandalwood encourage meditation.

Chamomile, Lavender, Sandalwood and Ylang Ylang induce relaxation because they make a warm and secure atmosphere.

Lemon and Rosemary will uplift mood, while jasmine will encourage self-esteem.

Basil calms and restores order to a mind where thoughts are confused, while Ginger will instil confidence.

Basil, Peppermint and Rosemary stimulate the memory centres, so they may have uses in reminiscence groups for the elderly.

Geranium and Lemon will reduce confusion, while Rosemary will affect disorientation.

A drop or two of Lavender, Marjoram, orange, Sandalwood or Sage under the pillow will help reduce insomnia.

It may be asked how can such a minimal quantity as six drops influence a clinical room. Experiments have shown that a subliminal degree of aroma causes the occupants of that room to subconsciously notice a difference, but to interpret it in terms of atmosphere rather than smells. (Tisserand, 1988). However, if the physiotherapist wishes to assist individual patients, they can immerse the hands or feet of the patients in warm baths containing the same six drops of essence or give hand and feet massages which will have a similar effect.

Fully qualified aromatherapists blend essential oils to suit the requirements of their individual patients and apply these blends directly to the skin with Swedish massage. Shiatsu and reflexology techniques can also be utilized if the patient is nervous about the undressing required for such massage. Mental health patients may be apprehensive of bodily contact and it is important that the physiotherapist approaches with tact and care and perhaps only treats such non-threatening areas as the hands or feet.

The advantage of foot and hand massage is that it is very non-invasive, and is a strong stimulus to reflex points throughout the body. Also in terms of clinical time, a benefit is felt without a great deal of preparation and clinical manoeuvres. The physiotherapist can teach the procedure to nurses or helpers, carers or relatives, not forgetting the patients themselves. It is surely a gesture of improving social awareness when patients show an interest and offer to help one another.

There are sufficient cosmetic creams sold on the commercial market which have an additional essence of, for example, lavender which is very safe. This will ensure that the physiotherapist does not get mixed up in the legal implications of using essential oils. (Lavender is one of the least toxic oils, but, commercially, Lavadin is often sold under the same name because it is cheaper to produce. It is distilled from a hybrid lavender and aspic. It has the same calming effect as lavender but not the same healing properties.)

Hand Massage

Remove all your jewellery and roll your sleeves up to the elbows. Position yourself comfortably on the same level to establish eye contact. This is especially important because you can observe changes in breathing rate and also it will encourage interaction. This may be the only close human contact people may experience in weeks.

Pour enough oil on your own hands to lubricate them well.

Enclose the hand of the patient. This is a very comforting gesture. Start massaging around the wrist and into the palm. In the palm massage deeply in the fleshy centre with alternating thumbs.

Progress down each finger, giving a robust tug to the tips. Pinch the finger web gently and rotate the metacarpal joints, supporting the proximal joint with your other hand.

Rotate the wrist three times and gently stretch it into extension. Support the elbow while doing this.

Gently bend the metacarpal joints into the palm to encourage finger flexion.

Turn the hand over and massage accordingly its dorsal surface. The skin is less dense, so take greater care.

Supporting the wrist, gently stretch all the fingers into extension.

Softly pinch the edges of the hand from wrist to fingers. Clasping gently at the wrist with flat hands, brush your hands to the tips of the fingers in a brisk way for the final invigorating stimulating gesture.

Encourage conversation, eye contact and observe behaviour before and after. Use a towel to clean up residual oil and establish an agreement as to when the massage will occur again.

Self-massage

Depression may be based on considerable self-dislike. Patients have to learn to love themselves. Sometimes this dislike extends to inflicting self-harm on the forearms, or to suicide attempts which leave scars of laceration on the wrists or broken limbs from aborted jumps from high places. A lavender cream can be utilized to encourage the patient to massage their own wounded areas to reduce swelling, encourage flexibility and just enhance physical awareness.

Some chronic illnesses also cause bouts of depression, which can spread to carers. Would it not mutually enhance the relationship between carer and the cared for if the cared for was taught to carry out a gentle aromatherapy massage on the back of the person who lifts them or the hands of the person who tends to them? And if such a justification is needed, is it not also a practical exercise?

Was aromatherapy always such a minority treatment?

Records from ancient Egyptian times tell of the use of aromatics for medicinal and cosmetic purposes which was passed on to the Greeks. Hippocrates mentions vast numbers of medicinal herbs in his writing. Circa AD 1000 an Arab doctor named Avicenna is credited with the discovery of distillation, beginning with the rose. The Crusaders in the fourteenth and fifteenth centuries brought this Eastern European knowledge of herbs and oils to England. Aromatics were used as a defence against the Black Death and continued in use against various plagues throughout the sixteenth and seventeenth centuries. These 'pestilence prophylactics' were held as perfumed balls, or scattered on warm coals, or two or three drops were placed at the temples and nostrils. But as Culpeper says: 'Yet it must be done with discretion, for it is very quick and percing' (N. Culpeper, *The English Physician*, London, 1653). Both on the Continent and in England oils were taken internally as well as by inhalation. From about 1650 there was a split between those who used natural herbs and those who used chemically synthesized drugs which formed the foundation for the modern industry of today. in the Twentieth century a chemist named Gattefosse began a revival of herbal remedies by promoting commercially the folklore knowledge of the benefits of lavender. During World War II, a French army surgeon called Valnet used oils to treat wounds and published his findings in 1964. On the Continent there is still more actual intake of oils, but not in the UK.

What is an essential oil?

An essential oil is one which is extracted from a plant source; prior to that they are known as essences. All odorous plant matter contains an essential oil, usually in some part of the plant. Contrary to their name, essential oils are non-oily, highly volatile and leave no stain on paper when they are heated.

Extraction is usually by distillation and only citrus oils are removed by extraction. The result is usually a clear, pale yellow liquid which dissolves in pure alcohol, fats and oils but not in water. Essential oils are highly flammable and are damaged by the effects of light, heat, air and moisture. Storage should always be in a dark glass bottle with a good seal at a cool temperature, e.g. 5°C (40°F) in the refrigerator.

Once an oil has been blended, i.e. mixed with a carrier oil, its shelf life decreases rapidly to around 3 months, but if wheatgerm is added, it will preserve to about 6 months. Essential oils should never be used neat on the skin.

Qualified aromatherapists can do a body massage where the essence will pass into the intestinal fluid and lymph system 4–6 hours after application.

And its carrier oil?

Fine vegetable oils are ideal for penetration of the skin and purity of quality. Mineral oils may have trace elements in them and do not penetrate so well.

Vegetable oils can be used 100% or as an addition of 5–10% to another carrier oil.

Types of blending oils

Many aromatherapists use a blend which is 2.5% essential oil to 97.5% carrier, This is suitable for adults in good health, but it must be remembered that essential oils will only be taken up by the skin for a period of about 7–10 minutes and will not be absorbed well if applied when the body is eliminating – when sweating through anxiety, heat or the menopause – or too soon after exercise. An obese person will not absorb the oil as well as a slim person, nor will those with water retention or poor circulation.

Sweet almond. One of the oldest cosmetic oils obtained from the almond kernel, it is rich in protein, minerals, vitamins, etc., and is pale yellow in appearance. It is good for all skin types and can be used as 100% base oil. It is the most commonly used by aromatherapists and can be obtained from any good local pharmacist.

Apricot kernel oil. Pale yellow in appearance, it is extracted from the kernel and again is rich in minerals, vitamins etc. It can be used for all skin types and is a natural moisturizer with high penetrative qualities. It can be used as 100% base oil.

Evening primrose oil. Pale yellow in appearance, it is especially good for skin regeneration and contains the vitamins E and F. It can be used as 100% base oil, but is rather more expensive than the other choices mentioned.

Grape seed oil. Pale green in appearance, it has good penetration and is used for a cleansing tonic effect, especially for oily skins. It can be used as 100% base oil.

Soya bean oil. Pale yellow in appearance, it is extracted from the bean and contains many minerals and vitamins. It can be used as 100% base oil.

Avocado. Viscous dark-green oil very rich in vitamins A and B and is used for all skin types, especially eczematous and dry skins. Often recommended for stretch marks in pregnancy. Because of its viscous nature it is used as an addition to the base oil in a 10% jojoba.

Jojoba. This yellow oil is extracted from the jojoba bean and contains waxy substances that mimic collagen, protein and minerals. It is a very good conditioner for the hair. Its uses are on inflamed skin, such as in psoriasis, eczema, acne and in hair care. It is a highly penetrative oil. It also can be used as an addition to base oil in a 10% solution.

Wheatgerm. This oil, which is a yellowy orange in colour, is viscous and contains vitamins A, B, C and E, minerals and protein. It protects the skin from blemishes, reinforces and strengthens capillaries and is said to help premature aging and keep the elasticity of the skin. Its most important quality for the aromatherapist is an antioxidant and it is thus used to preserve base oils. It is recommended for eczema, psoriasis and aging skin. It is used in addition to a base oil in a 10% solution and will enable a longer shelf life to be given to a blended oil.

Hazards regarding essential oils

The great majority of essential oils are non-toxic and perfectly safe when used sensibly, that is to say in small quantities and low dilutions. There are, however, some which are highly toxic, even in small amounts, and others which may give rise to toxicity if they are used over a longer period of time, and as mentioned earlier, some people are more vulnerable to damage from essential oils than others.

Toxicity is dose dependent, i.e. the greater amount of essential oils used, the greater the risk of poisoning whether by external or internal use. Almost every kind of medicine has a dosage level above which it becomes toxic. In the case of essential oils, liver and kidneys are the primary organs that are affected. The toxicity may be acute or chronic. Acute toxicity is usually the result of oral use; chronic toxicity may occur with multiple applications. There is a group of essential oils known as the abortifacient group which if used could cause a fetus to be aborted. However, some other oils are also thought possibly to be abortive, for example sage, basil, clove, myrrh, thyme etc., and therefore these oils must never be used during pregnancy, although they may be used for other clients at different times.

Uses in clinical practice

Essential oils can be used for many different complaints, ranging from skin problems and wounds through to respiratory and musculoskeletal problems and mental fatigue. Dependent on the problem that needs to be addressed, so the choice of oils will match what is required. Some oils will have properties that will make them antiseptic and muciliptic and thus will be used for respiratory conditions. Others that are antispasmodic and calming will be of help for gastrointestinal problems.

However, because some oils possess several characteristics, they are not all mutually exclusive to one condition. A good example is lavender whose primary property is that of a good balancer with sedative and tonic properties and yet it is cytophylactic which means it is good for cell regeneration. Hence it is a skin oil excellent for healing minor burns, but is also good for insomnia because of its calming sedative qualities. It is indeed the most versatile of all oils and the one of which the lay person is most likely to have heard.

Conclusion

Increasingly, complementary therapies such as aromatherapy are being used in many health care settings, both in acute care and in the community. It is the author's view that as physiotherapists, with our skills in touch and handling, we are ideally placed to take advantage of this therapy. Our training lays much emphasis on the therapeutic use of touching our client. It is apparent that there are many other care workers who would be only too willing to take this role from us if we allow them to do so. It is time that these therapies are brought into clinical practice in order that the effectiveness of them may be properly investigated, not as an alternative to our wide scope of practice but very much as an adjunct.

However, it is extremely important that any physiotherapist wishing to use this therapy must obtain a high-quality thorough training from a reputable training establishment.

Appendix 1

Case Study 1. Extreme anxiety/aversion to touch/low self esteem

Miss A, who is 42, was referred by the team at the Day Unit as they felt that aromatherapy might help her with her extreme anxiety problems. She had an aversion to being touched and found it difficult to form relationships; she also felt very tense and wound up. Initial treatment began with a full assessment, explanation of the therapy and her consent. A blend of oils was chosen that would help with the problems she was experiencing: anxiety, loss of self-esteem, and difficulty in relaxing. It was explained that therapy would commence with a hand massage only and she could withdraw at any time.

For the first few sessions the oils were massaged into the hands and then both arms. She then consented to a neck and shoulder massage of 10 minutes, the time being extended to 20 minutes. Gradually over a period of 3 months she was able to enjoy and relax in the sessions, even tolerating a back massage. Staff reported that she was interacting more in the various groups she attended. She was able to progress to joining activities/clubs in her area and the therapy stopped when she was discharged from the Day Unit.

Case Study 2. Bereavement/depression

Mr S., aged 72 is a recently bereaved gentleman who was referred to the Day Hospital by the CPN for support and social contact following the death of his wife of many years. He was depressed and lonely and due to arthritis of hip/knees had become increasingly isolated at home. He presented with difficulty in sleeping, poor appetite, was tearful and apathetic, preferring to sit alone. After the team had assessed him, he was referred for aromatherapy, although he was somewhat sceptical. He agreed to a first appointment and after a detailed case history it was decided to start with offering him a massage of oils blended to give some help with his painful joints, most especially his knees. Oils were chosen from those with a pain-relieving and circulatory effect and Mr S. was given a bottle of oil to use at home himself.

He was very resistant to any suggestion of using other oils to help him with his depression, but over the course of the month a good relationship built up and Mr S. reported that he felt better after the sessions. He began to interact in other activities in the Day Hospital and always came regularly for his 'massage' sessions as he called them. It would have been of interest to use some oils which are of use in depression and post-bereavement, but the client did not wish for this.

Appendix II   Useful addresses

Professional organizations
International Federation of Aromatherapists, Room 8, Department of Continuing Education, The Royal Masonic Hospital, Ravenscroft Park, London W6 0TN

British Association of Beauty Therapy and Cosmetology
2nd Floor, 34 Imperial Square, Cheltenham, Glos

Training Centres
London School of Aromatherapy
PO Box 780, London NW6 7DY

Raworth College
South Street, Dorking, Surrey

Tisserand Institute
PO Box 746, Hove, East Sussex BN3 3XA

Equipment manufacturers
Micheline Arcier Aromatherapy
7 William Street, London SW1

Baldwin and Co.
171-173 Walworth Road, London

Body Treats Ltd
15 Approach Road, Raynes Park, London SW20 8BA

Aromatherapy Products Ltd
The Knoll Business Centre, Old Shoreham Road, Hove, East Sussex

The Fragrant Earth
PO Box 182, Taunton, Somerset

References

Arcier, M. (1990) *Aromatherapy*, Hamlyn, London
Davies, P. (1991) *Aromatherapy: An A–Z*, revised edn, C.W. Daniel Co., Saffron Walden, Essex, UK
Tisseraud, R. (1991) *The Art of Aromatherapy*, 12th impression, C.W. Daniel Co., Saffron Walden, Essex, UK
Tisseraud, R. (1988) *Aromatherapy for Everyone*, Penguin, Harmondsworth, Middlesex, UK
Van Toller, C. (1988) Emotion and brain imaging of reactions to smells. In *Perfumery: The Psychology and Biology of Fragrance* (ed.), London
Warwick, and Williams, (1973) *Gray's Anatomy*, 35th edn., W.B. Saunders, Philadelphia

Aromatherapy publications
Aromatherapy Quarterly, 5 Ranelagh Avenue, London SW13 0BY
International Journal of Aromatherapy, PO Box 746, Hove, East Sussex BN3 3XA

C. Reflextherapy

Christine Jones

Reflextherapy is an exciting, holistic, readily available method of assessment and treatment. It is useful in the treatment of both mental and physical problems, providing a safe, gentle and cost-effective means of reobtaining and maintaining health.

Historical development of reflextherapy

Reflextherapy is a development of an ancient art of healing which has a recorded history of over 5000 years, appearing at various times in many parts of the world. An engraving found in Egypt in the tomb of the physician,

Ankhmahor, depicts practitioners treating the hands and feet of their recipients in 2500 BC. The therapy was also used at this time in India and in China, where it was recorded in the Chinese medical book, *The Yellow Emperor's Classic of Internal Medicine*. Later, further works were written in Japan and were brought to Russia and Europe adding more information. In Russia, in the early twentieth century, Dr Natalia Bekhteneva founded the Brain Institute in Leningrad and to this day the principles of reflex therapy are used in the treatment of both psychological and physiological conditions while scientifically researching the effects. Reflextherapy is well established in Russia.

An American ENT specialist, William Fitzgerald, worked both in London and Vienna at the time that a German Physician, Alfons Corneluis, published a paper on Pressure Points (Corneluis, 1902; Bekhtereus, 1932). Fitzgerald researched and documented his findings at his clinic in Connecticut, USA. He theorized that the body could be divided into 10 longitudinal zones in which the health of all tissues within the same zone were related to each other. Any organic disturbance was seen to affect all linked tissues. Manipulation or pressure in the zone caused a reflex response which reduced pain in the original trauma site. Fitzgerald and Edwin Bowers (1917) had several articles and books published on this zonal body work. Fitzgerald taught this approach to pain relief (Figure 16.2) to many physicians amongst whom were Jo and Elizabeth Selby-Riley. They extended zone therapy, also documenting their clinical findings (Selby-Riley, 1919, 1924).

In the early 1930s Riley taught a therapist, Eunice Ingham, who extended the therapy to the feet and hands, calling it reflexology (Ingham, 1938, 1945). She developed a specialized alternating pressure technique which was found

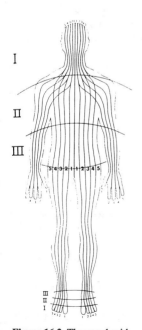
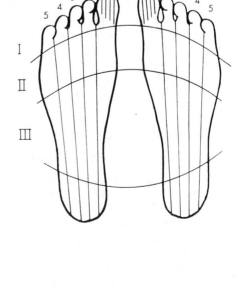

Figure 16.2 The zonal grid

to promote symptomatic change in the associated tissues. Usually the patient experienced a sensation of relaxation, decongestion and renewed vitality. Ingham wrote and taught reflexology to both health care professionals and lay persons. Her preferred action of using thumb and finger in a walking movement along the zones is a technique used by many reflexologists in Europe and America. Other schools use differing techniques and variable pressure.

Today, zone therapy, reflexology and reflex therapy are practised throughout the world by doctors, dentists and health care professionals. In Britain, non-medical practitioners should comply with EEC directives. Physiotherapists can train with schools recommended by the Association of Chartered Physiotherapists in Reflex Therapy (ACPIRT).

There are many schools, some teaching the original concepts, while others, particularly those working within specialized units, find that the patient only tolerates a more gentle approach, such as those in intensive care, in paediatrics or for the heavily traumatized patient, those in terminal care and the mentally and emotionally unstable.

The Midland School of Reflextherapy (MSR) has developed a gentle approach over 25 years and continues to adapt and extend according to patients' needs. This particular method will be described in the latter part of this chapter (Jones, MSR, 1976 to date).

Principles of reflextherapy and reflexology

Reflextherapy is a manual skill of applying specific finger and thumb pressure to the feet, hands, ears or spine. Each area is said to be a microcosm of the macrocosm of the total human body. Imbalance or congestion of energy in a system or part of the total body will be represented by altered sensitivity or pain in these corresponding parts (Figures 16.3 and 16.4).

The physical disorder may arise from imbalance of vital energy which is also dependent upon factors which include the basic genetic disposition, environmental input such as diet, atmosphere, solar energy, the frequency of sound and colour and mental health. Trigger spots along the energy pathways are found to connect and monitor associated imbalance.

Effects of reflextherapy

The following are the principal effects of reflex therapy:

- Pressure on these distal areas is seen to cause a reflex response in the original trauma site. This will either stimulate hypoactivity or sedate hyperactivity via the autonomic nervous system.
- More detailed examination will locate other reflected areas of local tissue tension which may similarly be affected during the course of treatment. The general and local reactions will constantly be assessed during the course of the treatment session.
- The resultant response of either stimulation or relaxation is seen to promote an increased flow of body fluids which will assist decongestion and

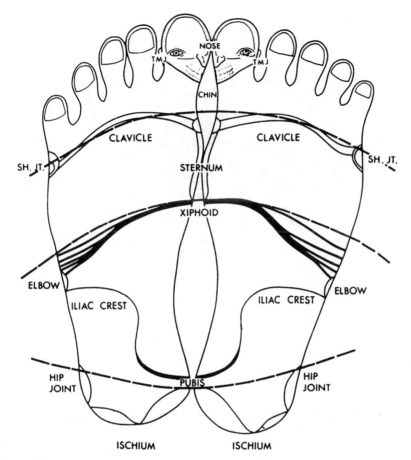

Figure 16.3 Dorsal aspect

elimination of waste and toxic material from the affected areas. The organs of elimination should be monitored and their function improved using reflex-therapy to accomodate the increased activity.

- Increased blood supply brings nutritional and healing requisites (subject to availability) to improve tissue repair.
- The patient often feels relief after the first session, but after 3–4 treatments there should be an overall improvement. If a plateau of benefit is reached, there may be a need for a fundamental change in diet or lifestyle.

The aims of reflextherapy

The aims of the therapy are therefore:

- to examine, observe and palpate areas and trigger spots of reflected hyper- or hypoactivity in the physical body or within the micro-organs in the feet, hands, ears or spine

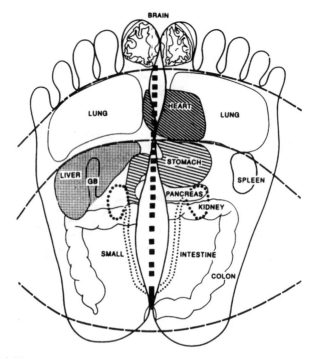

Figure 16.4 Plantar aspect

- to use appropriate sensitive pressure or manipulation to these reflected areas to affect the original trauma site
- to consider the history of the whole person, and to give further professional support and counselling
- to recommend changes in lifestyles which may be contributing to physiological or psychological imbalance within the scope of expertise of the individual practitioner
- to recommend consultation with an appropriate practitioner if necessary.

Development of reflextherapy

Reflextherapy is usually applied to zones within the miniature mirror image found in the hands and feet (Figure 16.5). The treatment usually consists of 'working' the feet or hands in a definite order along the reflected zonal pattern; usually one foot is treated completely, followed by the other, so the entire one side of the body is treated and this is followed by the second side. The areas located for treatment are worked on by an alternating pressure using the specialized walking technique with a firm pressure.

Following the author's training in this approach in 1970, and during the first year of clinical application, the response of patients was usually exciting and encouraging. Their symptoms were of a wide and varied nature. Reflexology presented an accurate assessment tool as well as a holistic mode of treatment.

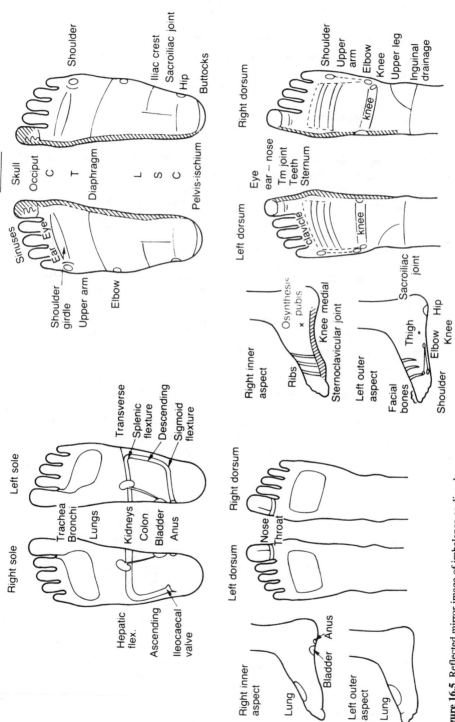

Figure 16.5 Reflected mirror image of imbalance or disorder

Contraindications to reflextherapy

The following are contraindications to therapy:

- deep vein thrombosis and acute inflammation of the lymphatic or blood circulation
- gangrene of the feet (careful treatment via the hands)
- melanoma
- at risk pregnancies
- any intuitive doubts

Special precautions are necessary for those patients on drug therapy, those with diabetes, those having pacemakers and/or implants, and those with low blood pressure. Experience with working in mental health is recommended when treating those with psychotic or schizophrenic disturbance. Lack of such experience is not a contraindication, but experience is advisable when assessing reaction to treatment.

However, as well as these precautions some of the author's patients were unable to tolerate the degree of pressure or reacted uncomfortably to the effect. There were also those, usually children, who were unable to take a full treatment. An adapted procedure and much reduced pressure was well tolerated not only by these groups but by an increasing number who preferred the new approach. This is now the established method of reflextherapy used by the Midland School of Reflexology (MSR). These findings, however, are in no way intended to detract from the developments and approaches of other well-founded and established schools.

Reflextherapy incorporates naturopathic principles which recognize and adhere to holism and the laws of natural healing. Naturopathy considers the holistic assessment, function, healing ability and treatment of the health or disorder of the interwoven mechanisms of body and mind. The principles have been utilized for thousands of years and are the result of trial, experience and common sense. The Hippocratic oath undertaken by medical practitioners expresses the value of natural medicine and the holistic approach. The laws of natural healing should form the basis of physiotherapy practice.

Reflextherapy incorporates scientific reasoning, particularly that postulated by quantum physics in the 'observer principle'. This acknowledges the influence of the mind of the observer (here, the therapist and the patient) on the behaviour of sub-atomic particles and the movement and change which accompanies the healing process (Gerber, 1954; Chopra, 1989; Wolf, 1987). The observer/therapist should therefore act as a facilitator while supporting the natural process of healing. This requires free movement and should not be interrupted or confused by the will or expectation of the therapist.

Procedure

An extensive case history is taken, in order to appreciate the total function of the patient. A detailed examination of the feet is carried out, noting temperature, texture, swellings, shape, skin blemishes and tension.

During healing the body attempts to rid itself of the wastes of cell metabolism and toxins via the lymphatic system, the venous circulation and the organs of elimination. The reflected pathways of these systems are investigated and treated in the early stages, treating the body as a whole using both feet or hands to normalize the body systems. A further aim at this stage is to calm the sympathetic nervous system if it is overactive, so allowing the parasympathetic system to exert its influence. Diaphragmatic breathing is taught and the patient advised as to the benefit of this during their everyday living.

Further holistic implications

Reflextherapy also acknowledges and considers the empirical teaching of ancient wisdom postulated in the 'Law of 5 elements' or 'stages of transition'. These recognize as 'the interconnectedness of nature' the interconnections of the universal energy, now supported by modern science (Capra, 1975; Kushi, 1977; Kaptchuk, 1983).

In acknowledging the organ relationship so postulated, the treatment may be also adapted to those with acute trauma inflammation. The stimulation or sedation via the reflected pathway of one organ will alter the quality of energy of the other; for example, a person with acute bronchitis, particularly if a heart condition has been diagnosed, is more safely treated via the reflected pathways of the colon and small intestine to 'reduce the fire' (acute inflammation) in the lungs.

The Law of 5 elements also acknowledges that the entirety is related to the twenty-four hour clock and to the seasons and planetary aspects. Each person has their own tendency to imbalance, being more subject to that both physically, mentally and emotionally at certain times and seasons. Mankind is included in this universal energy.

When treating the reflected imbalances of the organs, the therapist appreciates the paired and interrelationships of organs and the locomotor system, and also the interwoven emotional and mental imbalances which may occur when organ dysfunction is present. We acknowledge the 'irritable liverish' person and use expressions such as to 'vent one's spleen'. Eastern medicine details the links in the Law of 5 elements and sees fears and phobias of insecurity when the kidney and bladder energy become unbalanced. Also, it is aware of the possible suspicious nature of the person with unbalanced stomach and spleen energy, the excessive and inappropriate laughter expressed in the heart–small intestine imbalance, and the excessive grief as a disturbance in the lung and colon energy balance.

The general overall effect of reflextherapy may therefore have far-reaching implications in alleviating emotional and mental imbalances and may assist patients with anxiety, panic attacks, hyperventilation, phobias and fears and many other imbalances and disorders of the mind.

To complete a full reflextherapy treatment, the central nervous system is investigated and if appropriate, suitable treatment is given by gently massaging the toes, thus influencing sensitive areas within the brain structure, enabling free flow of cerebral spinal fluid (when the primary respiratory mechanism can be detected by the most subtle touch). If the patient has an acute trauma, such as a recent cerebral haemorrhage, this part of the treatment is omitted until the response to the early part of the procedure is considered safe. Touch to any area of skin is relayed immediately to the brain, and gentle treatment is essential.

The procedure is from the external to the internal structure – to ensure that the increased activity is not obstructed by tension or congestion of the channels through which it will proceed. The action is then to encourage flow. The essential balance of the endocrine system is investigated and treated and the autonomic nervous system balanced, encouraging the whole to be more harmonious and giving the benefit of complete treatment which is essential for the maintenance of health.

Balancing sequences, e.g. by gently holding the heels, provides opportunity for the realignment of the physical structure.This is sometimes preceded by deeper relaxation or the release of some stored emotion held within the linked tissues or in the conscious or subconscious mind. The therapist must be observant as to the true needs of the patient.

Harmonizing strokes in the direction of the flow of vital energy and foot movements complete the reflextherapy treatment, unless the therapist assesses that other more subtle methods are necessary. Not only will the physical mental and emotional aspects have the opportunity to heal and balance, but also that of the vital energy network – essential to achieve homoeostasis.

To obtain the greatest benefit, reflextherapy should be administered as a full treatment, but it can be adapted to local tissue trauma such as sports injuries or local musculoskeletal disorders such as 'frozen shoulder' if only the local tissues are involved. In more chronic disorders, the more extensive approach should be used if time allows.

Prenatal patterns

Empirically it is seen that the spine holds the memory of fetal development in which lies the ability to establish the self, the degree of development of which may influence the ability to form balanced relationships and may affect attitudes to life scripts. (Figure 16.6) The spinal memory of imbalance relayed into the feet, hands and head offers opportunity for a subtle unobtrusive approach of reflextherapy in which the person may mature further in these important aspects of a healthy approach to life. This may be in physical, mental or emotional need, resulting in an improved function, self-development, learning ability, social behaviour and communication. Robert St John, a naturopath and reflexologist, used this observation to develop Prenatal Therapy, now also known as the Metamorphic technique, where only the spinal reflected pathways are gently worked (St. John, 1980; Saint-Pierre, 1989) using the feet, hands and head.

The therapist must allow the process of change to come from within the patient acting as a facilitator and support for the natural process of healing. This supportive, caring, non-invasive attitude may allow an unexpected response totally instigated by the inner healing mechanism of the patient, such as memories and recognition and opportunity for healing of shock, grief, fear or guilt which may have been the origin of the presented physical or mental symptoms. It is vital that the practitioner recognizes the process of change and acts as a support especially when such a reaction is apparent.

In mental health, this gentle and adapted form of reflextherapy provides a most useful tool in relaxation and to access and heal obvious or hidden anxieties

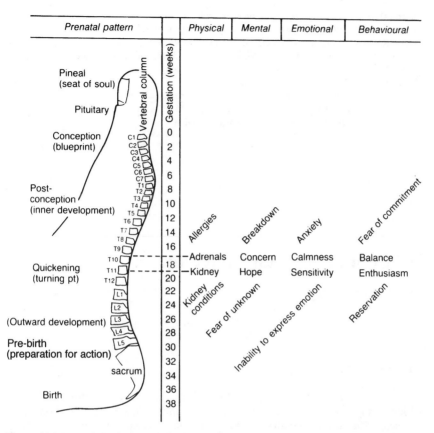

Prenatal pattern		Physical	Mental	Emotional	Behavioural

Figure 16.6 Prenatal development, indicating possible imbalance and corrected potential (MSR, 1989)

phobias, etc. or subconscious traumatic memories. The patients usually becomes more confident and secure, responding gently and safely to this subtle healing procedure.

Conclusion

Reflextherapy is a holistic, in-depth approach and should be regarded with respect, with suitable training, continuing education and support. For the therapist it provides a rewarding approach to treatment, where the practitioner grows in awareness, sensitivity, skill and satisfaction, seeing the benefit to the total health of the patient.

References

Capra, F. (1975) *Tao of Physics*, Fontana/Collins, London

Chopra, D. (1989) *Quantum Healing*, Bantam, New York
Cornelius, A (1902) *Pressure Points: Their Origin and Significance*,
Gerber, R. (1954) *Vibrational Medicine*, Bear and Co., Santa Fe
Jones, C. (1976–1995) Course Manual, Midland School of Reflextherapy, Warwick
Kaptchuk, T. (1983) *Chinese Medicine*, Rider House, London
Kushi, M. (1979) *Do-in*, Japan Publications
Saint-Pierre, G. (1989) *The Metemorphic Technique*, Element, Shaftsbury
St. John, R. (1980) *Metamorphosis*, R. St. John, OJAR, CA
Wolf, F.A. (1987) *The Body Quantum*, Heinemann, London

D. Connective tissue massage

Elizabeth A. Holey

Introduction

Connective tissue massage/manipulation (CTM) is a manual therapy technique which was developed by a German physiotherapist, Elisabeth Dicke, from 1929 onwards. She discovered that stroking thickened tissues over her lower back and sacrum relieved the back pain which accompanied her severe circulatory (endarteritis obliterans) problems. As Frau Dicke continued this manipulation with the help of a colleague, a surprising effect was achieved – the circulation in her legs improved sufficiently to enable her to avoid amputation. She was eventually able to return to work (Ebner, 1985).

The technique appeared to have a localized mechanical effect, reducing the tissue thickenings and decreasing pain, and a reflex effect which improved peripheral circulation and even reduced visceral symptoms.

The manipulation

The manipulation is one involving a 'hook-like' stroke, performed with the tip of the middle finger, which is reinforced with the fourth finger. Once contact is made between the therapist's finger and the patient's skin, tension is taken up in the skin by flexion at the therapist's distal interphalangeal joint and then a further pull exerted which creates a shear force at the interface between the skin and the fascial layer. A more superficial stroke can be carried out whereby the shear force occurs at the dermis/hypodermis interface.

Effects

The localized mechanical effect produces a stretch on the collagen fi
the application of an angulatory force at the tissue interface. This stretches the
elastic component of the tissue, thought to straighten out crimping in the fibres.
This effect is temporary. A stronger force breaks intermolecular bonds joining
crosslinks between fibres, in a permanent plastic effect. It is thought that a strong
effect can be produced by CTM because of the specificity of the stroke. Thus
remodelling of the shortened tissue is facilitated, reducing areas of thickening,
and re-establishing strength within the tissue and mobility at the interface
(Evans, 1973; Tillman and Cummings, 1992; Grodin and Cantu, 1993). In
addition, CTM possibly reduces viscosity in the ground substance by improving
fluid flow through tissues.

The mechanical effect will be of benefit where postural changes have
influenced tension in tissues. Posture is often a reflection of the psyche. 'Body
language' is a manifestation of personality, feelings and non-verbal communication. Where it is fairly static, it becomes held by fixed muscular patterns –
hence the ease at which an individual is recognized at a distance by unique
subtleties of gait or posture. This has been recognized by Reich (1949), and
practitioners such as Meziere, Rolf, Kurtz and Prestera treat the patient's
emotional condition by attempting to influence this body language. Emotional
factors make attempts to improve an individual's posture by purely physical
means less likely to succeed. Postural control is therefore much more effective if
the emotional aspects are simultaneously addressed. These practitioners attempt
the opposite – to influence emotional aspects via posture and movement. Meziere
uses open, relaxed, abduction and lateral rotation movements to correct muscle
imbalance and emotional imbalance, which are believed to coexist (Bertherat and
Bernstein, 1977). Rolf (1978) uses a manual therapy technique similar to CTM
but less anatomically based and specific, to normalize tissue tension throughout the body in a series of 10 treatments. Release of emotional tension is also
encouraged. Kurst and Prester (1970) have developed these principles in their
practice of body-centred psychotherapy.

Without such therapies, the muscles and connective tissues eventually
shorten, making posture less mobile, but fixed. The tightness is typically in the
tissues of the back due to the dual consequence of a tendency of the anti-gravity
muscles to shorten and emotional tension to manifest itself in the posterior
muscles of the neck, back and shoulder girdle. The tissues eventually can
become tender, painful and adherent. The situation is then self-perpetuating as
movement and exercise cause pain, since muscle contraction increases tension
on the adherent areas. A similar sequence of events occurs in patients suffering
chronic pain. The localized, mechanical stretching of CTM can reduce these
specific problems, reduce tissue tension and stimulate the autonomic nervous
system to achieve a sympathetic/parasympathetic balance. This latter effect
usually results in a significant feeling of well-being.

The effect of most interest in a psychiatric context is the reflex, autonomic
effect produced predominantly via the sympathetic nervous system. Dicke's
experience showed that CTM produces a reflex effect which occurs at some
distance from the point of stimulus. The previous work of Head (1898) and
MacKenzie (1917) elucidated this. Head discovered that visceral pathology
causes skin surface changes in areas sharing the same segmental nerve supply,

while MacKenzie found the same phenomena altering the tone of muscles sharing the same segmental innervation.

The skin areas were identified and named Head's zones and are recognizable as areas in which skin changes can be seen and palpated. These are found in the dermatome which corresponds segmentally to the sympathetic innervation of the affected structure. Haas (1968) differentiates the superficial zones between the dermis and the hypodermis, occurring in acute states and disappearing as the condition improves, from the fascial zones which appear in more chronic states and are palpable. The tissues exhibit an increased tension and may have an increased or decreased fluid balance with or without thickenings or indurations. When the stroke is effected in the region of a fascial zone, a sharp, 'cutting' sensation is felt by the patient (Ebner, 1985). Recognition of these zones forms part of the examination prior to treatment (Figure 16.7). They are used in treatment if the intention is to normalize all connective tissue tension. This is Ebner's (1985) ultimate goal of treatment, but usually CTM is more specifically focused. Also, the changes occurring in the zone areas may cause musculoskeletal symptoms themselves, so treatment may predominantly aim to have a localized mechanical effect in the zone areas. Head's zones identify visceral or systemic problems which may be treated via the connective tissue. Finally, and of most

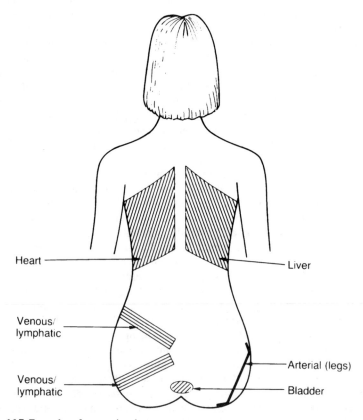

Figure 16.7 Examples of connective tissue zones

relevance here, is that the connective tissue can be stimulated to produce a general effect on the autonomic nervous system and lessen increased sympathetic activity occurring as a result of adverse neural tension in the autonomic nervous system or even an altered psychological state.

Assessment and treatment

A CTM assessment involves a detailed subjective assessment, followed by a visual examination of the patient's back and an assessment by palpation of tissue tension. Treatment with CTM must always start in the 'basic section' which is the area around the sacrum and buttocks. It appears to be necessary to stimulate the autonomics via the sacral area initially, in order to produce a controlled, satisfactory circulatory response. It is important that tissue tension is reduced and that a sharp sensation and triple response is produced in the basic section before proceeding. Where the therapist is unable to produce these effects, treatment must not be progressed. Undesirable side effects (such as faintness and palpitations) may otherwise be produced, although reasons for this are little understood at present.

The strokes are applied in areas where fascia occurs more superficially, where it joins muscle to bone or overlies anatomical spaces, or on intermuscular septa.

In the treatment of psychiatric patients, the aim is to induce the viscero-cutaneous reflex response. It is thought that CTM stimulates the sympathetic terminal reticulum in the skin (Bischof and Elmiger, 1963) and produces an autonomic balancing effect. The clinical application of this is perhaps best discussed by focusing on a specific study (see below).

Patients presenting for treatment who appear tired, listless, lethargic and depressed often respond to CTM by increased energy and enthusiasm for life, becoming more positive in outlook. Those who have a tendency to be anxious often become more calm and relaxed. In both types of patients, the sleep pattern becomes more normalized. CTM is described as having a tendency to stimulate the autonomic nervous system towards the parasympathetic side (Bischof and Elmiger, 1963; Ebner, 1985; Roozeboom, 1986), but clinical experience shows that if one system is more dominant at the commencement of treatment, CTM initially stimulates the opposite side until a more normal balance is achieved. A cathartic emotional release can occur.

The autonomic effects of anxiety are well known. They include: dizziness, palpitations, sweating, shaking, pins and needles (Lawler, 1990; Warren, 1992). CTM can reduce these sympathetic effects, inducing parasympathetic dominance and lessening the physical feelings associated with anxiety. The expected effects would be slowed heart rate, increase in skin resistance (lower levels of arousal), lower levels of muscle tension and a feeling of relaxation (Ebner, 1985).

Research findings

The observation that some patients experiencing a chronic anxiety state also present with poor circulation, muscular tension and pain (McKenzie *et al.*, 1983) prompted an investigation into the use of CTM in this condition, in the form of a pilot study. The subjects were 3 men and 2 women, age range 26–56 years, whose minimum duration of symptoms was 18 months, and who had all received anxiolytic drugs. Each subject received 10 treatment sessions of CTM, after having stopped drugs for 3 days prior to commencement. Heart rate, frontalis electromyographic (EMG) activity, forearm extensor EMG activity and skin resistance were recorded before the first and after the tenth treatment session, as measures of somatic 'tension' and 'relaxation'. Recordings were sampled at 1-minute intervals during a 12-minute rest period and immediately prior to each stimulus during a subsequent stimulation period. In the stimulation period, 20 noises of varying intensity and duration were played at random intervals, as described by Blackburn and Bonham (1980). Four out of five subjects experienced a significant (P=<0.0001) reduction in heart rate response after treatment, two experienced significant results with regard to skin resistance, another two with regard to frontalis EMG activity and two with regard to extensor EMG activity. Unfortunately, data for two subjects in skin resistance and extensor EMG parameters were incomplete and excluded from statistical analysis. All subjects showed a significant response to treatment in one or more of the parameters. Following treatment, two reported a reduction in symptoms and three discontinued drugs. Two physiotherapists assessed them and found a reduction in tension in all subjects.

Thus, responses compatible with a reduction in anxiety were significant in the majority of parameters. The anomalous EMG results were explained by the possibility that the frontalis muscle may be more reactive in depressive illness, but the xtensors more reactive in agitative states.

The number of patients included in this study was clearly too small to provide any firm evidence of the effectiveness of CTM in the treatment of anxiety. As a pilot study it does, however, offer some confirmation of clinical observation (Ebner, 1985), and suggests a trend in response, indicating the value of further study. It is suggested that the difference in the parameters by which each patient responded to treatment confirms the theory that individuals have a unique pattern of response to stress and that CTM helps 'unlock' this unique stress response pattern, sometimes producing a cathartic reaction. Many patients sleep following treatment.

Patients experiencing CTM often report a feeling of deep relaxation and well-being following a treatment, and sleep patterns are often inadvertently improved. Clearly this would benefit patients suffering from a range of psychiatric disorders. Where localized musculoskeletal problems coexist, the benefits would be multiplied.

Ebner (1985) describes the treatment of a depressed female patient, aged 32:

...headaches daily for the last one and a half years, complains of pins and needles in left arm and leg. Has been fully investigated for headaches. No obstetric abnormalities. Gives account of broken marriage. Has a history of depression. Sleeps very badly. ...Back inspection: Arterial area + (suffers from cold feet). Interscapular area ++ (headaches for $1\frac{1}{2}$ years daily).

Within five treatments, progression had been made to the interscapular area and the patient's sleeping pattern was improved. By treatment six, she had been free of headaches for two days and by treatment 11 they had become occasional and slight. The pins and needles in the arm and leg had also practically disappeared by treatment 11. On discharge after treatment 16, she 'sleeps well and is cheerful, no arm or leg complaint'

Conclusion

It is hoped that a case has been presented for a more extensive use of CTM in the treatment of patients with psychiatric disorders. The treatment is not always tolerated, as it is desirable to treat the patient in a sitting position and a degree of discomfort can be produced by the stroke. An opportunity is presented for the physiotherapist to treat the sympathetic symptoms of anxiety or to induce a feeling of well-being in those with depression, while symptoms of localized soft-tissue changes are lessened. Positive help is therefore offered to improve the subjective physical feelings of the patient, through which emotional responses may be 'unlocked' in catharsis. In some cases, it may be felt that clinical psychology back-up may be required for support during cathartic reactions.

Of course, CTM should be used in conjunction with other appropriate therapies such as relaxation, exercise and counselling, rather than replacing them. CTM should prove to be a vital component of the repertoire of physiotherapists who work with psychiatric patients, adding a powerful dimension to the ability to meet these individuals' needs.

Acknowledgements

The author is grateful to Hilary Lawler and Richard Stephenson who demonstrated the benefit of their psychiatric experience in constructive comments on this contribution.

References

Bertherat, T. and Bernstein, C. (1977) *The Body has Its Reasons*, Cedar, London

Bischof, I and Elmiger, G. (1963) Connective tissue massage In: *Massage, Manipulation and Traction* (ed. Licht, S.), Waverley Press, Baltimore

Blackburn, I.M. and Bonham K.G. (1980) Experimental effects of cognitive therapy technique in depressed patients. *British Journal of Social and Clinical Psychology*, **19**, 353-363

Ebner, M. (1985) *Connective Tissue Manipulations*, Kreiger, Malabar, Florida.

Evans, J.H. (1973) Structure and function of soft connective tissue. *PhD thesis*, University of Strathclyde, Scotland

Grodin, A.J. and Cantu, R.I. (1993) Soft tissue mobilisation. In *Rational Manual Therapies* (eds Basmajian, J.V. and Nyberg, R.), Williams and Wilkins, Baltimore

Haas, H. (1968) Bindegewebsmassage. Wirkunsphysiologische grundlagen unf methodik. *Zeitschrift Artzl. Fortbild*, **62**, Jg. H. 13 (English translation by Mrs Steiner)

Head H. (1898) Die sensibilitaetsstoerungen der haut bei viszeral erkrankugen. Cited in Ebner, M. (1985) *Connective Tissue Manipulations*, Kreiger, Malabar, Florida

Kurtz, R. and Prestera, H. (1984) *The Body Reveals*, Harper and Row, San Francisco

Reich, W. (1949) *Character Analysis*, Orgon Institute Press, New York

Rolf, I. (1978) *Rolfing: The Integration of Human Structures*, Barnes and Noble, New York

Roozeboom, H. (1986) Connective tissue massage: a review. *Journal of the Hong Kong Physiotherapy Association*, **8** 26–28

Lawler, H. (1990) Psychiatric illness. In *Cash's Textbook of General Medical and Surgical Conditions for Physiotherapists* (ed. Downie, P.A.) Faber and Faber, London

MacKenzie (1917) Krankheitszeichen und ihre Auslegung. Kabitzsch, Wuerzburg. Cited in Ebner, M. (1985) *Connective Tissue Manipulations*, Kreiger, Malabar, Florida

McKechnie, A.A. *et al.* (1983) Anxiety states: a preliminary report on the value of connective tissue massage. *Journal of Psychosomatic Research*, **27**(2), 125–129

Tillman, L.J. and Cummings, G.S. (1992) Biological mechanisms of connective tissue mutability. In *Dynamics of Human Biological Tissues* (eds Currier, D.P. and Nelson, R.M.) F.A. Davies, Philadelphia

Warren, E. (1992) Psychological treatment in physiotherapy practice. In *Physiotherapy: A Psychosocial Approach* (ed. French, S.) Butterworth–Heinemann, Oxford

Part III

17

Child psychiatry

A. Physiotherapy in a children's psychiatric unit

Janet Ward

General introduction

It is rare for physiotherapists in the UK to work in the field of child mental health. When the physiotherapy authors of this chapter were invited to work with children, there was very little literature to follow and few with practical experience to consult. It is inevitable, therefore, that the treatment approaches evolved out of specific working situations. What follows are personal accounts of work done and they are not in any way prescriptive or posed as expert opinion. If the future opens the way for more physiotherapists to work in this field, it is hoped that a more extensive body of knowledge and experience will develop.

The first section of this chapter describes physiotherapy with children in an inpatient psychiatric unit, while the second section describes the work of a physiotherapist in a child guidance clinic. In the final section, a psychologist writes about the child's world of internal pictures and the technique of creative visualization used to explore and understand these images, in order to relieve children's conflicts and help them to relax.

Introduction

Children admitted to residential psychiatric units have multiple problems. For example, the child may be an elective mute or a verbally and physically abused or abusive child. The child may have received physical and verbal abuse from adults at home or have an obsessive routine that inhibits normal family life.

In recent years there has been recognition of the fact that many of the children admitted to residential psychiatric units have difficulty in motor co-ordination out of proportion to their general abilities. These children may be called clumsy. The level of clumsiness can be from mild to severe. The child works hard to mask his/her clumsiness or avoids taking part in any activity where there is a chance of failure. Occasionally the child will deliberately court failure.

Children admitted to these units usually have poor social skills, low self-esteem, poor peer relationships and abnormal relationships with the adults with whom they regularly come into contact. If the child feels under pressure – real or imagined – their anxiety level will rise, resulting in disruptive behaviour or opting out. The unit provides a controlled environment, with specialist care provided by nurses trained in mental health, suitably trained care assistants, occupational and speech therapists and physiotherapists. Team work is essential to provide the consistent care required to allow the child to gain the maximum help and opportunities during the period of assessment.

General assessment

The task of the physiotherapist is to assess each child, devise an individual programme based around their particular problem, and then to reassess at regular intervals as the child gains in both skill and confidence. While most of the children may exhibit clumsy traits, only a small proportion will be diagnosed as truly clumsy.

Physiotherapy sessions are still valuable in building up a child's self-esteem, even when no clumsy traits are exhibited. A major factor in planning the programme is the estimated period of treatment/assessment on the unit. This may be as short as 6 weeks or as long as 2 years, depending on the policy of the unit, the child's problems and the suitability of a placement following assessment.

Before beginning an assessment it is prudent to check footwear, feet and clothing. Toenails that are too long damage the nail bed and cause pain, while badly cut, bitten or torn off nails can result in ingrowing toenails, giving severe pain and a reluctance to take part in any activity. Clothing and footwear that are too large or too small hamper freedom of movement and can make the child appear to be more ungainly than is the case. As the children bring in their own clothing and shoes, the nursing team's help must be sought to ask parents to ensure that the child has clothing of adequate warmth and comfort. The child can then proceed to gain the maximum benefit from the sessions.

Gross motor assessment

Fine motor assessment is usually carried out by the occupational therapist, who will use structured play therapy sessions to enable the skills to be practised. Therefore, the physiotherapy assessment is of gross motor movements. The age range in a children's unit is between 5 years and 13 years. Children 14 years and over are admitted to adolescent units.

It is important throughout the assessment that the child is encouraged to perform all the tasks to the best of their ability, even if the movement performed is clumsy. As a guide I have included a checklist of basic gross motor movements used in assessing children on admission. This is not a comprehensive list and physiotherapists wishing to progress further should read widely and develop their own assessment schemes.

The assessment area can be indoors or outdoors, but must be spacious and comfortable for the child and the therapist. The therapist begins an assessment by asking the child to stand. First, a large ball and then a small ball are thrown and the therapist notes balance, eye–hand co-ordination, a wide or narrow base and the degree of accuracy obtained in receiving the ball, be it thrown in the midline, or to left or right. Provided that concentration is maintained, the child can be asked to bounce the ball, beginning with the large ball and, if successful, progressing to the small ball. Balance and ability to gauge the push required to bring the ball back for the next push and stay more or less on the same spot is difficult for a child with clumsy traits. Most children are happy to show off their running ability and this can be followed by hopping, using alternate legs. The hopping is first in a straight line, then in a zigzag pattern. The normal pattern of movement is to withdraw the other leg behind the balancing, hopping leg. The clumsy child finds this difficult due to poor hip control. If there is a fixture point for a large skipping rope, the child may skip on the spot and then be offered a small rope to attempt to skip by themselves after which skipping, including forward movement, can be introduced. The therapist watches for associated movements, facial gestures as the child concentrates and the co-ordination needed to time the jump to clear the rope. Dribbling the ball in straight and zigzag lines shows balance and eye–foot control, together with foot dominance, while walking forward and backwards along a line using a heel-strike pattern is helpful in showing up defects in gait. Laterality is important and many of these children find it difficult to know left from right. The sequence of body patterns and games involving standing and lying, supine and prone, will help. Clapping rhythms encourage concentration and focus hearing for those children who 'switch off'. Finally, the Fogg test is used indoors and should be carried out with socks and shoes removed. The child is asked to stand on the outer border of the foot and then to walk towards the therapist. Inversion of the hands, mirroring the feet, suggests developmental delay in children over 8 years.

Aims of treatment

The aims of treatment are as follows:

- to provide an individual treatment plan for each child
- to promote skills enhancing feelings of self-esteem and confidence
- to enable the child to become a valued member of their peer group
- to enable the child to be at ease with themselves on discharge.

In simple terms this means that the child should be able to kick a ball with direction and accuracy, and to throw a ball and succeed in catching it every time regardless of the speed or direction from which it is thrown.

Treatment

Treatment is initially on a one-to-one basis, so that time can be spent on specific areas of difficulty. The environment is controlled, minimizing distractions and thus encouraging self-esteem and self-confidence.

Having gained the basic skills, the children are encouraged to display their new skills in more realistic situations. This may be football in the playground, throwing and catching games, hopscotch, skipping to increase stamina in the overweight child, playing tag or climbing on frames in the playground.

Suggested areas of specific skills to be covered

- balance
- eye–hand and eye–foot control

- movement
- body and space perception.

All treatments aim to equip the children with the basic skills on which they can build when they reintegrate into normal life.

Balance
Task. To improve balance statically and actively.

Equipment. Mats, tape, balance-beam, planks and bricks, beanbags, balls.

Exercises:
(a) Graded balance exercises in lying, kneeling and standing.
(b) Working in pairs at balance.
(c) Walking along tape.
(d) Walking along balance-beam.
(e) Handstands and cartwheels.
(f) Walking with beanbags on heads.
(g) Carrying objects while on the beam/planks.

Eye–hand and eye–foot control
Task. To develop the skill of catching and throwing with direction, force and accuracy; to develop the skills of striking and kicking with direction, force and accuracy.

Equipment. Streamers, beanbags, balls of varying sizes.

Exercises:
(a) Use of ribbon streamers to encourage eye–hand control and to gain relaxed head movements.
(b) Roll balls between a pair.
(c) Bounce ball between two.
(d) Throw beanbags/balls into box.
(e) Control ball/beanbag with hockey stick.
(f) Football with soft balls.

Movement
Task. To improve total body flexibility; to enable the child to roll, crawl, climb, run, skip.

Equipment. Mats, beanbags, hoops, balls, skipping ropes.

Exercises:
(a) Forward and backward rolls.
(b) Slow and quick walking.
(c) Funny walking.
(d) Jumping over rope forward, backward, diagonally.
(e) Hopping.
(f) Making shapes.

Games could include hopscotch, climbing over and under tables, jumping onto islands.

Body and space perception

Task. To gain knowledge of the body in space; to increase awareness of laterality; to stimulate body image.

Equipment. Large pieces of paper, pencils, blindfolds, sticker labels, fun glasses.

Exercises:
(a) Establish knowledge of right and left in supine and prone positions.
(b) Touch various parts of the body and name them.
(c) Draw around each other.
(d) Use arms in front, behind, under, over, through.
(e) Make funny faces.
(f) Mime and copy a partner.
(g) Trampolining (instructor must be registered).
(h) Sequencing – simple yoga movements.

Conclusion

It is always wise for physiotherapists to acquaint themselves with the restraint policy of their unit, and the Children Act 1989 for children's rights. Another important policy to know intimately is the loss of privilege policy. The child on admission is told about this policy and the therapist, as part of the multi-disciplinary team, follows a consistent approach.

As it is hoped that all the children will return to their homes and schools, it is vital to include some group work towards the end of the period of assessment. Group work, while offering scope for variety and team work, needs to be well planned and firmly structured. The element of competition and the prospect of failure mean that a dramatic fall in the level of behaviour can be expected. The therapist must be prepared for varying levels of behaviour as the child realizes it is safe 'to show some frustration', yet the therapist should firmly discourage unacceptable behaviour.

The rewards when a child succeeds and can put new skills into play, and when their self-esteem and self-confidence grows, make this tough and at times difficult job very worth while.

Further reading

Gordon, N. and McKinlay, I. (eds) (1989) *Helping Clumsy Children*, revised edition, Churchill Livingstone, Edinburgh

HMSO (1989) *The Children Act 1989*, Her Majesty's Stationery Office, London

Levitt, S. (1982) *Treatment of Cerebral Palsy and Motor Delay*, 2nd edn, Blackwell, Oxford

Tamsley, A.E. (1980) *Motor Education*, Edward Arnold, London

B. A physiotherapist's contribution to a child guidance clinic

Diana Beaven

Introduction

Children delight in kinaesthetic sensations, thus movement and touch can be potent interventions. Most children enjoy the acquisition of physical skills and provided that relaxation is taught using a method appropriate to their age group, youngsters will usually be receptive. Awareness of tension, posture and movement, learnt through relaxation, will act as a buffer against stress and ill health in later life.

Relaxation techniques can successfully be worked into physical education periods at school, but there is also a place for their application in the classroom, e.g. checking finger tension in writing, drawing and the playing of musical instruments. Older children can usefully talk about stress-provoking situations, e.g. bullying, parental rows and examinations. They enjoy taking pulse and breathing rate and other objective measures of human functioning and can master the Laura Mitchell method of relaxation (Mitchell, 1977).

Infants can feel overwhelmed by rage and need vigorous physical activity to release strong emotion. This activity needs to be followed by a slow and controlled task, e.g. walking along an imaginary tightrope or freezing when the leader, 'a witch', casts a spell over the group. It is necessary to have this quietening down time following the expressive activity, in order to ground children's energy and prevent them from feeling out of control.

Besides the teaching of relaxation to children in mainstream schools, there is an application to individuals with special needs. For one year, the author gave sessional input to a child guidance clinic, working closely with a multidisciplinary team. Children who demonstrated emotional and behavioural disorders were seen in the context of their family. A child experiencing difficulties may be reflecting problems within the family. In addition to the family receiving help from the multidisciplinary team, the team asked the author to become involved with children who were experiencing symptoms which were physical in nature or related to body energy. The problems included hyperventilation, migraine, bedwetting, aggression and hyperactivity. The approach involved relaxation, calm breathing and creative movement, supplemented by counselling of the child and family. The treatment of several children is outlined in the following examples.

Case studies

Example A

Jane was 14 and had experienced several panic attacks at school. She was frightened of the sensation of not being able to breathe and concerned by her sickness absence from school. I spent some time listening to Jane, which built a rapport

This helped in the next stage of teaching Jane the Laura Mitchell method of relaxation. In the third session I used diagrams to expand my explanation of the symptoms of hyperventilation and related this to her panicky feelings. Jane began to understand how the asthma she had largely outgrown had left her breathing with excessive upper chest movement which accelerated when she was anxious. The calm breathing she learnt helped her to feel more relaxed and she was able to tell me about episodes of bullying at school, which preceded the panic attacks. Jane was happy for me to pass on this information to our team psychologist who was planning a meeting with Jane's mother and her teacher. I taught Jane some stretching and shaking movements of her body to help her wind down after school. As muscular tension decreased, Jane found she was better able to discuss her worries with her mother. After five weekly sessions, Jane felt able to cope with school confidently and had learned to relax, breathe freely and express her difficulties.

Example B

Karen was a restless, overactive but endearing 6 year old. She was eager to please but could not keep still. The team psychiatrist, after meeting Karen and her family, was not able to identify any family dynamics or allergic food reactions that might be influencing the hyperactivity. Indeed the family seemed stable, loving and healthy. Karen was more at ease when allowed to move freely around the room, sometimes rocking and balancing on furniture or the floor. In her restlessness she appeared to be searching for rhythms. With her mother's assistance, we explored ways for Karen to enjoy movements which involved steadying rhythms. Sitting back to back on the floor rocking in different directions with me, then with her mother, helped her to settle. I mentioned the value of swings, hammocks and rocking chairs. I experimented with different pieces of music to find what rhythms encouraged Karen to express her restlessness in creative movement; slow steady music helped her to find calming movement rhythms for her body.

Dance type movement which brings a person's energy down into the lower limbs is useful. The position of hips and knees bent, as in a Zulu warrior's stamping and in Tai Chi, can be very grounding, i.e. can settle a person's energy. Karen enjoyed lunging and movement, performed very slowly and steadily in the skiing posture. At the end of each session, Karen and her mother lay down for a few minutes contracting and relaxing different parts of their bodies, then becoming aware of the contact of their floppy bodies with the floor. Karen was encouraged to think of stroking her cat and to capture all the details of this scene (children have a very good visual memory). I found that the stroking of Karen's forehead helped her to settle. This action is thought to produce alpha waves in the brain – the waveform related to relaxation and creativity.

As a result of the sessions with me, Karen and her mother found ways to channel and modify Karen's restless energy; however, I was unable to effect a permanent change. A break in the sessions was agreed while Karen's mother took her to a cranial osteopath. Five treatments proved dramatically helpful in relieving Karen's restlessness. Karen's birth was by forceps and, as a baby, she had been distressed and tearful, with an erratic sleep pattern. She had been happiest when rocked and carried around. The cranial osteopath defined the problems as a distortion in the cranium which was compromising the normal slight degree of mobility in the bones and meninges. The osteopath viewed this mobility as essential to health. With a very gentle hold of the head and a light use of pressure, the cranial osteopath worked to encourage tissue motion and improve fluid dynamics. Six months after the final osteopathic treatment, Karen's mother said her daughter had sustained the improvement in concentration and well-being and seemed much happier and less restless.

Examples of work with teenagers

An aggressive teenage girl presented with premenstrual mood swings and irritability leading to violent outbursts. I saw her for five individual sessions of relaxation and movement, weekly at first, then fortnightly. By the last session she described feeling calmer and her parents reported a decline in their daughter's destructive and abusive behaviour. Practical work with teenagers, in each case, included a counselling element. The release of muscular tension, brings to a person a greater awareness of feeling and willingness to discuss worries and conflicts.

A teenage boy who regularly wet his bed responded to a similar blend of relaxation and counselling. Although dialogue with parents is important, I found that teenagers benefited from having the majority of their sessions alone with me.

Several aggressive boys, aged between 9 and 13 years, needed a more robust treatment approach. Had the referrals been received around the same time, a group might have been effective, but this was not the case. A group would have allowed the boys to learn from each other in imaginative ways and pit their strength against equals. With the use of a creative movement approach, I explored strong but playful actions with individuals. Movements were chosen to provide controlled outlets for excessive energy, anger and frustration. The need to be masterful and expressive was also acknowledged. On one occasion, the youngster and I sat on the floor back to back, while we both tried to push the other across the floor. Pushing in pairs in the standing position with the back, the arms or the side and hips, provided opportunities to express strength and resistance. Where possible, siblings were involved in these games; stamping to African rhythms, punching pillows and using the voice, movement and breathing proved exhilarating and cathartic. After vigorous expression, it was sometimes appropriate to teach these youngsters a quiet relaxation technique. There was a need to explore opportunities, to express this unbridled energy at home and school; sport, drumming and the martial arts were found to be helpful, especially when these provided a context for father and son to be involved together.

Multidisciplinary approach

Multidisciplinary working can link together the psychological and the practical. For example, a physiotherapist and a psychologist jointly facilitated a group for three sexually abused teenage girls, sharing professional skills. The group dynamic developed from verbal disclosure of the problems to practical exercises chosen to provide the opportunity to work through the difficulties. Relaxation and breathing helped to release contracted pelvic muscles and to free diaphragmatic breathing when upper chest breathing was precipitating panic and insomnia. Creative movement in pairs was used to explore the roles of leading and following; this led to discussion of the girls' fear of being out of control when not being in charge of a situation. Assertiveness role-plays were enjoyed, with feedback given to the girls on voice and posture in order to help them understand the signals conveyed by their body language.

One of the main values of creative movement was to allow the girls to experience their bodies in a pleasureable way and to improve body image and thus self-image. Movement was at all times explored and not imposed. Emphasis was placed on sparking the imagination and encouraging acceptable playfulness, qualities which enhance mental health. The issue of correct boundaries was addressed using practical exercises and discussions in what is appropriate and inappropriate touching and play.

The kinaesthetic background of a physiotherapist can also be utilized in helping disadvantaged parents learn how to play with their young children when there is a failure in bonding. A Bristol dance therapist (Marie Ware, 1993, personal communication) described a group, for socially deprived mothers and children where there was little engagement of a physical or verbal nature between parent and child. After using movement, activities and games with this group, the children were spontaneously leaping onto their mothers' laps, giving eye contact, laughing and cuddling. The mothers felt delighted that they were learning parenting skills, something of which they had little experience during their own disadvantaged childhoods.

These children often came from families where there was unemployment and despair. Human interaction was replaced by the television; babies and young children were not being spoken to and not acquiring language skills. The constant high-decibel levels of video, hi-fi and television were replacing interpersonal contact. A speech therapist referred to this group children whose language was slow in developing. The speech therapist found that movement and body language skills preceded the development of verbal communication.

Conclusion

One of the exciting aspects of working with children experiencing difficulties is their responsiveness to help; small interventions in the family system and in the life of the young person appear to make significant and lasting change possible.

As the case studies demonstrate, a physiotherapist's expertise in movement and handling can make a valuable contribution to the overall care of children experiencing difficulties. In addition, groups led jointly by a physiotherapist and another member of the multidisciplinary team can open the way for new and imaginative approaches to treatment.

References and further reading

Bearan, D. and Tollington, G. (1994) Healing the split: a psychological approach to working with sexually abused teenage girls. *Physiotherapy*, **80**(7)

Foster, R. (1976) *Knowing in My Bones*, A. and C. Black, London

Madders, J. (1979) *Stress and Relaxation*, Acro, New York

Mitchell, L. (1977) *Simple Relaxation*, Pitman Press, Bath

Varma, V.P. (1990) *The Management of Children with Emotional and Behavioural Difficulties*, Routledge, London

C. Creative visualization with children

Brian Roet

Introduction

As youngsters, we have an ability that many of us lose on the way to adulthood. It is the ability to know the world, and our response to the world, by internal pictures. Adults call this inner world a fantasy world; to children it is their reality. We, as grown ups, do our best (worst) to reduce childhood imagery by commands such as: 'Don't daydream!' 'Come to your senses!', 'Stop imagining things!'

It is important to note that this internal world of pictures is as real to the child as the concrete material world outside, and the feelings created by these pictures as real as feelings resulting from external events.

We can make use of this knowledge to help children on a deep level by a technique called *creative visualization*, which enables the child to be in touch with his inner (real) world by way of pictures. As we do so, we help him to explore and understand his feelings, attitudes and behaviour on this deep level and change them if necessary.

The basic aim is to explore feelings (problems) and follow them by careful guidance to their pictorial representation, of which the child may or may not be aware. In this way we encourage (in a protective and supportive way) the child to explore the pictures and gain confidence in the process.

Example 1

Suzie is 9 and has been having problems mixing with the other children at school. She tells her mother she is frightened and does not want to go to school; her mother decides to explore the feeling she calls 'frightened'.

She asks Suzie where in her body the feeling is, and finds out it is in her stomach. She asks Suzie to 'go inside and see what it looks like'. Suzie sees a dragon and is frightened.

Her mother calmly and gently encourages Suzie in a supportive and caring way to learn about the dragon. Gradually Suzie approaches the dragon and pats it in her imagination. The dragon she feared becomes friendly and in time takes her for a magic ride on his back. Suzie now feels better because she has a powerful friend inside instead of a fearsome monster, and she is able to attend school with the help of this inner feeling.

The whole of this exercise took half an hour, helped Suzie and her mother to feel closer and was enjoyed by both as an exciting and joyful experience. Both felt they had achieved something positive and overcome a troublesome hurdle.

What had actually happened was that Suzie's mother had joined Suzie in *her* world, rather than dragging her to the adult world with words like frightened, tummy pains, naughty, resistant, school phobia and other words to describe our behaviour.

What are the benefits of creative visualization?

There are three principal benefits derived from creative visualization:

• We are relating to the child on his level. This has a very different feeling and response from trying to educate them to grow up. The child is really understood by their inner criteria, shares deep communication with the adult and feels happier, more secure and understood.
• Problems are dealt with in a creative, exciting and fun way. This appeals to the adventurous part of the child.
• Future difficulties are prevented, as the technique allows 'inner harmony' to build confidence, and mechanisms are set in motion to cope with future events.

The inner world of pictures is already there, it is not created by the technique. Adjustments and suitable alterations occur in the process, causing loss of fear and building self-esteem. This inner world may well go back to mythology or be related to learning experiences occurring at home or school. It is similar to the world of dreams, but is much more accessible and open to change.

Imagine sitting in a boat on the Great Barrier Reef off the Australian coast. The water is clear and your experience is of the sun, the breeze, the sound of the sea and seagulls and the gentle rocking of the boat. That is how you would describe how you felt with that perspective of your world.

Now imagine puting on a mask and snorkel and diving into the clear water to discover the magical world underneath. Your description now may well be of amazing colours, bright fish floating by, silence, perhaps an eerie feeling of weightlessness, excitement, perhaps fear or exhilaration.

Now imagine an experienced and trusted diver leads you through coral outcrops and helps you feel comfortable, confident and in control in this new underwater world, so that you are eager to explore more, learn the different dimensions of that area of the reef and combine your above-water activities and attitudes with your new underwater experiences.

In this way you gain the best of both worlds and are able to cope with experiences within the boat or under the surface.

Creative visualization is similar to the underwater guide. The inner world of pictures is already there, but competent, caring guides are needed to explore and enjoy it. The age most suitable for this technique is from 5 upwards. With patients younger than this it may be difficult to keep their concentration span long enough to focus on the inner world.

How do we go about creative visualization?

Example 2

Tony is 10 years old. He is an 'achiever' or perhaps an 'over-achiever'. He attends a school where excellence is demanded and competition very strong. He is captain of the swimming team; in the choir; practises martial arts; and learns a language all on top of pressurized schoolwork.

For a month Tony experienced illness in the form of abdominal pains, headaches and being very irritable with his friends and family. His doctor prescribed tablets for the abdominal pains, to no effect.

I asked him to 'explore inside' and see what he could find. He said, 'My brain says I'm not ill, but I need more rest'. He found a 'worrying part' in the back of his head which was a *'blue ball'*. This ball had, inside it, 'rest, ill, school' as things to worry about. He explained this as his worry about missing school and illness being interrelated; the concern about rest was to balance things.

He explored further and found a part of the right side of his head in the form of a *'yellow cube'* which kept telling him 'you can win, you can do it'. When he told this yellow cube he was being sick from this, the yellow cube replied, 'I don't care'.

He decided to replace the yellow cube, which was directing him to worry in case he did not win, with a *'green triangle'*. The green triangle was to continue telling him to 'do your best, be happy, have a good time, it doesn't matter if you do not win'. It was to continue telling him, 'you are OK even if you don't win'.

The 'internal Tony' (a part he had previously found) took responsibility for making sure the 'green triangle' remained in charge and the 'yellow cube' did not return. Over the next few days his pain, headaches and mood settled and he felt in control again.

Clean language

Clean language is important. In order to explore the world that is already there, it is important not to 'contaminate' it with our own personal comments, ideas or advice. Hence, the use of language which is not coloured or moralizing supports the child in his own exploration.

Supporting words such as 'Is that so?', 'Would you like to explore more?', 'I wonder where that could lead?', 'That sounds interesting', etc., focus the attention on the child and internal activity rather than bringing him 'out' to conscious logical thought.

One way of looking at what is happening is by viewing it on different levels. On the superficial, 'conscious' level the child has a symptom, feeling, attitude. This is mirrored by the internal world of pictures and if this world is altered there will be parallel alterations at other levels.

Example 3
Laura's daughter Joan, aged 7, was upset by being constantly left out of play groups. Laura decided to explore visualization as a method of understanding her daughter's plight.

She asked Joan about the feelings she had when left out and Joan indicated a 'sad feeling' in her tummy. In a supportive way Laura guided her into the feeling in her tummy (imagining she was inside her tummy) to see what it looked like.

Joan described a dark cave with a tunnel leading from it. With Laura's gentle, caring support Joan went on a journey along pathways, over waterfalls and through forests. At one stage some children were playing around a maypole and invited her to join. For some reason she was unable to do so.

After some minutes Joan sat there with her eyes closed describing the journey; sometimes she cried, other times she smiled, after a little while she decided to lie down in some grass and doze off. When she opened her eyes she said, 'I love you Mummy. You understand me so well'.

The next day when Joan was left out of a group she came running to Laura exclaiming, 'I now know why I'm left out!'

'Why is that?', asked Laura.

'Because I really want to be on my own.'

From then on there were no more problems when Joan was not included with her friends.

At no stage did Laura 'interrupt' the fantasy or tell Joan what to do. Occasionally, if Joan was frightened of the dark, she would offer the comment, 'Would you like a torch?', as there are no limits to the imagination's provision of things to help. Her main contributions were:

'What shall we do now?'

'Isn't that interesting.'

'I wonder what will happen next?'

The aim was to encourage Joan 'to face' whatever occurred on her journey and overcome fears in the process. In every instance, when a dragon or waterfall presented itself it changed in a positive way when not avoided. The dragon took Joan on a magic ride and the waterfall led her to a lake with fairies.

Often the pictures are purely mechanical, as illustrated below.

Example 4

Anne, aged 10, had been through troubled times with her parents divorcing. For four years her tension had been reflected by screwing up her toes in her shoes. This led to callouses on the ends of her toes, which worried her.

She sought help to stop the habit, which she explained as follows: 'My toes feel itchy, I screw them up against the end of my shoes, which stops the itch for a few seconds, then I relax them and they itch again, so I screw them up. This goes on all day and only stops when I go to sleep at night.'

I asked her to 'go inside' to look at the mechanism involved and, with some gentle guidance, she saw nerves taking messages from her toes to her mind carrying the 'itchy' message – these were coloured red. Other nerves came down from her mind to her toes carrying the message to 'screw them up' – these were green nerves. Between us, we worked out a way of blocking the green messages so the itchy message had no return vehicle to complete the habit loop.

Almost immediately she was able to have her toes at rest. I made her a tape with our discussion on it, so she could repeat the internal message and block the 'screwing' messages to her toes.

In two weeks the habit had been reduced by 80% and in a month it had gone altogether. Anne was delighted by the adventure, as was her father, who had sat in during the session.

Conclusion

In summary, creative visualization is a fascinating and rewarding way of helping children with their problems. The process enables child and adult to enjoy the experience and places the emphasis on a completely different plane from that of logical discussion or medical intervention.

18

Eating disorders

Kirstie Davison

Introduction

This chapter is concerned with a range of distressing conditions which have been increasingly publicized in the media over the last few years.

The effects that these conditions have on a sufferer's body and physical health are consequential to the way that the sufferer thinks and feels about herself and how she copes with problems. It is therefore quite natural for physiotherapists to find themselves included in the range of professionals who might be involved in therapy and rehabilitation.

Since the great majority of sufferers of eating disorders are women, feminine pronouns are used when talking generally about patients and in specific case examples.

Definition

Eating disorders are manifested when a person, at a conscious or subconscious level, first uses and then loses control over their eating in an attempt to cope with their problems. This process can result in life-endangering situations and grossly interferes with the individual's ability to live a full adult life, integrating self, family, work and social life. It affects their mental, physical and emotional health in a negative way. The two main diagnoses are anorexia nervosa and bulimia nervosa.

Anorexia nervosa ('want of appetite', OED) is characterized by weight loss in the absence of any other disease that might explain loss in body weight. The diagnostic criteria for anorexia sufferers are:

- an intense fear of gaining weight which does not diminish as weight is lost
- weight loss of at least 15% of original body weight
- disturbance of body image, claiming to feel fat even when emaciated
- amenorrhoea in women, of at least three consecutive cycles.

Bulimia nervosa is characterized by binge eating that is experienced as being out of control. It was described by Professor R. Palmer as 'total dietary chaos syndrome' (Palmer, 1979). The thought processes are similar to those of anorexia, and they have been called failed starvers, as opposed to the straight starvers (anorexia nervosa) and would-be starvers (Welbourne and Purgold, 1984). The diagnostic criteria for bulimia sufferers are:

- recurrent episodes of binge eating
- feeling of lack of control of eating behaviour during the binges
- regular self-induced vomiting, use of laxatives or diuretics, strict dieting or fasting or vigorous exercise in order to prevent weight gain
- minimum average of two binge episodes per week for at least 3 months
- persistent over-concern with body weight and shape.

Compulsive over-eaters may be seen as people who regularly and continually over-eat and are unable to control the weight gain by any means.

Epidemiology

Figures for sufferers of eating disorders are extremely difficult to establish with any degree of accuracy. They are differently quoted in every book or article published. The ones quoted below are those presented in a recent proposal to establish an Eating Disorders Service in Gloucester, and were provided by the Consultant in Public Health. Anecdotally the Royal College of Psychiatrists say that 1 in 10 women will be affected in some way during their lives. Clinical evidence is that the numbers are rising, both for women and men, but those for women are rising faster. As public awareness has arisen, so have the numbers of young women and girls presenting at the GPs surgery requesting help. This will have a positive effect in that help offered early can prevent years of suffering followed by years of therapy with a reduced prognosis.

The ratio of occurrence of anorexia nervosa is 10 females : 1 male. For bulimia, the occurrence ratio is approximately 20 females : 1 male. The peak incidence occurs in 15–16 year olds for anorexia and at 23 years for bulimia.

The incidence of anorexia nervosa is as follows:

- full syndrome: 1% of 12–18-year-old girls
- partial syndrome: 2–3% of 12–18-year-old girls
- rate of admission: 14–20 per million women.

Outcome of the severe syndrome:

- 50% recover spontaneously
- 15% become chronic but recover
- 5% die – half due to suicide and half from starvation.

The average duration of illness of those going on to the chronic stage is 4 years.

The incidence of bulimia nervosa is as follows:

- full syndrome: 2% of 15–45-year-old women
- partial syndrome: 4–5% of 15–45-year-old women.

Social and cultural context

Women with eating disorders are presenting in ever increasing numbers and over a wider age range; male presenters are also increasing but not so fast. Studies have shown that a gender conflict over homosexuality preceded the disorder in over 50% of male cases (M. Laing, personal communication). Cases of pre-pubertal boys and girls are being reported, all having potentially long-term physiological complications because of the delay in major sexual developments that are inhibited while they are undernourished. The social pressures on young people to conform with their peers are well documented. Probably none of us lives through a single day without being conscious at some time of a reference being made to weight, diet or food. To a person with an eating disorder this compounds their torture.

Many more families are experiencing separation and the consequent pain of hurt and loss. The children in those families may wonder whether they are the cause of the separation, and through their eating disorder draw attention to themselves in the hope of keeping the parents together. There may be family expectations of high achievement that make 'good enough' not acceptable, and perfection the only success. This black-and-white thinking when applied to eating patterns can have disastrous results. Parent–child conflicts over food challenge the very essence of parenthood, which is seen as the nurturing, caring, protective role. Thus parents find this particular challenge to their authority an impossible one to accept and will do all they can to encourage the child to eat. They bend over backwards to cook tempting dishes, buy the 'correct' food and become increasingly frustrated as their efforts fail. Refusing food is one of the strongest weapons a child can use to demonstrate power over parents.

Physical, verbal and sexual abuses are experienced as degrading behaviours leading to a sense of low self-worth, of lack of respect and hopelessness. The sufferer will attempt to restore the balance by struggling to control the last remaining area of her life left to her – her diet.

As healthy eating has been promoted nationally, so have the benefits of regular exercise. Over-exercising is not uncommon, particularly in the young.

Mary is a PE student at college in her second year, and living away from home for the first time. She comes from a large, close, sporting family who go swimming and play tennis together regularly. It became Mary's habit to cycle to a pool three miles away, swim 50 lengths and then cycle home again. This would be in the evening after a full day's work at college which would certainly have included at least one session of exercise. She was never able to go out with friends, only had time to pick at food and found herself increasingly isolated and unhappy. She found eating at home during the holidays very difficult and would make excuses to be out at meal times. Finally her weight loss became all too apparent and her worried parents took her to the doctor. Mary's initial reaction was to deny there was a problem. She felt very fit and she ate when she was hungry. It took several weeks of therapy before she began to accept that her tall gangling body was severely undernourished.

Jane had felt good wearing shorts last summer. She went jogging regularly but kept it within sensible limits, and she was happy at school and with her boyfriend. When her final 'A' level year started her studying increased, the evenings got darker and so she stopped jogging; she also broke up with her boyfriend. She began to feel 'out of shape', and decided to diet to remedy the situation. This illustrates the link between *feeling* in shape and *looking* in shape. Once Jane started to *feel* out of shape she equated this to *looking* out of shape and began to diet.

While coping with personal problems and their everyday life, patients with eating disorders are also living in the real world. They are being bombarded with TV film of Somalia starvation victims on the one hand, and slender models, male and female, on the other. How can they possibly eat when so many people are starving, and the desirable shape is slenderness? The sufferer's own body image may be distorted and she may see her emaciated body as fat, but she can recognize thinness in other people. Part of her feelings about her fat self are to do with her ego which feels incredibly small; and how can she fit a small self into a fat body? No amount of reasonable intellectual discussion will be able to persuade her otherwise. The therapist needs to accept rather than deny the value-belief-system in place and work with the patient to change it, reframing ideas by suggesting there could be alternative perceptions.

The media also floods the market with contrasting messages about food and diets. The swing to healthy eating has been a positive step, but there are still a host of articles and books on self-help methods of losing weight. It is obviously desirable and healthy to be thin.

Gender differences provide a fascinating contrast in perception. While non-bulimic women find bingeing and vomiting totally unacceptable and disgusting behaviour, participants at a young male rugby club dinner may, without a qualm, indulge in group overeating and drinking, be spontaneously sick and start all over again.

It is therefore apparent how pressures at national, family and peer group levels can fuel a weight-loss in a vulnerable personality.

Nature of illness

It is well documented that the key feature of eating disorders is control, or lack of it: 'Preoccupation with weight control and the all-pervasive fear of weight gain is the single most important and most characteristic symptom of anorexia nervosa' (Welbourne and Purgold, 1984).

Where does this preoccupation come from? The correct answer is probably different for each individual sufferer. To explore the enigma is the role of therapy, so that each patient acquires insight into her own set of problems and by understanding them begins to change her response to them. Eating disorders can be seen in behavioural terms as maladaptive responses to stressful stimuli; and cognitive behavioural treatment can be an effective therapy, particularly with bulimic sufferers.

Another key feature is low self-esteem which may have its roots way back in infancy or childhood and be based on the sufferer's experience of herself through other people's eyes. Her place in the family, her ability to be heard, to feel valued, to be praised and have achievements acknowledged, to be included in family discussions and decisions, i.e. to be accepted as a person on her own merits is crucial to her mental and emotional well-being. Anorexics and bulimics strive for perfection and are obsessional in their quest. Only 100% success is good enough – anything less is total failure. Perhaps this is a necessary personality trait for anorexia to develop? Perhaps the pursuit of thin-ness as a means of being in control automatically leads on to compulsive obses-sional behaviour? Whatever the answer, the compulsion to lose weight, and the feeling of success that comes from being in control of this, become the trap into which an accomplished anorexic falls. For the irony is, that from a starting point of being in control, the tables are turned and the anorexic becomes driven by the compulsion. She needs to see the weight falling off almost daily in order to feel successful, which leads to increasingly rigorous self-control and denial. The whole of each and every day will be preoccupied with food – the thought of it, the desire of it, the denial of it. To be totally successful is to die!

mics, while striving for the same goal, are unable to exercise the same .scipline. They fail, then succeed in a repetitive pattern that further under-mines their already fragile self-esteem. Every failure, i.e. binge, has to be punished by starvation or self-induced vomiting or using laxatives. When they have failed to be in control, these are the methods sufferers use to feel good again about themselves. Some bulimics will remain at a fairly average weight, others will be maintaining a low weight by this process. The physiological implications of all these behaviours are discussed below.

The trigger into anorexia or bulimia may be as serious as sexual abuse or as light-hearted as teasing about puppy fat. It does not follow that those triggers automatically lead to an eating disorder but once the control over food or weight is seen to be an effective method of coping with problems it begins to take over.

Alex is a young woman who had a responsible managerial and academic job following a successful career at university. She is the eldest of five siblings and had been a conscientious nanny to her brothers and sisters at her mother's request. But she had felt taken for granted; her intellect and academic achievements were seen as being what was expected, nothing special, and she became increasingly introverted following several incidents of sexual abuse by her favourite uncle. Her distress was identified by a teacher at school, but not her parents, and feeling unable to talk to him about it she told no one. Problems over her abstinence from food presented while working for her 'A' levels, and her mother seems to have spoon-fed her back to reasonable health. The time at university coincided with her best health, the lapses during vacations being made good once term started again. And so she continued underweight but holding her own and able to mask her thinness with loose clothes and at least an evening meal at home. Her mother by this time had developed cancer for which she was treated successfully but subsequently became increasingly alcoholic, which she has always denied and in which denial her husband has colluded. Alex became more enmeshed in the dynamics between her argumentative parents, feeling she could protect her mother from the alcoholism, while accepting that her eating disorder was, as she was accused, the cause of her mother's problem. The final straw came when Alex was raped by a discharged psychiatric patient whom she had been asked to befriend. The subsequent discovery that she was pregnant, the termination and finally the court case all served to add weight to her feelings of inadequacy and low self-worth. The only role of any value she could see was that of protecting her mother from drink. And so she felt trapped into a situation that intellectually she could see was very damaging to her, but in which she felt obliged to remain. This is not an unusual scenario; its complicated and tragic components will take years of therapy to work through. A combination of psychological counselling and day-to-day re-education of a healthy diet will be the key to ultimate success only if Alex is encouraged and motivated to work hard.

This case history illustrates the key features of anorexia – control and self-esteem – and demonstrates the interrelationship of all the varied dynamics in a person's life.

Pattern of illness and movement through it

Every person experiences their eating disorder in a unique way, dependent on their own set of circumstances. There are common themes, shared descriptive phrases of feelings, similarities in painting or pottery style. A psychoanalytical discussion of these might reveal an inability to separate from the mother and become an independent functional adult. At some point there is a trigger into this dysfunctional behaviour and from that point on the scene is set. It may be that some adults always maintain a low weight that will never be recognized as unhealthy or limiting, and with which they feel safe enough to live as they choose. The opposite end of the spectrum is the extremely rare incidence of a young girl of 9 years retreating into an infant state of total dependence for several months before spontaneously emerging and coming back to life again.

The different manifested behaviours are broadly categorized, but sufferers slide from one to the other and back again. Figure 18.1 illustrates this movement as a

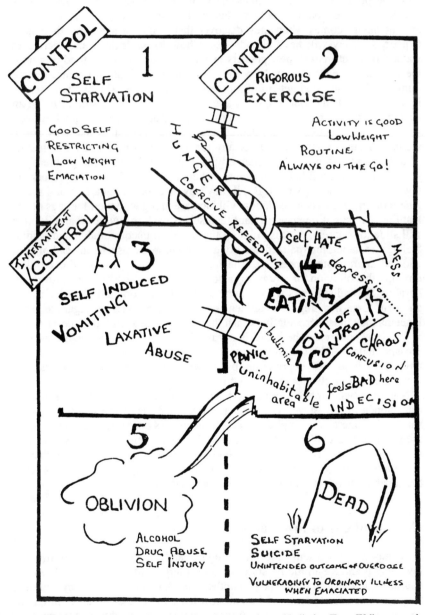

Figure 18.1 The deadly 'board game' played out by anorexics and bulimics (From Welbourne and Purgold, 1984, by permission)

board game, but it is no game – the currency is food and weight, conflict and unhappiness, and there are no winners. The only way to succeed is by getting off the board.

Entry to the board is by picking up the food/weight value belief token. Squares 1 and 2 are where the sufferer feels safe and good about herself. However, continuing to achieve in these squares leads inevitably to further weight loss, until the point comes when either the sufferer collapses and is rushed to the doctor or moves on to another square. For some people the moment of enlightenment comes when they discover that vomiting meets all their needs (square 3). They will have already learnt how to be devious and secrete unwanted food into envelopes, pockets or bags, or how to move food around on the plate and seem to eat it. Now they can eat as much as they want, reassure family and friends, and get rid of all the food afterwards. This is the next stage in their coping behaviour. Using laxatives and diuretics has a similar result and leads them to feel temporarily in control again. But it is a short quick move to square 4. Self-disgust, shame, depression, and the realization that they are the victims of their behaviour and not any longer in control of it, lead to feelings of desperation. They feel so ashamed that they cannot share the problem with anyone. This dreadful behaviour must be kept hidden at all costs to preserve the few friendships they have left. But if they stay on either of squares 3 or 4 for any length of time their social isolation will increase along with their feelings of self-loathing. Some will manage to haul themselves back to squares 1 and 2, others will slide to square 5. At this point on the board all uncomfortable and painful feelings are being internalized and contained within the psyche instead of being allowed appropriate expression. The intense emotional pain is relieved either through the oblivion of drugs or alcohol or by self-harm, e.g. cutting and burning. Several sufferers with whom the author has worked have hideous scars on their forearms, thighs, abdomen, even faces, as well as cigarette burns. It seems they must perpetually punish themselves – that is all they deserve.

The final square on the board is not reached very often, although how some grossly underweight sufferers survive is amazing. The body has incredible powers to adjust to deprivation by slowing down the metabolic rate and metabolizing muscles for energy, but it can be pushed too far.

Not all patients move around the board; the moment when they ask for help can happen at any stage. The sooner it does, the better the outcome and the shorter the illness. The heightened public awareness does mean that more people are seeking help earlier, and even those who have been in the illness for many years and felt totally trapped by it feel encouraged to try and make changes. A complete cure may not be possible, but a more acceptable lifestyle is within the capabilities of most people, given appropriate therapy.

Complications of low weight

It is important to discuss the physiological and intellectual complications of low weight and a bulimic lifestyle because a large part of therapy is health re-education and reassurance. The physiotherapist, if involved in therapy, will need to know both what to look out for and how to tailor the therapy according to the complications. Some problems will need referring on to the doctor medically responsible for further investigation and monitoring.

There are intellectual complications as weight is progressively lost. It is usual to take standard height and weight charts for men and women, with precise weights for each sex according to each half inch of height and age band. Thus the recorded appropriate weight is seen as being 100% average expected body weight (AEBW). Because on average the general population is overweight, 90% of that could be accepted as an ideal. However, once 85% of AEBW is reached the effects of starvation begin. From that point to 70% AEBW, the patient is still able to work intellectually and benefit from counselling, but communication becomes increasingly difficult. Their ideas become more rigid and black and white. Opinions that might be quite bizarre are stubbornly sustained, and although any other number of topics can be discussed rationally, no sensible connections can be made over food and weight. Once the weight has dropped below 65%, particularly if it is still falling, hospital admission for refeeding is probably essential. At any weight below 50%, death is imminent. It is necessary to know the age of onset and the AEBW at that time, because any target weight will be related to that point and not to the patients' current age and weight. Formula to establish % AEBW:

Actual weight/AEBW $\times$ 100 = % AEBW

Stringent refeeding measures using a section of the Mental Health Act, if necessary, may be called for once the weight is dangerously low and insight has been lost. Nasogastric feeding may be offensive but it ensures safety, although maybe not without a struggle if the tube is repeatedly removed and replaced. Even so, there are specialist units who prefer to maintain the patient as an outpatient and manage to hold and support for several months, gradually building up a trusting relationship that will enable weight gain to take place slowly. There are many studies and anecdotal evidence which show that weight gained too rapidly in hospital is just as quickly lost on discharge.

The physiological changes of starvation affect all the body systems. Body mass index (BMI) is arrived at by dividing weight in kilograms by height^2 in metres. A BMI of under 18.9 suggests undernourishment, while an index of less than this suggests the sufferer is at risk of symptoms of starvation. The BMI scale is as follows:

< 15   = emaciation
15–18.9 = underweight
19–24.9 = normal
25–30 = obese

Therefore an average 1.69 m (5 ft 6 in) woman weighing 59 kg (9.5 stone) has a BMI expressed thus:

59 kg ÷ 1.69^2 = 59/2.85 = 20.7
   BMI = 20.7

However, if her weight were to drop below 54 kg, i.e. 8 st 10 lb, she would become undernourished.

Any of the effects of starvation can be serious and threaten life, but all are reversible, particularly in the early stages. Giving information to patients detailing the damage that starvation can do to their bodies should not be used as scare tactics, but more as an incentive to encourage them to eat healthily again. The body has amazing capacities to perform, even when severely under-weight. There is anecdotal evidence of women driving cars and holding down challenging jobs at 60–65% AEBW. This is largely due to the release of endorphins that occurs with starving or fasting and over-exercising. It results in a chemical 'high', with the patient feeling charged up, elated and full of energy. Most of us will have experienced this at some time after an aerobics session or a game of squash. To the eating disordered patient it has a potentially addictive effect which they will be loath to lose.

If weight loss continues, the patient will herself notice and become concerned about the obvious changes in her body. She may feel faint, suffer from oedema and have cold hands and feet. Her hair will become thinner and more brittle with split ends, her fingernails will crack and split and her skin look unhealthy and flaky. She may be aware of uncomfortable feelings of fullness when she does eat because her stomach will retain the food for longer to maximize the digestion. If she has been using laxatives, then food will also be delayed in the intestines, causing constipation. She will feel tired and listless, have poor concentration and find sleeping difficult. Her thoughts will be preoccupied with food, to the exclusion of other things, and this will lead her to isolate herself, thus excluding social contacts which could otherwise have been a source of support. The deviousness and secret behaviour of bingeing and vomiting will lead her to feel disgusted with herself and further increase her social isolation. Repeated vomiting causes erosion of dental enamel and is worsened by immediate teeth-brushing. It also causes partial salivary gland enlargement, leading the patient to think that her face looks fat and to respond to this by losing more weight. She may experience oesophageal and gastric pain caused by ulcers, which could lead to rupture in extreme cases. She can find herself trapped in a vicious circular pattern of behaviour that can be extremely expensive, lead her to break the law (shoplifting) and run up enormous debts. It can be a realization of the hellishness of this situation that finally moves people to seek help. By this time, the patient may also be suffering from clinical reactive depression.

The unseen complications of anorexic and bulimic behaviour need medical screening, and this should be a routine procedure. Electrolyte levels need to be checked, heart rate and blood pressure monitored, and obviously the patient needs to be weighed regularly. Blood tests should also cover haemoglobin levels and red and white cell counts, with appropriate measures taken to restore the balance where necessary. In large specialist units it may also be a routine pro-cedure to do a bone scan and ovarian scan. The risk of polycystic ovaries is not uncommon when there is ovarian shrinkage and amenorrhoea. The risk of osteo-porosis is high, with only a relatively short period of weight loss (months) necessary before the bone mass, particularly in trabecular bone, decreases. The main cause of trabecular bone osteoporosis is oestrogen deficiency, and it affects the vertebral bodies in particular. These may suffer spontaneous fractures and become wedge shaped leading, in combination with a myopathy, to anorexic kyphosis. Palliative treatment is all that can be offered. Table 18.1 gives the medical symptoms of anorexia.

Therapy in general: principles and aims

The reader will by now have a broad idea of the possible causes, course and

Table 18.1 Medical symptoms of anorexia nervosa (Courtesy of Dr J. Mackie, Cullen Centre, Edinburgh)

PHYSICAL EFFECTS OF STARVATION	SIGNIFICANCE
Cardiovascular system	
Reduced heart rate and blood pressure	Can cause postural hypotension and fainting
Conduction abnormalities/ECG abnormalities	Prolonged Q-T reported as present before sudden death
Oedema	Perceived weight gain might drive further fasting
Cold peripheries	Probably adaptive response conserving heat
Electrolyte disturbance	
K abnormal worsened by purging and diuretics	Can cause cardiac arrhythmias or fits, depends on rate of change. As guide: 3 abnormal, 2.5 needs urgent Rx
Na abnormal associated with abnormal fluid intake	Deaths have been reported mainly connected with water intoxication
May be abnormal if Na or K abnormal	
Mg	Can cause tetany and arrhythmias
Zinc	Has been claimed to be causative, but trials of replacement disappointing
Metabolic disturbance	
Hypothermia	Depends on rate of change. As guide: 37°C abnormal, 35°C requires urgent Rx
Hypoglycaemia	Can cause coma and death
Hypophosphataemia	Described as serious/fatal complication of refeeding too fast
Liver dysfunction	Raised transaminases seen in a minority of patients
Blood	
Anaemia – increased tiredness	RBC <11 abnormal, <7 requires urgent Rx
Leucopenia – increased liability to serious infections	WBC <4 abnormal, <2 requires urgent Rx pneumonia and other infections can be fatal
Gastrointestinal system	
Slowed gastric emptying	Discomfort on eating normal portions of food; gastric dilatation a rare but dangerous complication
Slowed intestinal transit, constipation	Serious complications mainly in laxative abusers
Bones	
Decreased mineral density	Pathological fractures
	Osteoporosis in later life
Skin	
Colourless unhealthy complexion	Due to poor circulation
Flaky dermatitis	Reduced skin collagen
Lanugo hair	Cause unknown
Loss of scalp hair	Nutritional
Endocrine	
* (Amenorrhoea, ovarian shrinkage)	If prolonged may lead to permanent infertility
In men, reduced levels of testosterone	Reduced libido
Low T3 syndrome	Largely adaptive change
Mildly elevated cortisol	Probably response to stress
PSYCHOLOGICAL EFFECTS OF STARVATION*	SIGNIFICANCE
Preoccupation with food	Can drive binges
	Become frightened to reduce control
Narrowing of interests	Social withdrawal
Restlessness	Compulsive exercising more likely

* Not simply secondary to starvation.

effects of eating disorders. This section on therapy begins by talking in general terms and then moves on to discuss the role of physiotherapy in particular. What is the purpose of therapy? Who initiates it, who ends it, how long can it last? The answers to these questions could be different for each individual and depend very much on the initial presentation. Has the patient asked for help because she knows she has a problem, or has she been brought under duress by her family, in a state of denial? Does the acknowledged problem encompass disordered eating or is it quite unrelated? It is essential when working with these clients that no attempt is made to 'get them better', either in response to their request to do so or to the therapist's need. The therapist is there to facilitate change in a healthy direction; the patient is the only person who can effect that change and she will do it best in a non-threatening, non-judgemental, understanding, empathic and information-giving environment. At no time can the therapist collude with the patient in unhealthy or unhelpful activities, nor can she tell her what to do or what not to do. They may together explore the possible consequences of hypothetical courses of action to enable the patient to make an informed decision. So the role of the therapist is to work with the patient, alongside her, seeing things from her perspective, and gently working towards reframing her thoughts about herself and her value belief system. Ultimately she is enabled to become an independent, autonomous and functioning person. The therapist and client will negotiate their working relationship which will include confidentiality issues, time boundaries and the professional boundaries of the therapist.

There is a great danger, when counselling someone who has been abused, of the therapist repeating the pattern. Two girls with whom the author has worked recently have been abused in different ways by members of their family and friends, both directly and indirectly. Indirect abuse can take the form of severe verbal criticism when the patient feels continuously put down and comes to expect that treatment; it can come from friends who have been supportive suddenly backing off, seemingly in frustration because their efforts have not been very successful; it can come from a therapist who also 'does to' the patient by directing the counselling and not encouraging the patient herself to initiate the discussions. The previous experiences of being 'done to' may make it extremely difficult for the patient to switch from passive to active participation in her life; the role of the therapist is to facilitate this change.

Two things are essential when working with a client with an eating disorder. The first is to engage in a trusting therapeutic relationship, and the second is to complete an accurate assessment of the problem. In the course of making this assessment, engagement may well take place, especially if the therapist is *respectful*. This is emphasised because it is crucially important to listen to what the patient says, and not pre-empt or presuppose what she might say. Essentially the patient is going to tell a story – her personal story – and in the course of telling her story she will reveal important evidence that the therapist can use to build up a picture. In the first instance, it may be helpful to give the patient an assessment form to be completed at home. This will cover basic information on height, weight, age of menstruation, presence/absence of periods, eating patterns, use of vomiting, purging, and laxatives and exercise. The therapist also needs to know how the patient understands her condition, and from where she thinks the problems stem. Drawing a family tree and a personal lifeline are useful non-verbal techniques, as are using Russian dolls or small ornaments to do family sculptures. These techniques enable the patient to have a better grasp at a conscious level of how she sees the family functioning, which she can then verbalize and discuss. The telling of the story will not necessarily be chronological, and the therapist will soon realize at which point in each session the important matters are introduced. Silence during therapy can be very precious and need not be interrupted, reflection being an important part of discovery and decision-making. Therapy may take place over several years, particularly if the patient has suffered for years. At times it may appear that the patient is regressing, at others that no movement is taking place. Occasionally there may be a need to facilitate hospital admission, but most of the work will be done in an outpatient setting. Variable lengths of time are needed gradually to establish a therapeutic relationship in which it is safe for the patient to take risks. And risks she must take if she is going to change her psychologically safe but physiologically unhealthy lifestyle.

Therapy works on two different levels – the cognitive and the behavioural. It is not usually possible to effect a cure without working on both levels, sometimes simultaneously and sometimes with one or the other predominating. If the patient's weight is very low, the emphasis is on preventing further weight loss and then gradually gaining weight. This needs to be done at a pace that is psychologically acceptable. Too much weight gained over a short period is both medically unsafe as well as intolerable and may well be lost on discharge. The patient will need information and reassurance in order to take the risk of gaining weight and then feel confident enough to hold it. At a very low weight she will probably not be able to work cognitively other than understanding the health education and health promotion issues. Thinking becomes concrete, black and white, and rigid; abstract thoughts and lateral thinking are often impossible and the ability to work at these levels will not be restored until sufficient weight is gained. The patient may be labelled as stubborn and negative because of a lack of understanding of the restrictions placed on thinking by low weight. Likewise, understanding the psychodynamics within the family and close friends and making the connections with the illness can be tackled later when the physical health is more robust. So the nature of therapy is dictated by the patient's physical and mental state and by her current behaviour patterns. Habitual vomiting, purging and using laxatives need to be tackled very directly, with a gradual reduction in frequency. Weekly goals can be negotiated, and a daily diary kept of all food and drink taken. Weight-losing measures are recorded, along with the feelings before and after they are used, as well as feelings before and after a meal. Bulimics respond well to the support of group therapy.

Group work

A 12-week closed group has proved to be a successful package for bulimia sufferers. Patients work together to moderate the excessive and unhealthy behaviours, establish a healthy 3-meals-a-day diet and acquire stress management and assertiveness skills. Individual therapy can also be offered, with follow-ups at monthly, 3-monthly and 6-monthly intervals for up to 2 years. While a group of bulimics can be self-supporting, a group of anorexics can be self-destructive because of the sense of competition, of wanting to be the best anorexic. However, an education group explaining and discussing the effects of low weight, combined with shopping for, and cooking, a main meal, provides a safe environment for them. It will complement the individual therapy in which they will also be engaged.

Multi-abusers with a chaotic lifestyle need a tremendous amount of support to change their behaviour. There are a handful of specialist units in the country that offer a safe and structured environment where long-established and potentially dangerous behaviours can be reduced and eliminated. The support of specialist staff and a small unit dedicated solely to this purpose, with follow-up support on discharge, are the keys to any success.

When could a patient feel cured? The clinical criteria to be established are the restoration of periods, an ability to engage in all normal social functions including making new friends, and an acceptance that one's weight does not relate directly to one's self worth. During the course of therapy it is hoped that each patient will come to an understanding of why she began to use weight control as her *raison d'être*. She may also have developed other more healthy ways of coping with stress and be able to put these into practice if she finds herself falling back into old coping techniques. At the very least, the insight she has gained will enable her to ask for help as soon as she thinks it necessary.

Physiotherapy techniques

Most of the therapy with these clients is verbal. They have an ability to intellectualize, and are happy to rationalize their behaviour, the advantage being that this prevents them from getting in touch with their feelings. But as un-expressed feelings and emotions are often the heart of the problem, it is of paramount importance that these are recognized, identified and dealt with to achieve a resolution.

The non-verbal techniques of massage, relaxation, movement and exercise can be utilized to facilitate the client being in touch with her feelings. This in turn can lead onto verbalization of feelings, disclosures and ultimately an understanding of where the feelings are coming from. The sharing with an empathic trusted therapist of previously secret, dangerous and upsetting events or feelings that have been blocked in the subconscious, is a necessary step in therapy.

Lorraine was a young well-educated woman in her mid-twenties. She worked in a responsible managerial post with a national charity and she had been working for several months with a private psychotherapist before being admitted specifically to gain weight. (This situation in itself highlights a problem that occurs when therapy is switched from one agency to another overnight, when liaison between the two is minimal and when styles of therapy are very different. The patient can become the pawn in a game of professional rivalry between the two systems. Once recognized, this situation can usually be dealt with satisfactorily so that the patient benefits rather than suffers.) Lorraine responded successfully, though not always happily, and gained weight slowly but steadily. I was working with her twice a week, gradually building up a picture of her and her family in which conflict and cultural differences seemed prevalent. When I suggested we try some massage and relaxation with the intention of helping her feel more integrated, she responded positively. I used two massage techniques, eliciting different responses and thus producing different results. Lorraine was happy for me to give her a back massage in prone-lying on her bed, using oil. She could tolerate this level of touch in a position in which she felt safe and was soothed and also valued as a result. In contrast, I also massaged her through clothes and a light bed covering, using full-length effleurage strokes both from feet to shoulders and the reverse. The intention, as I told her, was to enable her to feel a whole person; to use this massage to integrate her whole body so that she felt 'joined-up' and together. While I was doing this, I encouraged her to feel each part of her: feet, legs, hips, trunk, arms and shoulders, to be in touch with them and acknowledge them as part of her, and not in any way separate from her thinking, feeling self. Using this technique with other clients I have found that some tolerate massage better in one direction than the other, so it is important to check with each patient which method they find most comfortable. It is also sensible to investigate why she does not like any particular part of the massage. Feelings long buried may have been aroused and will need dealing with. Having used massage as an ice-breaking technique, it can then be possible to suggest relaxation with the intention of teaching a self-applied stress-relieving tool. With Lorraine this produced an interesting result. She chose to lie on her back, although another patient might well choose prone-lying as being a much less vulnerable position. When I suggested that, similar to the full-length massage, she try to consciously feel each part of her body in turn, she told me that she could think down as far as her stomach, but was unable to go further and make the connections with her hips and legs. When asked to describe the block, she spoke of a dense black chaos that was her stomach, where eruptions would take place that seemed to want to get out.

Here we enter the range of symbolism, of feelings that have been internalized and need to be released, of a stomach that is so full of blackness that it throws up healthy food as if that will rid it of its unwanted contents, or that is so full of badness and pain that it cannot possibly digest anything. Non-verbal techniques of massage and relaxation can enable a patient to get in touch with deep feelings in the subconscious that need to be aired. A physiotherapist working in this way needs not only awareness of the psychodynamics of the subconscious but also, and most importantly, the counselling skills to handle a situation like this and see it through to its resolution. At no time does a physiotherapist in this dual role attempt to do things without the necessary skills; if caught unawares, the best advice is to listen, check out by reflection what is being said and let the patient say as much or as little as she wants. Patients in the author's experience instinctively know how much they can safely say, and if in doubt, will not say it. The importance of complete trust cannot be too strongly emphasized, and it may take weeks of therapy before it has developed enough for confidences to be shared.

The use of movement and exercise as therapy tools promotes some interesting discussion. There are some who feel that contact with a physiotherapist is contraindicated because the patient will abuse the therapy and use it to burn off unwanted calories. However, other professional colleagues working in psychiatry will have a more accurate knowledge of physiotherapy skills and how they can be applied. The accuracy of this knowledge relates directly to the contact with the physiotherapist in the team: her ability to promote her skills, and her confidence in proposing usage and application. The author would argue strongly that the patient who has compulsively and obsessively exercised her way to emaciation needs to reintroduce exercise and demonstrate to herself that she is in control of how much she does, and not vice versa. This should not be done too soon, but it needs to be part of the re-education of the diet : activities/input : output equation. It may be helpful to start this stage of rehabilitation while in hospital, when support is at hand, and continue it after discharge. While daily circuit training or indoor sports may be available, a couple of sessions a week combined with other group activities such as relaxation would be suitable initially. The physiotherapist taking such a group will be aware of the temptation to over-exercise and should check this out with the patient. Equally the patient should be encouraged to share her feelings about exercise in an open way, so that she is able to identify honestly and then resolve any tendency towards compulsion or obsession.

Another use of exercise is to teach static contractions of postural muscle groups to facilitate the patient's acceptance of her body and help her feel 'in touch'. Most underweight anorexics express feelings of panic connected with being flabby or ballooning as they put on weight and these fears are so strongly held that no amount of logic and reason can reassure them. They are caught in a conflict of head versus intuition. The intuition is illogical and anorexic but very powerful, and an incredible amount of courage and strength of character is needed to take even small risks that might result in weight gain. Muscles that have shrunk because their bulk has been metabolized into energy, and through dehydration, will only be restored to normal size, strength and function by food (protein) and exercise. An anorexic needs constant reminding of all the physiological changes that take place during the course of the illness, in order to have enough intellectual ammunition to fight the instinctive irrational fears. A physiotherapist can give this information as well as anybody else and also, through teaching and monitoring static contractions for postural muscles, provide the patient with a prescribed activity that is both reassuring and positive in outcome. There is no point in shying away from using exercise sensibly. As always in therapy, the patient is responsible for what she does to her body; she needs to own that responsibility and not delegate it to nursing staff, or other therapists or deny it altogether. If she chooses to over-exercise and lose weight, then she has to live with the consequences. It is not that therapists are unaware of the difficulties and dangers, but they cannot do the work for the patient. So while the patient is trying to ensure that input verus output ensures a positive result, the therapist is balancing the amount of support given, with the level of reponsibility handed over to the patient to ensure growth and forward movement.

Physiotherapy skills can also incorporate movement techniques, specifically Veronica Sherborne techniques or, more generally, dance techniques. Movement or dance therapy sessions are not now uncommon in a mental health setting. Exercises that encourage trust, touch, mutual sharing and supporting, and that explore personal space and allow spontaneous expression of feelings, can be very valuable tools in enabling an anorexic or bulimic to reintegrate into the society around them. Her illness will have isolated her, made her introverted and introspective, and part of the healing process is first to find and integrate herself and then to come out of herself. Dance and movement therapies, under skilled leadership, provide a medium in which a non-verbal technique can lead to verbalization of feelings, and a deeper awareness of where one is at. They can facilitate the identification of relationship problems, of fears that threaten security and privacy, which once realized may be able to be resolved.

Having extolled and explained the benefits of applying generic physiotherapy and specialist movement techniques in the rehabilitation of patients with eating disorders, these now need to be set in the context of the overall therapy package.

Most physiotherapists will come into contact with these patients in an inpatient facility. They are unlikely to meet them as outpatients unless working in an adult mental health resource centre, or are known to have special expertise and take referrals. Inpatients will be the most seriously affected, either in terms of weight loss or in using self-abusive behaviour to resolve their feelings.

As in all inpatient scenarios communication, planning and liaison between team members are of paramount importance and particularly so as the patient with anorexia is able to use people and situations to her own advantage. A written and agreed contract is a most useful tool, whether or not the patient is admitted under a section of the Mental Health Act. It will need regular updating, and any unacceptable parts of it need to be renegotiated. It needs to be seen and presented as a positive aid to therapy rather than a negative restriction of activity. Gone are the days of token economy when privileges were the reward for pounds gained. A contract will give a secure framework in which recovery can take place, and should include details of diet, activity and visitors, as well as guaranteed sessions with the key worker and other therapists. At all times the emphasis is on working with the patient, helping her to solve the problem and understanding things from her perspective. Any sense of conflict or of being 'done to', tends to be counter-productive, but this does not mean that challenges cannot be made in a constructive way to encourage insight. Each therapist needs to have a clear understanding of their role in the therapy, with regard to other therapists and the patient. There may be occasions when a key therapist in the community requires admission for their patient and will like to feel included in the team while unable to be a key worker during the inpatient stay. Continuity of care, allowing the initial therapeutic relationship to be maintained and then continued after discharge, is essential.

Members of the multidisciplinary team involved in the therapy of eating disordered patients will need to meet regularly and offer each other support. Clinical supervision with a team colleague outside the team will enable the therapist to gain insight into the dynamics of the therapeutic relationships and so work more effectively. There are times when one can feel chewed and spat out in the same way that anorexics can treat food; it is not uncommon to feel drained and starving hungry after a session, and clinical supervision is an essential support to recharge the batteries and maintain an objective view of the therapy.

Conclusion

Physiotherapists who are well integrated into a multidisciplinary team have the necessary structure in which to work with this clientele. They have both generic and specialist psychiatric skills that enable them to make a valuable contribution to the rehabilitation of sufferers of eating disorders. The challenging nature of the therapy can result in the therapist as well as the patient realizing their potential.

References and further reading

Bass and Davis (1991) *The Courage to Heal – A guide for Women Survivors of Child Sexual Abuse*, Mandarin

Bruch, H. (1978) *The Golden Cage*, Open Books

Cleese, J. and Skinner, R. (1983) *Families and How to Survive Them*, Methuen, London

Crisp, A. (1980) *Anorexia Nervosa, Let Me Be*, Academic Press, London

Dana and Lawrence (1988) *Women's Secret Disorder – A New Understanding of Bulimia*, Grafton

Duker, M. and Slade, R. (1988) *Anorexia and Bulimia – How to help*, Open University Press, Milton Keynes, UK

Kano, S. (1990) *Never Diet Again*, Thorsons

Orbach, S. (1978) *Fat is a Feminist Issue*, Hamlyn Paperbacks, London

Palmer, R.L. (1979) Dietary chaos syndrome, *British Journal of Medical Psychology*, **52**, 187–190

Palmer, R.L. (1980) *Anorexia Nervosa – A Guide for Sufferers and their Families*, Penguin, Harmondsworth, UK

Welbourne, J. and Purgold, J. (1984) *The Eating Sickness*, Harvester Press, Hemel Hempstead, UK

19

Substance misuse

A. The medical approach

Maureen Dennis

General introduction

This chapter on the physiotherapist in the addiction team details two approaches to the problem of substance misuse – the medical model and the Oriental method of natural health care. Neither approach is mutually exclusive and it is hoped that in the future modern enlightened methods will permit an integration of the two.

The problem

Society's attitude towards the consumption of drugs is ambivalent. Some drugs are actively promoted and sold by the free market system. Others are promoted for their medicinal purposes and prescribed by a monopoly, namely medical practitioners, under licence. A third group are actively banned, and promotion or possession of these drugs is considered illegal.

The overriding concern of society is that drugs from all three categories by their nature and content are addictive. The compulsive need to acquire and consume a drug or several addictive substances can lead to irrational behaviour, criminal activity, physical illness and social disruption on both the personal and public levels. The causes and progress of addiction are poorly understood. It is made up of a complex process of biological toleration, psychic compulsion and social demand. Addiction is more easily acquired than discarded; it has many victims and its social cost is enormous.

This social ambivalence to addiction has been manifested either by tolerating it or criminalizing it. Only since the 1960s has society sought to approach the problem by medical means, that is to state in principle that the addicted person is suffering from an illness caused by the compulsive consumption by eating, drinking, inhalation or injection, of a substance or substances (Glatt, 1982). Sudden separation from this substance or substances will cause a massive reaction within the autonomic nervous system with consequential effects on liver function, cardiac output and cerebral working, known as 'withdrawal symptoms'. It can make people who are withdrawing feel so dreadful that they will easily relapse into pursuit of the very substances from which they are withdrawing.

Behind every addiction to a drug, however, is a physical, psychological or social problem or problems not directly related to the drug problem but provocative to it. These can be related to upbringing, self-esteem, sexual and social identity, quality of personal relationships, social environment, and a host of political forces over which the individual has very little control.

Added to this will be a multitude of problems directly caused by the addiction. These will be a breakdown of family and social relationships, unemployment, debt, homelessness, and perhaps involvement in criminal activity as a means of financing the addiction. In addition, the element of self-abuse which reaches almost death-wish proportions will override all rational argument that people must take responsibility for themselves. It denies logic, can lead to impulsive self-destructive behaviour and prove the biggest challenge in the behaviour modification of addicts.

Types of addiction found in a substance misuse clinic

Addiction *per se* can take many forms of compulsive behaviour, from smoking to eating disorders. This chapter will confine itself to three main groups of addictive chemical misuse – prescribed drugs, illegally acquired drugs and alcohol.

Prescribed drugs which become addictive. Benzodiazepines were freely prescribed for anxiety in the 1970s and 1980s without much concern for their addictive properties. Doctors are now much more aware of this problem and prescribe minimal doses with caution. Patients who are admitted to the unit may have a long history of addiction supported by 'repeat prescriptions', but little social or criminal disruption to their lives. Abusers, however, can inject the drug as temazepam and can give themselves an overdose, which can prove fatal.

Barbiturates act as a sedative or a hypnotic and excess consumption can lead to depressed respiration, cyanosis, disorientation and coma. They too can be injected. Their use is now considerably diminished.

Illegally acquired street drugs. Heroin comes under the category of opioid drugs and is only available as an illicit drug. Drug and detoxification units prescribe methadone, an analgesic which does not produce euphoria, sedation or narcosis, as a substitute permitting withdrawal without the acute symptoms. Heroin abusers are less likely to be hospitalized because groups form their own sub-culture which is counter-productive.

A further group of patients who are also more likely to be found in the community rehabilitation programme are those who consume stimulants such as amphetamines, cocaine, crack or ecstasy.

Alcohol. The final group is the largest – those who abuse the sedative effects of alcohol and who present with considerable physical deterioration as well as the social complications of addiction.

Within all these groups there may be found people who present with an underlying mental illness or personality disorder which underpins their resorption to substance misuse. There are also sadly those who manifest psychosis as a result of continuous substance misuse. Early signs of Korsakoff's syndrome (alcoholic dementia) can be manifested by confabulation, i.e. the creation of credible stories of misfortune which are believed by the patient himself (Glatt, 1982). The earlier therefore that rehabilitation can take place, the better is the prognosis for recovery.

Physiological effects of substance misuse

This chapter can only indicate those physical complications which physiotherapists should be aware of. Detailed explanations can be found in, for example, Glatt (1982) or Sherlock (1982).

Common withdrawal symptoms from benzodiazepines include anxiety, sweating, insomnia, headache, shaking and nausea. Changes in body physiology will cause a sense of unreality both in sensation and movement. Patients are hypersensitive to stimuli.

Heroin causes equally intense anxiety, insomnia, amorphous pains and gastrointestinal upset.

Excessive alcohol consumption causes the following:

- Physiological changes to the liver, pancreas, gastrointestinal tract and heart leading to inflammation, chronic tissue changes, such as cirrhosis, and pancreatitis, and a predisposition to cancer in all tissue actually exposed to the substance.
- Vascular and physiological disorders: hypertension, anaemia due to toxic damage to bone marrow causing fatigue, vitamin B deficiency (all groups) leading to macrocytosis and hypoglycaemia. The malformation of platelets causes easy bruising, a tendency to bleed internally (e.g. gastric ulcers) NB. Alcohol reduces the capacity to metabolize glucose in red blood cells so that exercising after having taken alcohol may lead to hypoglycaemia (Glatt, 1982). Exercising during detoxification should therefore be gentle and moderate.
- Acute or chronic myopathy of the musculature can cause pain, tenderness or weakness. Ataxia may also be present.
- Cortical atrophy causes initially 'memory disturbances' (Glatt, 1982).
- Neurological disorders. Withdrawal from excessive alcohol consumption can precipitate epileptiform fits, subdural haematoma and polyneuritis. Insomnia, a mentally confused state and loss of memory are often present. The sympathetic nervous system and the adrenal medulla are stimulated by alcohol, so that after the initial sedative effect, reactions can become depressed and physiologically equitable with anxiety.
- Korsakoff's syndrome or alcoholic dementia. Visual-motor and visual-spatial functions may be damaged before this condition is diagnosed, but higher cortical functions deteriorate irreversibly as part of this symptom. Individual susceptibility, nutrition and age are obviously contributory factors.

Detoxification

Understanding the predicament of the patients

Patients admitted for detoxification have usually been drinking or consuming addictive substances even up to the morning of admittance. Alcoholics in particular have two patterns of drinking – 'binge-drinking' and 'topping-up' drinking. Binge-drinkers can have periods of abstinence and then relapse into excesses that can lead to unconsciousness or at least episodes of behaviour which are violently antisocial. Topping-up drinkers misuse alcohol on a more regular basis and have subtle methods of appearing not to drink excessively, but they are constantly maintaining their alcohol level through all their waking hours.

Women are often 'secret drinkers', being constrained by social prejudice or domestic circumstances from drinking in public but they may follow either pattern.

Both men and women can compound the problem by combining alcohol with prescribed tranquillizers or antidepressants or illicitly purchased street drugs. This is usually aggravated by poor nutrition and heavy smoking. The body has become tolerant of the narcotic substances being consumed. Usually larger and larger doses are required to reach the former intoxicated effect. Admittance into hospital has necessitated withdrawal from these substances. Detoxification is a much longer process when a compound of substances has been abused, especially if the chemicals have been synthetically manufactured. Medication cushions the shock, but patients do not sleep, may be prone to epileptic fits, and suffer deep depressions.

It is therefore important that the patient is vetted by the doctor upon admittance for suitability for any activity more than gentle exercises. In the department there must also be additional nursing support. It must be remembered that the amount of alcohol consumed which can damage health is much lower than the amount needed to induce dependence.

When is the best time to intervene?

Some people are able to modify or withdraw from their addictive behaviours without any assistance from professionals. Others adopt the patient role and are processed repeatedly through the system as they relapse into the chronic state.

In the late 1970s, a theoretical model was devised in an attempt to discover what is common to all processes of recovery from addictive behaviour. At what point will people be able to decide to and maintain a decision to change? McConnaughy *et al.* (1983) defined four components in this process of change (Figure 19.1):

- *Precontemplation*. Addicts at this stage do not reflect on the consequences of their behaviour. Their health beliefs successfully mask a realistic appraisal of the consequences.
- *Contemplation*. People are admitting to the self-destructiveness of their behaviour and begin to re-evaluate themselves.
- *Action*. People 'need to believe they have autonomy to change their lives in key ways'. It is the most stressful time in a process of change and much support is needed to overcome habitual behaviours.
- *Maintenance*. Once a change of behaviours has been achieved it has to be sustained or there is a relapse. Sustained change raises self-esteem as former addicts resist temptation.

Relapse at any stage of the last three phases does not necessarily mean a return to the precontemplation phase. People may rerun through the process many times before a sustained change is achieved.

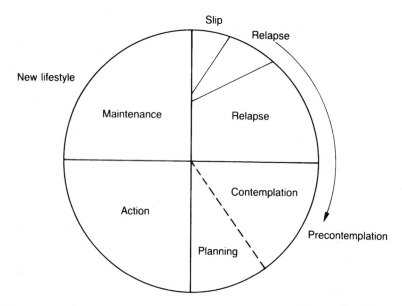

Figure 19.1 Stages of change in recovery from addictive behaviour (From McConnaughy *et al.*, 1983, by permission). Different strategies should be used by the therapist for different stages and transitions:

Stage	Models/methods	Therapist's tasks

Precontemplation	Health Belief model
	Health as a Resource model
	Theory of Reasoned Action
	  motivational interviewing
		Raise doubt – increase the client's
		  perception of risks and problems with
		  current behaviour

Contemplation	Personal responsibility
	Decision Matrix
	  motivational interviewing
		Tip the balance – evoke reasons to
		  change, strengthen the client's
		  self-efficacy

Action	Contracting
	Modelling and shaping
	Goal-setting and self-monitoring
		Help the client to determine the best
		  course of action to take in seeking
		  change

Maintenance	Behavioural Self-management
	Behavioural Analysis and
	Behaviour model motivational
	  interviewing
		Help the client to take steps towards
		  change

Relapse prevention	Skills training, e.g. – time management – assertiveness	Help the client to identify and use strategies to prevent relapse

	Explore high risk situations
	Relapse fantasies
	Anticipatory coping
		Help the client to renew the processes
		  of contemplation and determination
		  and action without becoming
		  demoralized because of relapse

All therapists have to be aware of these stages, otherwise they may create a mismatch between the cognitive awareness of the addict and the instructive aims of the therapist. During precontemplation they can only raise awareness of the risks involved. Contemplation calls for moral support in the decision to make a change. At the action stage, guidance to self-monitoring is needed in order to avoid habitual behaviours and to maintain the change. During maintenance the former addict should experience the benefits of the lifestyle changes.

After any relapse the patient must receive support to try again, knowing they have not returned to the precontemplation stage.

The addiction team

In the UK, physiotherapists may find themselves part of a team treating addiction within a hospital of trust status within the National Health or of private status in the free market system. Increasingly, rehabilitation is taking place within the community, where physiotherapists may support the Community Psychiatric Nursing team. Finally, as general practitioners widen their scope of services on a budget-holding framework, lifestyle clinics may include groups for those who admit to alcohol dependency, as opposed to abuse, or for those who are dependent on tranquillizers.

The multidisciplinary team may consist of a consultant psychiatrist, registrar, psychologist, psychiatric nurses and social workers, occupational therapists, physiotherapists and counsellors. Art and movement therapists may also be part of the team and hopefully complementary therapists will be included.

Aims of the team

The approach of the team will depend at what stage in the model of addictive behaviour modification the patient has reached.

At the precontemplation stage

Has the patient been persuaded by spouse, employer, social worker, doctor or law courts to attend? Patients who deny they have an addiction are usually very preoccupied with blaming circumstances or other people for causing their problems. The aim of all professionals is to:

- form a working relationship with that patient
- raise doubts concerning the Health Belief model which the patient holds, but not confronting the patient, which can have negative results. Liver tests can prove convincing, dire warnings are not
- indicate the positive benefits of making a change
- encourage self-esteem and discussion of those factors which undermine it.

At the contemplative stage

- educate and discuss the physical, psychological and social effects of drug addiction relevant to the particular addiction of the group
- seek agreement on targets and specific behaviours which will bring about change

- discuss relapse prevention which is to enable patients to be aware of those situations, habits and cognitive failings that trigger a return to former escape behaviours
- create opportunities for self-reflection by permitting the discussion or writing of autobiographies.

At the action stage

The patient has made the decision to change and is attempting to maintain it. Therefore:

- the greatest support is necessary to help target those behaviours which may create relapse – this may be caused by lack of confidence or over-confidence (i.e. the patient may feel they can handle a drink)
- support and reinforce the will to change during maintained abstinence; sustain support if there is a relapse, in the knowledge that the majority are only temporary and that insight can be gained from them
- assess the patient's coping skills relevant to either discharge or maintained support for meeting future problems
- reinforce the confidence gained by overcoming opportunities to relapse.

Role of the physiotherapist

The team may not be aware of the advantages of having a physiotherapist among them. It is important therefore that the physiotherapist relates well to the team, and informs them of the services that can be offered rather than waiting for referrals.

In sum, the physiotherapist has a role to educate patients into the physical processes which will enable them to feel better. This is to counterbalance the emphasis on medical and psychological intervention. It is one thing to tell the patient that they should feel better, but it takes skill to be able to make them feel better by therapeutic techniques and exercise. No other member of the orthodox team has the skills to create holistically that 'feel-good' factor which is so important if people are to make constructive changes to their lives.

There is a heavy emphasis within programmes on cognitive and social adjustment, with the physical problems treated symptomatically by prescription. The physiotherapist can widen the perspective of this adjustment by education and practical exercise, to demonstrate the need for greater insight and awareness into physical resourcefulness. Mind and body are indivisible and physiotherapists with a holistic understanding of their skills can do much to alter the perspective which perhaps imbalances the treatment of addiction within the medical field.

Secondly, the physiotherapist can focus upon and reduce those physical symptoms which come to light upon withdrawal. Often, clients have a chronic history based on a chaotic lifestyle and create aggravation and tension:

- neuropathy and ataxia
- old musculoskeletal problems aggravated by lack of care and poor lifestyle
- hyperventilation, palpable anxiety and panic.

There is no stock treatment for a stock set of symptoms. The physiotherapist must have a wide repertoire of massage techniques, e.g. connective tissue massage, shiatsu, acupressure, reflexology, craniosacral therapy. It is important to treat the person who has the symptoms and not just the symptoms. Also, it is helpful to have a wide repertoire of exercises from Qi gong, yoga, simple non-aerobic stretch exercises, to the aerobic and sporting type, all of which are helpful to motivate patients at various levels of ability.

The use of technology is not recommended. These damaged people need caring touch and the physiotherapist must have confidence in traditional skills.

Attitude of the physiotherapist

It is important when dealing with any patient with a history of addiction to remain non-judgemental. To adopt the high moral ground will be quickly sensed by people. It is better to cultivate a sense of empathy and humour, to remember patients' names and to show concern during those days when withdrawal symptoms strike. Close observation of patients' notes may sometimes make objectivity difficult. Some may have committed violent crime to finance their addiction. Women may have so neglected their children that they are taken into care. Cultural biases exist in all of us and we may dismiss members of certain ethnic groups as so prone to excessive drinking as to be beyond hope.

Empathy implies the ability to acknowledge feelings in a sympathetic and non-judgemental way. Humour is very necessary to cope with the mixed reactions people present when they are coming to terms with the fact that they are addicts. Body language will speak volumes to the patient. It is important to have good eye contact, a patient manner, to show a concerned interest in whatever communication is made by individuals and yet to be able to hold the group together in a cohesive whole. Individual patients may appear to try to dominate or disrupt a group, but one must never respond with anger. People must be listened to, but it does no harm to calmly indicate the priority of group discussion.

Aims of the physiotherapist

Other members of the team understand the psychological stresses which a detoxicating patient is experiencing, but who can explain the consequential physical stresses that they experience? The eight principal aims of the physiotherapist are as follows:

- *First*, to educate in simple non-medical terms the patients into the symptoms and processes of anxiety and its physiological effects.
- *Second*, to explain the process of panic attacks and especially hyperventilation, their relationship to addictive behaviour and of methods of dealing with them.
- *Third*, to indicate that confusion in thinking may contribute a great deal to the anxiety they are experiencing. Psychologists call the method 'cognitive skills', but it is simpler to indicate that clear reasoning can greatly help us to stand apart from our mixed up emotions and help us decide what is important and what is not.
- *Fourth*, to indicate that there are ways of helping themselves and to seek counselling is one very important source of help. It is not automatically offered to this group of patients, but they should be encouraged to seek it out. Patients greatly underestimate the importance of confiding as a very necessary human activity for coming to terms with painful events in their lives.

Unresolved emotional conflict will create havoc with any attempts at rehabilitation.

- *Fifth*, to stress the importance of lifestyle changes, mindful that many patients are living on financial support of very limited means. For example, they do not have the resources to visit sports centres or to buy expensive equipment.
- *Sixth*, to stress that the resources come from within the patient themselves and that the physiotherapist can assist the patient to get in touch with those resources.
- *Seventh*, to demonstrate that one way to obtain those resources is to experience the 'feel good' factor. By the simple process of persistent exercise, breathing control and meditation, they can actually experience a physiological benefit and a better sense of emotional balance and a relative sense of calmness.

It is important to reassure those who have difficulty with this last aim that success is always relative, and failure to experience physical and emotional benefit just means they are not ready and does not indicate personal inadequacy. Physical exercise is not part of the culture of the majority. Walking to overcome anxiety is one of the simplest options. Exercises must be simple, slow, enjoyable and not aerobic. Discussion and re-experience of lapsed sports activities is sometimes possible.

Knowledge of local complementary resources is always useful and arouses curiosity, e.g. local yoga and shiatsu classes.

- *Finally*, a physiotherapist can help those individuals who seek help for their extreme anxiety, somatic pain or disabilities caused by their accident-prone lifestyle.

Exercise class for the 'feel good' factor

There will be reluctance on the part of some patients to participate in an exercise class and it is important to set out the ground rules of participation from the start. It must clearly be negotiated with the nursing staff when and where the class will take place, so they can add their support.

The class is not energetic and is within the capacities of all ages and abilities. It involves exercise, education in stress management, breathing instruction and meditation. It can be given to patients who are detoxifying or who are on a rehabilitation programme, in addition to more energetic activities. Patients can be seated or can use mats.

It is important to give initial explanations as to the purpose of the group, if only to dispel the image that a physiotherapist makes people leap about in an energetic manner. The majority of the exercises that the author uses are borrowed from the Chinese. This is because the Chinese had such a profound understanding of the effect of exercise not just on 'muscles' and 'strength', but on the whole energy system of a person (Brown, 1989).

To simplify, one can explain that relaxation is the aim of the class, but to lie or sit down with all the accumulative tensions still within the body and mind would be a great pretence. (It often is!) We have to literally shake or loosen out these tensions by the simplest of shaking and swinging of limbs, percussion, stretching and finally breathing exercises.

Dao-in exercises

The gentle touch of a human hand has been instinctively accepted as something that eases pain and comforts. The Chinese capitalized on this fact with dao-in exercises which are simply the use of our own hands on ourselves in an energetic but gentle fashion to stimulate and relax our bodies' energies.

The exercises are listed below. For those familiar with the Chinese approach to body energy through the meridian system, they will be aware that the simplest of acupressure techniques is being used percussively to balance 'Qi' (chi) or body energy flow (Brown and Fletcher, 1989).

Start in the seated position
Recognize that some participants may have neuropathies and be unable to stand for very long – acknowledge this fact and allow them to remain seated.

1. Rub your hands together vigorously and squeeze the sides of each finger before pulling the tips, again vigorously.
2. Use your hands energetically to tap the scalp.
3. Tap the cheeks and gently stroke the nose downwards.
4. Use the index fingers to massage the coin size area at the end of the eyebrows. Stroking the forehead from midline to temple will relieve cranial tension.
5. Hold the whole external ear and bilaterally pull downwards and away. Massage the immediate external auditory shell with the fingers.
6. Grasp the main muscles of the back of the neck with the palmar surface of the hand and massage them vigorously.
7. Continue this along the triangular area of the upper trapezius with a kneading motion (if the arm gets tired, it can be supported at the elbow with the opposite hand).
8. Massage vigorously the upper arm and shoulder joint bilaterally. Tension causes respiratory stress and consequential connective tissue stress which may be said to contribute to all the neck and shoulder problems.

The group can stand at this point
9. Form two soft fists and vigorously thump the upper chest with one's hands which will invigorate the apical lobes of the lung and the thymus gland.
10. Continue the thumping to the stomach to stimulate the digestive organs.
11. Turn the knuckles to the back and massage the kidney area, the sides of the ribs and sacrum area.
12. *Be seated* – slightly forward on chairs. Place a leg out straight with the heel resting on the floor. Vigorously tap the muscle groups on all sides. Massage around the knees and then at their posterior surface.
13. Make vigorous long strokes downwards on the outside of the leg from hip to ankle.
14. Make vigorous long strokes upwards from the ankle to the groin.
15. Remove shoes and massage the soles of own feet deeply with the thumbs.
16. Vigorously rub the forefoot between two hands and turn the forefoot into inversion and eversion.
17. Pull and circle the toes individually. Vigorously tug the tips.
18. *Standing* – the following are to relieve general tensions within the body:
    (a) Keeping the feet and hips still, swing the upper body to left and right, not bending forward. Allow the arms to be so relaxed that they flap like 'wet

washing' against the body. Arms which are held out in a rigid fashion only show that the individual is having difficulty letting go (many will).

(b) Shake the body with a loose bouncing motion from the heels, knees and hips. Allow the shoulders to shake and concentrate on breathing out.

(c) Swing the arms individually in a circular fashion as if trying to throw away the hand.

19. *Stretches*. Take the left arm right across the front of the body to the right shoulder. Assist with the right hand at the left elbow to give an extra stretch, and vice versa.

20. Hold hands behind the back. Bend forward and stretch hands to ceiling. (Not for the very sick!)

21. Place right hand behind back. Legs astride, slide left hand down side of left leg to obtain a good stretch all the way down the right side, and vice versa.

22. Still standing, raise the arm to the ceiling and stretch, at the same time pushing the left arm towards the floor. Reverse the arms to give a stretch in the opposite direction. The instruction 'Push the floor and ceiling away!' helps.

23. Start with the hands facing the front of the thighs. Slowly raise the hands with the arms slightly curved to make a bowl shape in front of the chest. As the arms reach the level of the forehead, turn the hands outwards and upwards towards the ceiling. On the return, turn the hands back to their bow-shaped form slowly return to the starting position.

Do not do all these exercises at once.

Measure the tolerance of your group. Repeat each one at least three times.

At the conclusion of the class have a pause for thought. Allow people to sit and sense how physically more comfortable they feel. Do not suggest that they ought to feel so changed, because this will increase the sense of inadequacy of those who do not. Let them discover it for themselves.

Shiatsu or simple acupressure techniques

Patients are in need of touch in a non-invasive caring manner. Shiatsu techniques can be taught to a group of patients, working only on the back, hands and arms or feet. No undressing is required, only 'safe' areas of the body are touched and it can be given in the sitting position. Women help women, and only very rarely will men not wish to help each other. Preference not to take part must always be respected.

1. Stand at the side of your partner, facing the shoulder. Place one hand on the bony sternum to support. With the palm of the other hand, vigorously rub the area of the upper back.

2. Give brisk strokes down the total back, from neck to shoulders, and down the arms. Use the little finger edge of both hands to percuss either side of the bony spine.

3. Thumb massage the upper trapezius area.

4. Hold your partner's hand with one hand. With your other hand, gently squeeze the muscle groups down to the wrist.

Aromatherapy and hand or foot massage (see also Chapter 16)

Patients who have become addicted to tranquillizers have greatly suppressed the functioning of the limbic system in the midbrain, which affects emotional and imaginative functioning. The olfactory centre has special connections with the limbic centre. Aromatherapy is therefore a useful procedure, especially if given to such safe areas as the hands or feet, for these clients.

Directions

A towel is given upon which the hand or foot rests. We will assume the hand is being massaged. The masseur puts a little oil between their hands and rubs it over their own hands. They then gently hold the wrist and massage from the wrist to the fingertips. They bend their own index and centre fingers in order to squeeze each finger, from base to tip at the sides, with these bent fingers. Thumb and index finger are used to give firm tugs to the very tip of the fingers – this, in Chinese terms, stimulates meridian energy. Turning the hand over, the palmar surface is massaged with the thumbs and then the masseur makes a fist with their own hand. Supporting their partner's open hand with their other hand, they firmly place their fist into the palmar surface and knead the soft parts of the hand. They can also give soft stimulating pinches to the outer edge of the hand. They can end with vigorous whole-hand strokes from wrist to fingertip.

Visual display material (see illustrations)

Members of the group will be of all educational standards and mental abilities. A group which is detoxifying is unable to absorb too much information, so do not overestimate the amount that you can get across. It is helpful to have a placard with the simplest of diagrams, to illustrate the physiological process of stress and to emphasize the physical changes which take place.

The anxiety spiral (Figure 19.2). Explain the physiological basis of stress. It has to be indicated that addicts are caught up in a double spiral because their bodies have become accustomed to the substance they are taking. When it is withdrawn, the body goes through a massive alarm reaction, i.e. withdrawl symptoms caused by sympathetic nervous system arousal and parasympathetic suppression.

'Help, doctor!' is to explain the suppression of the immune system and the breakdown of health. It is useful to use the imagery of 'all accelerator and no brake' regarding the nervous system.

Hyperventilation (see also Chapter 11). It is useful to identify those in the group who experience this problem and to allow them to recount the distress that it causes. From experience of these groups it appears to be epidemic within the population and considerably impairs social freedom in crowded public places. Also smoking is heavy among addiction groups, with its associated bronchial complications and postural tensions. Addiction patients are very resistant to any suggestion to renounce smoking as well as other addictions, and their health beliefs do not include a rational realization of the consequences of the nicotine habit.

Anxiety causes us to breathe in but to fail to breathe out and release at the end of inspiration. This has become an entrenched habit with many addicts who also fail to associate pace and quality of breathing with their emotional state. By 'release' is meant to entrust the situation enough to let go so that inspiration happens reflexly.

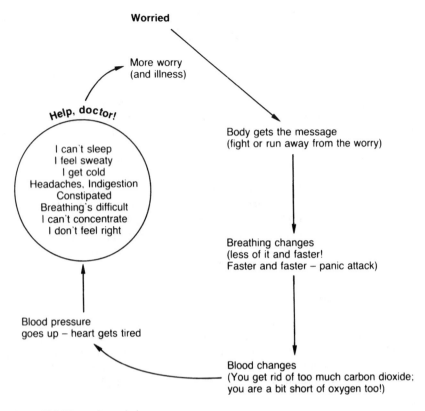

Figure 19.2 The anxiety spiral

The importance of correct breathing

Helpful hints towards teaching breathing control (Figure 19.3)
The subject of breathing exercises is enormous and should not be divorced from voice production. This in turn is a reflection of self-confidence and self-assertion.

1. Indicate which parts of the body are involved in the act of breathing – the diaphragm, the rib cage, the volume of the lungs (most people have a poor idea). Emphasize where the focus of our breathing should be – near the navel – and where it usually is – somewhere near the middle of the sternum.
2. Advise that if we are unfit it is difficult to feel any sense of control over our breathing, and if we want to triumph over panic attacks, we have to walk, sing, dance, practise breathing exercises or meditate when we do not experience anxiety, in order to be able to cope when we do.
3. Mind will triumph over matter, so it is very important to be aware of the power of our imaginations to reinterpret seemingly threatening situations. Also when it comes to the physical act of relaxing the body and breathing out, it is better to imagine it happen rather than making it happen. There is a subtle difference which prevents over-exertion to succeed.

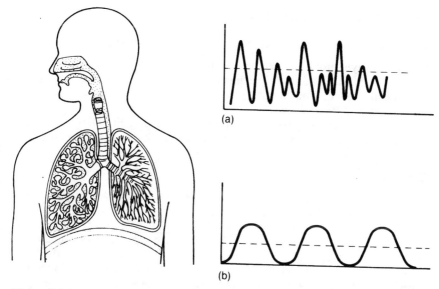

Figure 19.3 Emotions affect breathing: (a) high and rapid anxious breath; (b) low and slow calm breath

4. Poor posture and physical tenseness. Addicts have lived so long with both that it will take a great deal of re-education to change patterns of movement and stance. After exercise sessions, the following can be recommended:
   (a) Standing erect but with relaxed shoulders.
   (b) On breathing out, do not give way to gravity by slumping.
   (c) Relax the jaw and allow the throat to open.
   (d) Visualize a stretched spine.
5. Breathing exercises – *always start by breathing out*
   (a) Make 4 sighs of big relief; 6 sighs of contentment; 8 anticipatory pants; frequent puppy pants.
   (b) Breathe out – let go – wait – give an extra 'Huh' from the diaphragm, then *relax* to let the air come in *spontaneously*.
   (c) Pant 'Huh, Huh' sounds, bouncing them out to exercise the solar plexus!
   (d) Breathing in must be 'receiving' rather than taking in breath. Breathing out can be prolonged to reduce the number of exhalations to five or six a minute. At the end of breathing out we can pause, count to four and at the end of that pause, release from the diaphragm to 'receive' the breath.

Breathing and visualization
Anxiety makes us live 'too much in the head and full of monkey chatter' as the Chinese would describe it. Our breathing pattern follows suit. It is helpful to describe that the focus of our energy and breathing should be low, near our navel or diaphragm. We have an expression in our language of a 'gut feeling', which means that we feel intuitively about something. We should develop a gut feeling for our breathing and our physical and emotional energy will follow suit.

Lifestyle recommendations

There are two illustrations which can demonstrate important points:

- Is the lifestyle problem of attempting to cope with too much work or social responsibilities, instead of recognizing early the symptoms of breakdown (insomnia, loss of temper, failure to delegate, lunchtime drinking), persisting to the point of breakdown (Figure 19.4)?
- Are the necessary simple steps to a positive and coping lifestyle being taken? Figures 19.5 and 19.6 and Table 19.1 give some self-explanatory guidelines.

Cognitive skills – meditation

Physiotherapists can introduce patients to meditation if only to prove that it is simple, effective and an accessible process. Meditation has nothing to do with formal religious instruction or an ascetic cloistered lifestyle. It is simply a means whereby people focus their energy within, obtaining some contact with a calmness and silence of spirit, which enables them to function more effectively within daily life. It is important to acknowledge, however, that failure initially to experience such calmness is no disaster. It requires a certain degree of acceptance and tranquillity which will only come with practice.

The essence of meditation is that thoughts will come into our heads as we sit quietly, but the difference is that we do not let the content of those thoughts emotionally trouble us. If we follow the trains of thought, we will get lost among them. It is helpful to use the idea of looking through binoculars which are out of focus. Everything seems blurred, so we do not know what is important and what is not. Meditation helps us to get matters in focus. We must get in touch with our self, which is there, troubled and battered though it may be. Our essential self is a source of fundamental goodness and strength.

It is within the physiotherapist's capacity, therefore, to choose a method of meditative instruction with which he or she is happy and to introduce it

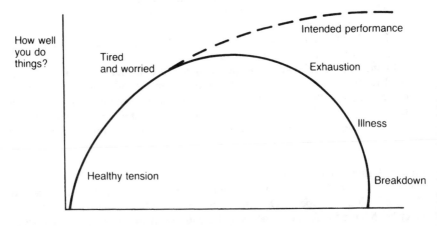

Figure 19.4 The stress curve, demonstrating that prolonged stress can create a mismatch between expected performance and maladaptive behaviours due to overload

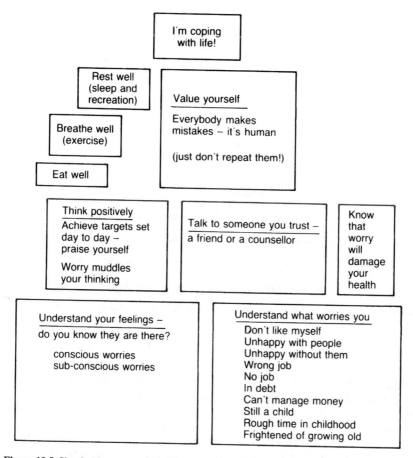

Figure 19.5 Simple steps to a positive lifestyle (see also Figure 19.6 and Table 19.1)

to patients. The author uses a method, described below, to which she was introduced by John Tindall.

Patients are seated with the chair fully supporting the back and the hands resting on the thighs, near the belly. In a quiet voice the physiotherapist asks participants literally to 'concentrate on the right foot'. The physiotherapist then names the body parts on the right side and uses words like 'heaviness, warmth, stillness, feel the weight, let it rest against the chair/floor' and progresses to the head. The same process is used for the left side. Finally the therapist asks participants to centre on their 'tummy', near the navel, and literally to focus on their breathing. What is this for? From the concrete and physical, the patients are guided to a 'metaphor of being'.

'The right side is the past and all the grief and remorse and anger which we carry with us. The left side is the future in which we continue to place anxieties and insecurities. Our minds, however, must focus on the present, on the very essence of being alive in the present. If we live for the moment and cope with the moment, our energies will be focused, we will be in touch with the possible.'

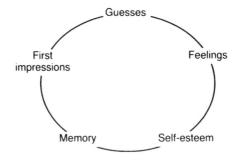

Do you value yourself?

Do you only remember the times when you failed?

Do you jump to the worst conclusions?

Do you guess the worst when you don't know?

Do you let your feelings colour your decisions?

Figure 19.6 The importance of thinking right (or do you have the habit of worrying?) (see also Figure 19.5 and Table 19.1)

Leave room for silence. The energy of the group will have changed considerably if it has been handled with skill. People need quietness within the reassurance of a group, rather than loneliness in a clattering world.

Mix and match
The contents of the group can vary according to what the therapist decides is the need for the group. Exercise, discussion as education, and meditation can all be intermixed.

Table 19.1 Ten simple guidelines for coping with stress (see also Figures 19.5 and 19.6)

1. *Recognise* that it is interfering with your life – to ignore it is to become more of a victim to its process
2. *Understand* the symptoms – mental, physical, emotional
3. *Decide* to do something about it – assert yourself – question life style – set limits
4. *Question* what are the real problems and what are not. We confuse the two – talk about them with a close friend or counsellor
5. *Acknowledge* the emotions that real problems create. They have to be recognized or they create trouble/illness
6. *Live* a lifestyle that helps you rebound from life's difficulties. Avoid or cut down on self-destructive habits
7. *Learn* to feel good – really good. That means eat sensibly – sleep regular hours – encourage friendship – and exercise for enjoyment
8. *Share* duties – in the family – in the workplace. Do not play the martyr – slice jobs into daily possible achievements and accomplish them
9. *Give* time to yourself – be kind to yourself – go easy on criticism – forgive yourself – meditate on good possibilities
10. *Enjoy* the physical – dress more comfortably – dance! – be alive – stretch – breathe and relax

Physiotherapy skills

Also, after a group, patients will approach with individual physical problems, insomnia being high on the list. The physiotherapist must be prepared to help and it is within these circumstances that complementary skills such as connective tissue massage, shiatsu and reflexology are immensely useful. For the acutely stressed individual, a few sessions of one of the above can give valuable help.

The above procedures, as described, can be modified for groups in hospital, the community or for 'abusers' identified within a group practice or occupational health. For groups who are proceeding through a more lengthy rehabilitation process within the community or within the voluntary sector, a more vigorous exercise programme is recommended in addition to the one described. However, education must have a high priority in the treatment of addiction, so it must be emphasized that repetition and discussion of the above programme must continue activities. To dash into high activity can cause injuries.

The physiotherapist should bear in mind the following

- when playing games, take into consideration the ability of the group, avoid contact games, e.g. American football
- never be fooled by people looking fit – they are not
- discourage weight training – it can cause tissue damage
- remember that participants are often experiencing considerable stress in the rest of their programme – the atmosphere must be positive, successful and happy
- a simple fitness test at intervals can aid motivation
- create a feedback session to hear opinions
- have local sports information to hand.

The physiotherapist is presenting an important counterbalance to the psychodynamic processes of other therapeutic groups by the emphasis on physical as well as mental well-being. Involvement of the patient in discussion or practical exercise gives the greatest hope for learning. It is only what the patients discover for themselves that will be retained. There are no quick fixes.

Patience, *practice* and *perseverance* are the three key words in the rehabilitation process from substance misuse.

Further reading

Brown, D. *et al.* (1989) Cardiovascular and ventilatory responses during formalized Tai Chi Chuan exercise. *Research Quarterly for Exercise and Sport*, **60**(3)
Brown and Fletcher (1989) *Vital Touch*, Community Health Foundation
Glatt, M. (1982) *Alcoholism – Care and Welfare*
Sherlock, S. (Ed.) (1982) *Alcohol and Disease*, British Medical Bulletin

B. The natural health care approach

John Tindall

The abuse of drugs in modern societies is reaching epidemic proportions possibly as a 'coping mechanism' to social psychological stress factors. Substance misuse is not a new problem, but has existed throughout the ages in all cultures. Medical practitioners over the centuries have developed treatments to help people deal with the problem. Natural health care in this field is an 'eclectic' approach that is able to draw on rich sources of experience from many countries.

Addiction

Generally, all the natural healing systems of the world recognize addictive substances as materials which will create a temporary 'illusion' of well-being whilst they suppress the body's natural instinct to reject them, thus causing the body to accumulate the 'toxic' waste from them undetected. This can be seen in the overall manner of many addicts according to their length of drug misuse history.

For instance, the young user is on the 'run' all the time chasing the drug and is up all day and night and seemingly extremely active. The addictive 'fire' is new and young and burning with a passion out of control. As the person is young the body is able to absorb a great deal in order to survive, as the drug switches off the natural rejection response. In comparison, the long-term user has accumulated a large quantity of toxic material internally, which helps to keep the body addicted, but the years of abuse have not allowed the person to age gracefully and so the body is frail, slow and without vigour.

Eventually, for all drug misuse clients the gradual build up of a 'toxic slag heap' leads to the person's decline. The essence of drug treatment is to descend from this slag heap and ascend to higher levels of personal awareness and functioning.

Withdrawal or detoxification

In orthodox medical practice the symptoms of withdrawal are often listed as 'purposive' and 'non-purposive'. Purposive symptoms, i.e. pain and anxiety, are subjective and can only be measured and reported by the client. Doctors fear they might be faked in an effort to get more drugs, so what the client describes is therefore deeply mistrusted. Non-purposive or visible symptoms, i.e. running nose, sweating or dilated pupils, are considered more authentic and reliable.

In natural health care, virtually all the body's responses during detoxification represent the body's efforts to cleanse the system and repair itself on all levels. Each of the eliminative channels of the body may go through this 'spring-cleaning' process. For example:

- the skin: sweating, spots, boils, rashes, etc.
- the lung: flu-like symptoms – cough, mucus, headache, running nose

- the liver and gastrointestinal tract: colic, gas, diarrhoea or constipation, pain, loss of appetite
- the kidney and bladder: dark cloudy strong-smelling urine, scanty or copious in volume
- the musculoskeletal system: muscle aches and pains, joints and bones heavy and tired
- the nervous system: dilated pupils, shaking and jerking at night, insomnia
- mental/emotional: irrational thoughts, quick-tempered, depression, fear, anxiety, paranoid, impulsive thinking, etc.

The picture is representative of the body's 'alarm system going off', now the drug is not suppressing it any more.

In any helping relationship you have to be able to relate to the client's immediate needs, no matter how trivial or insignificant they are, before progressing to deeper underlying issues. In natural healing we utilize the most effective health-giving source, the patient's own body. Methods of natural healing operate by releasing and encouraging the healing capabilities and energies of the body.

Methods of treatment

Acupuncture

In Chinese medicine, the lack of a calm inner nature in a person is described as a condition of 'false fire' because the heat of aggressiveness burns out of control when the calm inner tone is lost.

Chinese doctors have observed that the 'hot' nature of drugs like heroin, cocaine and alcohol damages the calm – yin – inner quality. It is easy to be confused by the false fire that many addicts present with and to conclude that the main goal should be sedation of excess fire or escape from its consuming attachment. the hostile, paranoid, hustling climate of modern cities demonstrates this energy-depleted condition with false fire burning out of control. Our clients seek greater power and control over their lives. The empty fire condition represents the illusion of power, an illusion that leads to more desperate chemical misuse and senseless violence.

Chinese medicine sees the need to clear away the impurities, replenish the yin and centre the mind. A simple and effective format of treatment developed by the National Acupuncture Detoxification Association (NADA) is the use of auricular acupuncture and is conducted in large groups in conjunction with counselling and other modalities. The pioneering work of Dr M. Smith and his colleagues from the Lincoln Clinic, New York, since 1975 has led to this approach being successfully employed in many countries throughout the world. Most of the research work has been based upon this protocol of treatment (Bullock, 1989). The basic protocol is that of applying five auricular acupuncture needles to the external aspect of both ears in the liver, kidney, lung, sympathetic and shenmen points (Figure 19.7). This is done on a daily basis and clients are requested to sit and allow the acupuncture to take effect. Many clients say they feel 'relaxed and alert'; this is a great contrast to orthodox treatment in which people say they feel 'drowsy and tired'. After 40 minutes the needles are removed and the client can go on to the next part of the programme.

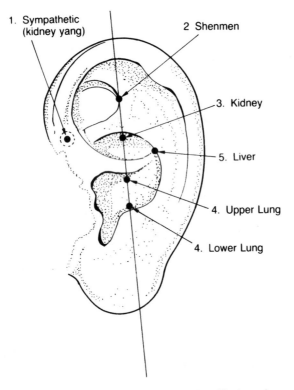

1. Sympathetic (kidney yang)

2 Shenmen

3. Kidney

5. Liver

4. Upper Lung

4. Lower Lung

Figure 19.7 Auricular acupuncture – the five detoxification points

Modern testing of acupuncture demonstrates that it involves the homoeostatic actions of the autonomic nervous system, neurotransmitters and elements in the pituitary subcortical axis.

The use of auricular acupuncture is much less frightening than body acupuncture to the addict, especially those that have had bad 'fix' experiences. As the whole body is being treated from one area which represents a hologram of the entire body, there is no need to apply body acupuncture for the greater part of the detoxification.

In some cases, when the client is down to low doses of drugs or off them completely, other secondary health problems emerge that require whole-body acupuncture. At this point, traditional Chinese diagnostic principles can be applied, i.e. pulse and tongue diagnosis, leading to the use of appropriate body points.

This approach to treatment allows the clients instant access to treatment. The acupuncture is blind to the client's level of recovery and so the fearful guilt-ridden initial encounters can be avoided. This sets the stage for more conventional treatments and is the foundation for psychological recovery.

Auricular acupuncture is efficient, effective and economical – in our unit, every member of the clinical staff can easily provide treatment for 20 patients each morning and still be able to complete their other duties.

Clients appreciate the service and the quiet space it provides to reduce their inner turmoil. This non-verbal approach helps break the denial and ambivalence in the early stages of treatment which usually would create miscommunications and more fear and confusion. The fact that most clients choose to come back for more treatment shows how powerful this tool is in helping clients gain autonomy and self-responsibility.

After the withdrawal process is completed, acupuncture is still effective in reducing craving, residual long-term drug effects and in rehabilitation to release tension and act as a further 'creative' coping mechanism.

Families and spouses can also receive treatment for stress management, harm reduction, relapse prevention and relaxation – this can create a community atmosphere that is supportive and helps to reunite societies.

Shiatsu and reflexology

Shiatsu is a Japanese system of massage which utilizes pressure on active acupuncture points. The practitioner may use their hands, knuckles, elbows, knees or feet to apply the pressure. There are many techniques which refine the process in order to redistribute the energy circulation of the body.

Reflexology's origin is Egypt and this system makes use of active pressure points in the hands, feet and head. The technique is performed primarily with the thumb and fingers. Through the stimulation of the end-points of the body's subtle systems, the internal organs are encouraged to reset the balance.

These massage techniques are a powerful tool for releasing pent-up physical and emotional blocks. The effectiveness depends on the ability of the therapist, and in many cases clients will be able to let go of the deepest imbalances with continuous treatment. It is common to observe that massage is not as quick or as effective for acute withdrawl symptoms as acupuncture and yet obtains good results with long-term problems.

The addition of massage to inpatient and rehabilitation programmes is very important for the following reasons:

- all members of staff and clients can learn these techniques together, as gentle methods of giving and receiving in a non-threatening way
- clients get to experience a nurturing process without having to 'psychologize' every step of the way
- self-help client groups provide an opportunity for non-verbal communication that brings people together and clients learn to deal with difficult issues through body-releasing and creative techniques
- clients like to learn more and often come back on a voluntary basis to help out, which fills the void once they are not using drugs any more.

These aspects help remind us and our clients of the purpose of treatment – to be drug free and able to cope with and enjoy life in a positive and creative manner.

Relaxation

There are many forms of relaxation one can use, some Western in nature, like contract relax, autogenics, Sylva mind control, which use a self-induction method and/or music, whereas others are Eastern in nature, such as T.M., Buddhist and Taoist meditations which use sounds, chanting and mental imagery, breathing techniques and hand postures. Generally, drug misuse clients get a lot of benefit from this treatment and it can considerably reduce withdrawal symptoms and craving and help people see their goals more clearly. Because many clients have had unusual mind/mood altering experiences, they can often make good use of this type of session in a way that a non-drug user cannot do easily.

Exercise therapy

Western approach
Using circuit training, weight training, swimming, rebounder work, basketball, volleyball, jogging, etc. the aim being to promote lymphatic and blood circulation and cardiorespiratory output. The more the body is able to keep the circulation active, the more easily it can clear waste debris and promote the release of natural opiates and internal organ function. Many drug users have not done any exercise since early school days and they enjoy the opportunities to let the 'inner child' free in play. The team spirit and competitiveness help develop determination and personal discipline in a 'yin' manner and create openings for interpersonal skills training. The recognition of personal limitations, abilities and goal-setting can, with very isolated individuals, begin on this basic physical level and progress from there. The use of exercise to release emotional frustrations and boredom is a positive coping mechanism that clients quickly learn to use appropriately to prevent relapse. Occasionally there is a need for specific corrective exercises for musculoskeletal injuries as a result of falls, etc., while 'under the influence' of drugs.

Eastern approach
Yoga. This Indian system is complete in itself and there are many varied forms, some very physical and others concerned purely with the mind and spiritual development. In substance misuse treatment, generally one needs to start with simple postures, and clients who find that static postures suit them soon find they are able to release physical stiffness. Some clients have a natural aptitude for yoga and are able quickly to learn how to use it to clear their mind and reach high levels of meditation.

Qi gong. This Chinese system is also complete in itself. There are many varied forms, some static and others moving. The focus of the practice may be to mimic animal movements and gestures or meditate on becoming an object like a tree or a rainbow. The Chinese concept is essentially to forget the body and everything else, in order to allow the natural healing process to take place uninterrupted by conscious thoughts. Qi gong can be practised by the patient following the therapists lead, or if the therapist is able to, they can set up an 'energy field' in which clients are led through the exercise by the healing field created by the therapist. This is a very popular activity, as both conscious and subconscious blocks can be released in a 'total body' experience. Many qi gong Masters are able to conduct sessions for hundreds of people at a time. Clients usually experience a natural 'high' and feel stronger and sleep more easily. For some clients, emotions will spontaneously emerge and they release them through laughter, crying, chanting, shaking or other physical reactions.

The Eastern systems of exercise are closely linked and require more mental focus than the Western approach. The main aim is to promote optimum health through mental, physical and spiritual harmony. The therapist needs to maintain a high level of awareness in order to be capable of assisting clients fully through this method. Detoxification means learning to cry and laugh again, experiencing all sorts of pent-up emotions and gradually releasing repressions and complexes built up over years of inactive psychic life. It is not helpful to 'psychologize' every step of the detoxification process. Teaching clients not to ask or worry out the 'cause' of the fears all the time is helpful and natural. Clients should expect to face the psychosocial problems gradually as they gain strength and after the basic cleansing and balancing process.

By having a broad approach to the physical dimension, one can meet the needs of a greater number of clients. There are, of course, many other modalities that can also be useful to provide an avenue for conscious and unconscious expression, e.g. art, music, dance, drumming, writing and chanting.

Herbal medicine

Historically throughout the ages when the local beverage ran out the herbalist was called upon to detoxify the drinkers safely. In China, the Imperial Court had many doctors to research herbal treatment to stop drug craving and experiencing any withdrawal symptoms.

The study and practice of these treatments is not just fascinating but very productive. NADA's 'mother clinic' in New York initiated the modern use of a 'sleep mix', to cleanse the internal systems and restore the nervous system. This consists of:

Camomile	2 oz (56 g)
Scullcap	1 oz (28 g)
Peppermint	1 oz
Catmint	1 oz
Elder flower	1 oz
Yarrow	1 oz
Hops	$\frac{1}{4}$ oz (7 g)

These are all mixed together in a container and shaken up thoroughly. The client then takes 1 teaspoon per cup of boiling water 3 times daily. In acute phases of detoxification it may be drunk hourly.

The Gateway Clinic, South Western Hospital, Brixton, London uses the above mix as the detoxification formulae and has the following formula for sleep:

Camomile	1 oz
Scullcap	1 oz
Damiana	1 oz
Passiflora	1 oz
Peppermint	1 oz
Motherwort	1 oz
Red clover blossom	1 oz
Lime flower	1 oz

This is mixed and taken in the same manner. It is a very effective treatment for the nervous system, headaches, insomnia, shaking, convulsions, fits, tension, etc. These herbal formulae are simple teas which can be used in the bath, as poultices and compresses as well as internally. Clients find them very easy to use and pleasant to take. Many clients have completed detoxification with orthodox methods and still have withdrawal symptoms. They then decide to use herbal treatment and the problem is rectified in many cases. The herbal treatment is like a 'superior' form of food to the body's internal chemistry which after years of abuse is run down.

Many of the dermatology problems, both acute such as abscesses from bad 'fixes' and chronic conditions such as in acne from a toxic internal system, respond well to external and internal applications which patients find remarkable, helping them break away from the 'drug'/'magic pill' culture. It is essential that the herbalist is fully qualified and has good clinical experience in this field in order to be both effective and safe.

The use of Chinese herbal medicine is another powerful tool and also requires careful diagnosis and thought before presciptions are written. In the treatment of the secondary problems of drug misuses, especially HIV/AIDS, this approach is proving extremely effective (Wu Bo Ping Tanzania, 1988–91). All stages of HIV/AIDS can be improved upon and there are essentially four tasks:

- to boost the body's immune system
- to inhibit the HIV
- to stop opportunistic infections
- to educate the clients how to use natural medicine safely and appropriately to improve the quality of their life to achieve longevity

Homoeopathy

This too is a complete health care system in which each remedy perfectly matches an individual's whole picture on all planes and the dose is diluted to such a degree that the resulting effect is subtle, safe, efficient and extremely economical. The Colombo Hospital in Sri Lanka has a good homoeopathy programme which is very effective.

Initial detoxification: nux vomica C30, dose 3–4 drops in glucose base daily for 3 days.

Symptomatic therapy
12–16 hours after last dose of opiates:
Yawning – Cicuta virosa
Rhinorrhoea – Nat. mur./Gelsenium
Lacrimation – Euphrasia
Sweating – Nat. mur
Piloerection – Tuglans regina
Restlessness – Aconite/Ars. alb./Rhus. tox.
Shivering – Carbo veg.
Exhaustion – Kahli phos./Arnica
Nervousness – Argent nit.
Flu-like symptom – Gelsenium/Nat. mur.
Poor concentration – Apis mel.
Confusion – Actaea rac.
Cramp in calf muscles – Arsen alb.
Watery eyes – Euphrasia

24–72 hours after last dose of opiates:
Muscular twitches – Gelsenium
Aches and pains – Arnica bryonia/Pulsatilla

Abdominal cramps – Nux vomica/Bryonia/Lycopodium
Vomiting – Kali bich/Ipecac
Diarrhoea – Argent nit.
Loss of appetite – Arsen alb./Ignatia
Agitation – Argent nit./Aconite/Rhus tox./Ars. alb.
Profuse sweating – Sepia/Thuja
Weightless – Vanadium
Insomnia – Aconite/Ignatia/Calc carb.

Bach flower remedies. These are remedies discovered by Dr E. Bach. Each one correlates to an exact emotional disharmony. The remedy is diluted according to homoeopathic principles and the liquid is taken in 3–6 drops either internally or externally. This treatment can in many cases help clients turn the corner of a previously intractable problem.

Example: walnut – protection from powerful influences; white chestnut – persistent unwanted thoughts; wild oat – helps determine one's path in life.

Cell salts. These are 12 tissue salts discovered by Dr Schuessler, each of which, if it is out of balance within the body, will create health disturbances. Taking these cell salts is not a supplement but rather a catalyst to reset the internal harmony. They are homoeopathically prepared and so very simple and safe to use.

Example: trembling hands – mag. phos.; irritable/impatient – kali. phos.; profuse sweating – calc. phos., kali. phos.

Essential oils

These are pure oils extracted from plants and trees. Generally they are used externally for massage in baths, inhalations, poultices, compresses, etc. However, provided that the oil is very pure, 1–2 drops can be used in water for internal use – this type of practice is more common in France than the UK. The neat oil is not applied to the body; instead it is mixed with a carrier oil, e.g. almond or wheatgerm.

Phoenix House, Forest Hill, London, which is a rehabilitation centre, has a good formula for helping clients who still might be experiencing withdrawal symptoms:

Lavender
Ylang ylang
Juniper (not if pregnant)
Rosemary (not if pregnant)
Four drops of each in the bath

Clients particularly enjoy this therapy because the smells are pleasant and the treatment is very relaxing. It can be a powerful tool, especially if combined with hot and cold foot baths to reduce acidosis, stop leg and back pains and improve circulation.

Vitamin and mineral therapy

It is well known that most addicts have vitamin and mineral deficiencies as a result of the lifestyle created from drug misuse. In many orthodox units clients are given a supplement for their first week of treatment. The following is a useful regimen:

- *Vitamin C*: 2000 mg daily. It is essential for detoxification and raising the body's immune response. It is rapidly depleted from the body by drugs. It counters acidosis, capillary breakage and assists adrenal and liver function. Organic form: fruits and vegetables.
- *B complex*. It is essential for nervous tissue, liver and skin. In some cases of severe nervous and emotional symptoms, additional niacin 150 mg daily will increase calmness and well-being. Organic form: brewer's yeast.
- *Vitamin E*: 400 iu daily. Prevents the destruction of vital fats in the body and helps production of fatty hormones which are depressed by drug use; improves liver function; dissolves scars and other deposits which interfere with micro-circulation. Not to be used if high blood pressure is present. Organic form: green leafy vegetables, whole grains and wheatgerm.
- *Vitamins A and D*: 10 000 iu (1000 iu daily). Vitamin A helps the eliminative functions of the skin and mucous membranes, improves liver function and tones dry, itchy skin. Liver deficiency causes decreased absorption of all the fat-soluble vitamins (A, D and E). Vitamin D improves the absorption of calcium and thereby aids the healing of nerves, bones and muscles. Organic form: cod liver oil.
- Calcium and magnesium: 600 mg and 300 mg daily. Stops bone pains and increases calmness of the nervous system. Organic form: dolomite tablets.
- Zinc: 30 mg daily. Improves the reaction to all types of stress, inflammation, low fertility and insulin usage. Organic form: wheatgerm, pumpkin and scuflower seeds, fish.

There are many more micronutrients and amino acids, etc. that clients may also need, but for the purposes of drug withdrawl the above is appropriate. Also, this type of therapy can be quite expensive and if one uses the inorganic form the client may not absorb the nutrient, in which case they create expensive urine. This is quite likely, as the intestinal function after prolonged drug misuse is poor.

Diet

This area is always a difficult subject to approach, as most people's eating habits are very personal, secretive and deeply rooted in their psyche and culture. In recent years there have been many different 'fad diets' that have emerged on the natural health market. However, for the purpose of drug treatment there are some very common guidelines that are logical, easy to follow and apply:

Detoxification phase – cleansing diet
1. Eat lots of fresh fruit and vegetables – cleansing function.
2. Whole grains, eggs and fish, more than meat and milk which burden the liver and kidneys.
3. Yogurt and cottage cheese rather than dairy products which produce mucus.
4. No greasy and fried foods which harm liver, skin and circulation.
5. No sugar or refined flour products as they leach vitamins and minerals.
6. Plenty of water and herbal tea.
7. No tea or coffee which leach vitamins and minerals.

Growth diet – after detoxification

1. Keep protein and carbohydrate separate, as in the Hay system.
2. 80% alkaline foods to keep the body's pH at the optimum level.
3. No fluid with meals, to prevent dilution of digestive enzymes
4. 75% of the meal should be water, e.g. fruit and vegetables, to keep the body at 75% liquid.
5. Chew well, to partially digest the food and create a better situation for digestion and absorption.
6. No emotional 'pigging out' – eat only when hungry.
7. Eat regularly and allow time for digestion.

These simple principles have proved effective over the years in many different cultures. Most people do not find them too difficult or restrictive. Once the results of improved digestion, vigour and health are experienced, clients are keen to continue and know more.

Conclusion

In our modern times we require treatment programmes that are cost effective, efficient, simple and that work without creating further problems.

In the study and practice of ancient natural medicine, it can be seen that throughout history man has managed to employ the products of his environment to help him survive in it.

The natural health care systems can be added to all types of drug treatment programmes to improve the results, the quality of care, the retention rate, relapse prevention, harm reduction and the long-term sobriety level.

Drug misuse is a worldwide problem – and as in all wars, in order to win you have to form a coalition. In order to deal with drug misuse we need a coalition of all health care systems, since no one method has all the answers.

References and further reading

Bullock, M. (1989) Acupuncture treatment of alcohol recidivism – a pilot study. *Lancet*, 24 June
Byers, D. (1983) *Better Health with Foot Reflexology*, Ingham
Chang, S. (1985) *The Great TAO*, TAO Publishing
Christopher, J. (1976) *School of Natural Healing*, Christopher Publications
Cummings, S. and Ullman, D. (1989) *Homeopathic Medicine*, Gollancz, London
Deal, S. (1979) *New Life through Natural Methods*, New Life
Diamond, H. and Diamond, M. (1987) *Fit for Life*, Bantam Books
Downer, J. (1992) *Shiatsu*, Hodder and Stoughton, London
Grant, D. and Joice, J. (1984) *Food Combining for Health*, Thorsons, Wellingborough, UK
Guorui, J. (1988) *Qi Gong Essentials for Health Promotion*, China Recantructs Press
Holford, P. (1983) *The Whole Health Manual*, Thorsons, Wellingborough, UK
Hyne Jones, T.W. (1976) *The Bach Flower Remedies*, C.W. Daniel
Jarmey, C. and Mojay, G. (1992) *Shiatsu: The Complete Guide*, Thorsons, Wellingborough, UK
Kaptchuk, T. (1983) *The Web that has no Weaver*, Rider
Kloss, J. (1939) *Back to Eden*, Eden Books
Lindlahr, J. (1981) *Natural Therapeutics*, Vol. II, *Practice*, C.W. Daniel, London
Maciocia, G. (1989) *The Foundations of Chinese Medicine*, Churchill Livingstone, Edinburgh
Masunoga, S. (1977) *Zen Shiatsu*, Japan Publications

Scarfe, C. (1989) How to *Improve Your Digestion and Absorption*, Ion Press
Smith, M. (1977) *Legal Heroin. A Problem Disguised as a Solution*, NDAC
Smith, M. (1988) Personal communication on the management and treatment of substance abuse
Smith, M. and Khunat, R. (1985) Acupuncture in the treatment of chemical dependency and violence.
    Presented at the Caribbean Mental Health Conference, Bahamas, July
Stanway, A. (1982) *The Guide to Biochemic Tissue Salts*, Van Dyke
Stephenson, J. (1976) *Helping Yourself with Homeopathic Remedies*, Thorsons, Wellingborough, UK
Tisser, R. (1990) *The Art of Aromatherapy*, C.W. Daniel, London
Valnet, J. (1990) *The Practice of Aromatherapy*, C.W. Daniel, London
Wahlstron, S. and Tindall, J. (1989, 1990) *Workshop Manuals*, Vols 1 and 2, Swedish Council on
    Alcoholism and Addictions
Wu Bo Ping (1992) Personal communication on the treatment of drug and alcohol abuse. Academy
    of Traditional Chinese Medicine, Beijing
Wu Bo Ping *et al.* (1988–91) Treatment of 158 HIV-infected patients with traditional Chinese
    medicine in Dar es Salaam, Tanzania
Yang Jwing Ming (1988) *Qi Gong*, Yang's Martial Arts Association
Zhi Xing Wang (1990) Personal communication on 'Qi field' therapy, by a Qi Gong Master

20

Post-traumatic stress disorder

Elaine Iljon Foreman and Alexandra Hough

History of the Disorder

Early reference to post-traumatic stress is found in the literature of Ancient Greece (cited by Niles, 1991), and is also described by Samuel Pepys when writing about the Great Fire of London in his diary in 1666 (cited by Daley, 1983). Shakespeare's 'Macbeth' contains clear reference to the phenomenon, in the immortal lines: 'Out, out, damned spot! out, I say!' (Lady Macbeth is suffering visual illusions of bloodstains on her hands and so troubled is she by all of her symptoms that she eventually is driven to suicide.)

The diagnosis 'post-traumatic stress disorder' (PTSD) first appeared in 1980 in the third edition of the *Diagnostic and Statistical Manual of Mental Disorders* (DSM-III) of the American Psychiatric Association. Prior to this, the symptoms were referred to under the heading of 'gross stress reactions' and 'transient situational disturbance' in DSM (1952) and DSM-II (1968). Examples of other terms for the disorder include physio-neurosis, hysteria, whiplash injury syndrome, effort syndrome, soldier's heart, shell shock, traumatic neurosis, combat exhaustion, battle stress, operational fatigue, survivor syndrome, concentration camp syndrome, rape trauma syndrome and gross stress reaction.

In the current classification of Mental Disorders, PTSD falls under the heading of an anxiety disorder. Gersons and Carlier (1992) add that with the introduction of the diagnosis 'PTSD' into DSM-III, it is possible to recognize victims of war and violence as psychiatric patients, without the stigma of their being classified among the more serious psychiatric conditions such as hysteria, depression or psychosis. It also allows the facilitation of compensation claims, they contend. However, Spragg (1992) points to the controversy over the application of the diagnosis, given that it depends on the reasons for making the diagnosis: these could relate to clinicians concerned solely with treatment issues, institutions assessing for compensation, forensic assessment preliminary to legal decisions, or for epidemiological purposes. Solomon *et al.* (1991) refer to the suspicions regarding malingering and the opportunity of secondary gain in compensation among PTSD patients.

Legal implications for compensation have led to a change in the 1977 legislation concerning statutory compensation for victims of civil violence in Northern Ireland. The Criminal Injuries Scheme now requires that people provide evidence of 'serious mental impairment', as opposed to claiming compensation for 'nervous shock'. The latter did not specify that the person had to be present at the time and place of the event, and thus claims could be received from people in another part of the country. The new legislation also requires that the person's life be changed for 'a considerable time', and that the condition is serious enough to warrant professional intervention, rather than be self-healing over time. Interestingly enough, there is a discrepancy between the minimal amount claimable for psychological versus physical injury, the former being £2500, and the latter £1000. This discrepancy does not apply to the Criminal Compensation Scheme operating in Great Britain.

Description of the syndrome

The DSM-III(R) (1987) has clarified five criteria for a diagnosis of PTSD:

- a history of exposure to severe stress
- re-experiencing the trauma through intrusive recollections, nightmares or flashbacks
- persistent avoidance of emotionally charged stimuli through numbing of responsiveness, avoidance of charged stimuli or psychogenic amnesia
- persistent hyperarousal, as indicated by insomnia, irritability, hypervigilance and increased startle response
- the symptoms must be of at least 1 month's duration; if the symptoms occur 6 months or more after the trauma, it is known as delayed onset PTSD.

In addition to the above, Miller *et al.* (1992) mention additional symptoms which commonly occur: depression, obsessive compulsive behaviour, dissociation, and a difficulty in concentrating.

Other features, such as identity problems and violent behaviour, are less constant, and relate to the premorbid personality (Spragg, 1992).

The physiological reactions to a threatening provocation, such as heightened perception, increased muscle tension and quickening heart beat, which are experienced by the individual as a feeling of overwhelming fear, are entirely appropriate responses to the preparation of dealing with danger. However, in PTSD, these symptoms also contain lasting features such as increased arousal, irritability, concentration difficulties, extreme alertness and excessive shock reactions. The individual seems to stay mobilized in a state of heterostasis, even when the outside danger has long passed. Thus, Gersons and Carlier (1992) comment that it is for this reason that PTSD has been called a 'physio-neurosis'. It is more than an adequate or inadequate psychic reaction to a frightening experience, as it also comprises a lasting physical and psychological reacting mechanism. Discussion continues to abound as to whether PTSD is in fact a normal reaction to an abnormal event, or whether it is an abnormal pathological reaction to an abnormal experience.

It is considered to be a process, not an illness, with a cause and effect. Mejo (1990) states that with PTSD there is no single cause that creates the disorder. Rather, the personality and the resistance of the individual, the strength and nature of the trauma and the individual's past and present environment all play powerful roles in PTSD's development.

PTSD may be explained, Gersons and Carlier (1992) suggest, as an initially adequate reaction to danger, which becomes pathological if it does not disappear after the danger has gone. PTSD, they continue, is the central syndrome at the junction between 'outside' traumatic events and the individual's capacity for adaptation to some horrific reality.

In addition to the above symptoms, a preoccupation with bodily function, where there are no demonstrable organic findings, is often noted in PTSD patients (Miller *et al.*, 1992). Such cases can well be misdiagnosed as primarily a physical disorder and be referred for physiotherapy.

The concept of 'somatic re-enactment' is put forward by Lindy *et al.* (1992), and can provide a way of understanding the lack of organic involvement found in certain ostensibly physical presentations. These somatic re-enactments are seen as physical representations of the intrusive symptoms characteristic of PTSD. Four case studies are reported, where persistent, severe physical pain and symptoms such as difficulty in walking were identified as paralleling incidents within a traumatic experience. Psychotherapeutic treatment enabled the link to be made, and the symptoms disappeared. The symptoms had repeated the actual memories with 'uncanny precision'. The way in which the symptoms themselves contain a somatic repetition of the trauma is also highlighted in the work with survivors of torture. The latter is discussed more fully in the second part of this chapter.

Diagnostic issues

The disorder is distinguished from other stress-related problems in that the diagnosis should only be applied to people who have experienced 'a psycho-logically traumatic event that is generally outside the range of usual human experience' (DSM-III-R 1987). It thus excludes psychiatric conditions precipi-tated by a divorce, bereavement excluding traumatic causes, loss of employment, chronic illness and marital conflict. The distinction between normal and patho-logical is not clear cut in all cases.

Lindemann (1944) suggested that grief reactions would normally be worked through in a period of 4–6 weeks. However, Parkes (1972) and others demon-strated that this 'normal' process could take up to a year or more, and it has been suggested that PTSD may be included as a possible component of pathological grief reaction (Parkes and Weiss, 1983). Likewise, Miller *et al.* (1992) suggest that in certain special cases of bereavement, separation or divorce, there can be traumatic elements which produce distinctive qualities consistent with PTSD.

Certain changes in the definition of PTSD are apparent in the revised edition of DSM-III (DSM-III-R, 1987); additional detail about avoidance response and a sense of foreshortened future are included, as is the recognition that PTSD can occur in children. 'Survivor guilt' has been deleted as one of the primary features, and the separation of acute from chronic PTSD has also been dropped. However, numerous authors report that the acute versus chronic PTSD distinction has both clinical and prognostic implications, and therefore it continues to be employed in many studies (Famularo *et al.*, 1990; Davidson, 1992). Likewise, a number of studies published since 1987 still refer to the feature of 'survivor guilt' (Spragg, 1992). Niles (1991) adds that many clinicians believe that helping trauma victims work through survivor guilt is often funda-mental to the intervention process.

Studies that employ the categories of 'acute, chronic and delayed PTSD' are generally in agreement with the following criteria. Acute signs usually develop within hours of the trauma, and persist for at least a month. They generally abate within 6 months. In chronic PTSD, symptoms persist for over 6 months and may continue for decades. Delayed PTSD refers to a delay in onset, such that the symptoms only surface 6 months or longer after the event, and once again can last for many years (Murray and Huelskotter, 1987). A minimal trigger can be sufficient for delayed PTSD to emerge. For example, Lovell (1991) describes an electrician who suffered severe injuries through an accident at work. No symptoms of PTSD occurred at the time, but 7 years later a minor incident in which a fuse blew, creating a small spark, resulted in a full-blown presentation of PTSD, requiring psychological treatment. Lim (1991) also cites a case where, following an accident, some avoidance and a degree of anxiety were experienced, but otherwise the patient showed no additional symptoms. However, witnessing a different trauma led to delayed PTSD emerging after a period of 6 years. Weisaeth, in 1985, cited by North and Smith (1990), states that such cases are relatively uncommon.

Nevertheless, Kaplan *et al.* (1992) emphasize that individuals who have apparently recovered from PTSD retain a heightened vulnerability to subsequent stress, and are more likely to suffer a reactivation of symptoms, even when the second trauma differs from the original event.

Distinguishing PTSD from other physical and psychiatric disorders

The first DSM-III-R criterion for the diagnosis of PTSD is that the individual has 'experienced' an extreme, or catastrophically stressful, life event. However, an interesting point is raised by Burges Watson (1990) when considering victims who are rendered unconscious by the trauma, and who suffer head injury. Given that certain survivors are rescued while unconscious, they have not in fact 'experienced' the event. This, he suggests, can explain the absence of flashback phenomena, given the amnesia that can surround the event. However, he cites two cases of victims of road traffic accidents who had total amnesia of the accident, but did show patchy awareness of their surroundings in the ambulance. Both had symptoms satisfying the criteria for PTSD, with the exception of re-experiencing the event. This report is supported by Baggaley and Rose (1990) and McMillan (1991) who each describe a single case study. Behavioural techniques, it is asserted, can be employed to ameliorate the symptoms of PTSD in such cases, despite amnesia of the traumatic event.

Looking at the ambulance crew, rather than the patients travelling in the ambulance, Kinchin (1993) refers to a British study which shows that 15% of London's ambulance crews suffer from PTSD. He suggests that PTSD can often be preceded by physical symptoms such as back pain, migraine or depression, and adds that if the underlying 'psychological injuries' are not addressed, PTSD may develop.

This issue is of central importance to the phsyiotherapist, who may have referrals for ostensibly physical treatments, but where the precipitating trauma has been overlooked. Patients can be reluctant to talk about the trauma, as doing so brings back the distressing, unpleasant and highly stressful event. The possibility of misdiagnosis is referred to by Choy and De Bosset (1992) who state that PTSD may be treated as another physical disorder, for example post-concussion syndrome.

Hickling *et al.* (1992) support this concern, reporting that of patients referred for post-traumatic headache following a motor vehicle accident, 80% had either full-blown PTSD or a subsyndromal manifestation of this diagnosis. They add that in order to treat post-traumatic headache successfully, attention needs to be paid to the post-traumatic stress disorder as well as the headache.

This point is emphasized by Davidson (1992) who reports that chronic PTSD often presents with non-specific symptoms such as headache, insomnia, irritability, depression, tension, interpersonal or professional dysfunction, and substance abuse. The latter is a common reaction to trauma, as people often attempt to dull their emotions and suppress the trauma using various drugs. The result can then be substance addiction, which can cause additional difficulties (Miller *et al.*, 1992). The need for careful assessment is stressed, as the underlying cause can otherwise remain undetected.

However, Solomon *et al.* (1991) query the much reported finding of the link between substance abuse, antisocial behaviour and PTSD sufferers. Their sample of Israeli veterans did not show this association, and it is therefore suggested that the findings may reflect trends among Vietnam combat veterans, rather than features of PTSD.

Famularo *et al.* (1992) warn that children presenting with possible personality disorder diagnoses should be reviewed carefully for any evidence of earlier history of maltreatment, and a diagnosis of PTSD.

Several studies have statistically examined whether PTSD is a separate diagnostic category that can be distinguished from other psychiatric disorders (Solomon *et al.*, 1991; Watson *et al.*, 1991). Despite a high degree of overlap (McFarlane, 1989, reports that 50% of persons with PTSD have a coexistent psychiatric diagnosis), the overall conclusion is that PTSD can be discriminated from other patient groups.

Davidson and Smith (1990) suggest that PTSD is not sufficiently recognized, even by psychiatric personnel. This view is supported by Kolb (1989), who states that many cases of PTSD go unrecognized by both medical and psychiatric communities. The reasons given are that PTSD is often confused with other anxiety disorders, alcoholism and depressive reactions. In addition, it is suggested that sufferers may wish to avoid all enquiries concerning the trauma, and seldom offer information. Ramsay (1990) states that a significant proportion of rape victims do not report the event.

Gersons and Carlier (1992) comment that the treatment and study of PTSD have generally been characterized by confusion and a failure to generalize from or elaborate upon earlier findings and clinical experience abroad.

Events which may lead to PTSD

Man-made disasters are thought to be more emotionally devastating than natural disasters (Table 20.1), given that the latter are out of human control and therefore outside human responsibility (Baum Fleming and Davidson, 1983; Beigel and Berren, 1985; Fisher and Reason, 1988).

It is suggested by Green *et al.* (1990) that witnessing another person's grotesque death is the strongest predictor of PTSD. North and Smith (1990) cite several authors who suggest that the elements of terror and horror contribute to

Table 20.1 Man-made and natural disasters which could lead to PTSD*

Man-made/technological			Natural
Accidental/error	*Deliberate*	*Byproduct*	
Ferry sinking	War	Hospital procedures	Earthquakes
Collisions	Concentration camp/	Dental procedures	Floods
(air, land, sea)	torture	Immigration	Bushfires
Fire/explosion	Violent crime		Tornadoes
Accidents	Rape/mugging/abuse		Volcanoes
(domestric/work)	Kidnapping		
Leakages	Terrorist attacks		
	Hostage		

Experiencing any of the above, individually or within a group.

Witnessing any of the above, especially if a loved one is involved.

* The population potentially developing PTSD can include all ages, those injured or involved, onlookers and carers.

the impact of disaster, providing the material for intrusive recollections of the trauma.

With this in mind, one of the most horrific forms of trauma must be that of deliberately inflicted pain and harm, as evinced in torture. Amnesty International estimates that brutal torture and ill-treatment have been practised by one out of every three governments in the 1980s (Allinson, 1991). Because of the deliberate nature of torture, it has been taken as outside the sphere of the first part of this chapter, and is discussed in detail in the second section.

PTSD can be an occupational hazard in such professions as firefighters, police, ambulance crew, soldiers, sailors, medical and paramedical staff, jurors and aircrew. The spouses and children of people suffering from the disorder can also be affected (Niles, 1991). A woman whose husband was sent to Zeebrugge to help assist in the disaster response described how her husband went away, but 'a stranger' returned (Iljon Foreman, 1991). Nevertheless, as recently as 1991, Duckworth reports that 'there is no shortage of experienced police officers who flatly refuse to believe that post-traumatic stress reactions are anything other than a sign of "weakness" in those who are affected'.

Incidence and predictors of PTSD

The incidence of PTSD occurring at some point in a person's life has been reported as 1.3% by Davidson *et al.* (1991) and as 1% by Helzer *et al.* (1987). Breslau *et al.* (1990) reported a prevalence of PTSD as 9.4% in young adults.

Looking at specific groups, the following has been reported: 3.5% in civilians exposed to an attack and non-wounded Vietnam veterans, 20% in wounded Vietnam veterans (Helzer *et al.*, 1987; Kinzie *et al.*, 1990). Thirty per cent of the 23 million Americans involved in motor vehicle accidents or indirect victims of homicide will develop PTSD (Choy and De Bosset, 1992). The incidence rises to 50% of the schoolchildren assessed a year after a shipping disaster (Yule, 1992), and to 50% in adult survivors referred for a medicolegal assessment following the Eniskillen bombing (Curran *et al.*, 1990), while 85% of Nazi death camp survivors developed PTSD (Kinzie, 1989), and 100% of children involved in the kidnapping of their school bus (Terr, 1981).

The attitudes of society, which tend to be positive towards hostages and victims of natural disasters, but somewhat negative towards refugees, may alleviate or exacerbate the original trauma (Kinzie, 1989). Likewise, the differences in the reception of soldiers returning from the Vietnam war, versus the Falklands conflict, are referred to by O'Brien and Hughes (1991). Despite the comparative heroes' welcome that the Falkland soldiers received, O'Brien and Hughes calculate that 22% of the veterans suffered from PTSD. This indicates that though there may be certain 'protective features' against the development of PTSD in soldiers (Spragg, 1992), in that they are fit, healthy men, who most importantly have been trained, and should not be particularly susceptible to PTSD, it nevertheless does arise.

Foa (1992), in a review of the treatment of PTSD in civilian contexts, cites 16 studies, 13 of which concern rape or sexual abuse. Sexual abuse has been reported to give rise to PTSD in 48.4% of children studied by McLeer *et al.* (1988). Donaldson and Gardner (1985) add that delayed PTSD may be more severe and long lasting when the abuser is not an anonymous rapist, but some-one presumed to be trustworthy and whose presence persists, i.e. when the stressor is part of the family.

It has been suggested that PTSD in both adults and children is more likely to be triggered if the person involved has experienced the precursors of domestic violence and child abuse (Speed *et al.*, 1989; Klusnick *et al.*, 1986, in Miller *et al.*, 1992). Likewise, Davidson *et al.* (1991) report that those who developed PTSD had frequently suffered from adverse events during childhood, early parental divorce or separation, parental poverty, and had been victims of abuse. They showed conduct disorder, had a higher risk of attempted suicide, and an increased likelihood of suffering from psychiatric and physical disorders. Some of the above childhood events can be seen as both predisposing risk factors to the later development of PTSD, following other traumatic events, or as traumata themselves, leading to acute, chronic or delayed PTSD.

Graziano (1992) points out that adult survivors of child sexual abuse may not necessarily present for outpatient psychotherapy related to the abuse, and for treatment of subsequent PTSD, but could appear in a variety of inpatient and out-patient, medical, psychiatric and community settings. Care needs to be taken, when offering treatment which includes touch, to ensure that it does not inadvertently give rise to memories of the abuse.

Solomon *et al.* (1989) report that following a traumatic event, subsequent negative life events increase the probability of developing PTSD, while positive events have the reverse effect. It was also reported that previous life events were unrelated to the probability of developing combat stress reaction, but that people who did develop combat stress after battle were more likely to suffer from PTSD (Solomon and Flum, 1988).

A study of psychological sequelae following accidental injury (Feinstein and Dolan, 1991) revealed that 66% of patients, within a week of the injury, reported sufficient symptoms to be rated as 'psychiatric cases'. Without inter-vention, less than 25% remained as 'cases' by 6 months. Physical morbidity at 6 months was minimal, and did not influence psychiatric outcome. Neither the nature of the stressor nor its perceived stressfulness influenced outcome, in contrast to the DSM-III-R view which correlates severity of the stressor with the development of PTSD. Reference is made to the lack of consistent findings in this area (March, 1990), and also to the view of Horowitz *et al.* (1987) in which the stressor is seen as a trigger to the development of psychopathology, rather than acting as an aetiological agent *per se*. The importance of constitutional and environmental factors is stressed, and the focus is shifted to the individual's subjective response to the traumatic event.

Supporting this, McFarlane (1988) reported that psychiatric impairment is more closely related to levels of distress following the disaster than to the victim's severity of exposure or loss.

Pre-existing pathological conditions may predispose to the development of PTSD (Thompson, 1989; Watson *et al.*, 1991), with premorbid depressive tendencies and neuroticism predisposing to the development of PTSD, and psychopathic traits protecting from it. Thompson and Solomon (in press) found support for the relationship between neuroticism and psychological distress, and for the protective effect of extraversion, but were surprised to find that psychoticism was a vulnerability factor. However, Allison (1991) stresses that the vast majority of cases of PTSD arise in 'perfectly normal individuals'.

Considering incidence and predictors, it is concluded by North and Smith (1990) that, despite the appearance of systematic studies, there is little agreement on the proportion of affected populations that can be expected to develop a clinically significant PTSD syndrome following a given disaster. Reported rates have ranged from 2% to 100%.

One way of reducing the likelihood of PTSD is the early identification of people who are likely to develop it. Yule and Udwin (1991) have developed an assessment battery, which appears highly predictive in identifying school-children who are likely to seek help following a trauma, and are at high risk of experiencing longer term psychological distress.

Looking specifically at the emergency services, Thompson and Solomon (in press) refer to the way in which effective management of the personnel involved in disaster work can reduce the likelihood of psychological problems being experienced. The main features highlighted in this effective management are: talking about the events, with high-quality social support available, praise from leaders, debriefing, appropriate training and education. They also point to the need for careful selection of stable and extroverted individuals.

An indication of the extent of interest in PTSD is shown by a bibliography from the British Library (1991) on 'Treatment of psychological aspects of war 1986–1990', which lists 379 studies. Of considerable relevance to therapists working with military casualties is the suggestion by Solursh (1989) that certain PTSD sufferers are actually experiencing 'combat addiction'. The intrusive memories can give a 'high' experience, so exciting that the person may resent and resist treatment, despite the other accompanying problems of PTSD.

Given the depth of study and interest that PTSD has aroused, it is easy to forget the point made by Choy and De Bosset (1992) that, apart from extremely prolonged catastrophic conditions, most who experience a trauma do not develop PTSD. Likewise North and Smith (1990) make the point that in spite of the fact that psychiatric distress often plagues the survivors of extreme traumatic events, the general mental health of a significant proportion, sometimes even the majority, of the subjects in most studies attests to the resilience and strength of the human mind to withstand even the most extreme stress.

Treatment

General considerations

The days of suggesting that PTSD is merely feigned, and that sufferers should be imprisoned or summarily executed, are fortunately past (Gersons and Carlier, 1992). Gone are the World War I days when the English psychiatrists working with soldiers in mental institutions, separated from the front line by only the English Channel, advised the soldiers to 'ignore it', and 'don't talk about it'. Unfortunately, but not surprisingly, this advice led to a consolidation of symptoms.

While one cannot expect to prepare the whole population for the experience of disasters, several studies, e.g. Thompson and Solomon (in press), Iljon Foreman (1991) and others, stress the need to provide appropriate training for personnel who are going to be working with disaster victims. This, in conjunction with many of the post-disaster therapeutic support mechanisms that the victims receive, can reduce the likelihood of the helpers themselves becoming victims of PTSD (Allinson, 1991).

Yet despite the increased awareness of PTSD, it can easily be overlooked by both the sufferer, friends and colleagues. Hinks (1991) describes his personal aftermath of the Hillsborough disaster, and how despite working as a mental health professional, it still took a year to recognize and admit to symptoms of PTSD and to seek help. He adds that therapy enabled him to identify the specific effects of post-traumatic stress, and to separate these from other painful aspects of his life. Previous to this, he had been blaming every negative aspect of his life on Hillsborough – from domestic arguments to minor illness.

The need for treatment is stressed by Kolb (1989), who suggests that it may prevent the long-term psychosocial problems of alcoholism, divorce, suicide, violence and difficulty in holding employment. Allinson (1991) stresses the need to highlight the lack of information available for the UK on PTSD. The potentially severe consequences of the disorder are given in the following grim summary: 'If untreated, PTSD can lead to prolonged distress, misery, and even death. It can have a devastating effect on children, and in adults chronic PTSD can predispose to major personality breakdowns.' Loughrey *et al.* (1988) and Kaplan (1989) also mention the increased likelihood of sexual and marital difficulties. On the more optimistic side, Duckworth (1991) asserts that there is great scope for preventative management following a specific disaster, and that satisfactory adjustment to experiences which have provoked strong initial disturbance is something toward which a person can be guided, from the very early stages.

The forms of treatment offered vary, and at present there appear to be no clearly agreed criteria for the choice of one over others. Ramsay (1990) suggests that in the first instance 'many of the symptoms of PTSD can be successfully self-medicated with alcohol'. While this may be so, the dangers of dependence are stressed throughout the literature. However, certain authors do have strong views as to which treatment should be initially offered, as can be seen within the various therapeutic approaches considered below.

It is suggested by Burgess Watson *et al.* (1988) that PTSD, with its multiplicity of diagnostic labels, can only be understood by an approach which takes into account biological, psychological and social factors, and that a single treatment modality is unlikely to be identifiable. Ramsay (1990) stresses the necessity of an integrated way of understanding the nature of the human response to trauma, in order to be able to provide a rational approach to the treatment of its casualties.

Certain controlled trials comparing different therapeutic approaches are being undertaken, such as the comparison of psychotherapy with exposure-based cognitive therapy, currently running at the stress clinic (Thompson, 1992).

There are, however, certain elements common to all the forms of treatment reviewed, such as the provision of information regarding the normal symptoms experienced after trauma. This normalizing of the experience can provide considerable relief to people, who can otherwise fear that the symptoms themselves are dangerous, and that having them is a signal of impending mental breakdown, that they will never end, and that they signify a 'weak personality'.

A study by Patterson *et al.* (1990) examined patients with burn injuries. The findings replicated that of Perry *et al.* (1987) that PTSD inpatients with burn injuries can be regarded as a non-pathological syndrome, unless symptoms are found to persist unduly. While PTSD appeared to resolve in most cases with standard hospital care, it is suggested that it may be preventable if those who are at risk are identified and receive appropriate psychological treatment soon after the injury. 'At risk' indices were related to total body surface burn area, length of hospital stay, sex (females more likely to develop PTSD) and lack of responsibility for injury. This finding replicates results of previous research (Perry *et al.*, 1990), and is consistent with findings with spinal cord injury which suggest that 'innocent victims' have more difficulty adjusting to the disability than those who were in some way responsible for their injuries (Treishman, 1980). It was also noted that patients with PTSD reported higher levels of pain than those without PTSD, despite receiving equivalent doses of analgesic medication. Detecting this disorder can therefore have important implications for pain control. Likewise, the need for training and awareness of this feature is important for phsyiotherapists, who may be working with these patients.

Sturgeon *et al.* (1991) give a case report of burn injuries sustained during the King's Cross fire. The patient required skin grafts to her back and legs, which caused her considerable physical discomfort, and this was exacerbated by her physiotherapy. In addition to several symptoms of PTSD, she also developed intense anticipatory anxiety before her dressings were changed, which necessitated further treatment with morphine compounds to contain her distress.

Psychological first aid

Rose and Richards (1991) provide the following list of the principles of 'psychological first aid'. They are of relevance to all professionals who may be involved in the treatment of the patient.

1. Reassurance that stress symptoms are normal, will pass, and are not signs of 'madness'. This can be given both verbally to patients and staff, and also as printed leaflets for later reference.
2. Rest and sleep, preferably without medication as far as possible, although this may sometimes be necessary.
3. Recall of traumatic experiences and personal injury with other patients or

staff – gentle encouragement to talk and sympathetic listening. This can initially take place at a 'psychological debriefing' (Dyregrov, 1988; Allinson, 1991) soon after the event, and then within therapy sessions. Yule and Udwin (1991), however, point out that the assumption that debriefing sessions significantly reduce later clinical morbidity has not yet been empirically tested, though a later study by Yule (1992) does indicate that early intervention, including psychological debriefing, group support as well as group and individual therapy, appears helpful in reducing reported levels of psychopathology. Both intrusive, painful, traumatic memories and feelings of loss and bereavement require addressing.

4. (Truthful) reassurance concerning personal medical condition, with, where possible, news and information on friends, comrades, relatives (killed, wounded and survived).

5. Rehabilitation by encouragement in self-care tasks, activity and mobilization as soon as possible. This is clearly an area for involvement of the physiotherapist.

In addition, McFarlane (1989) stresses the need to encourage reduction of social isolation.

Warning is given of the danger of therapist overkill, whereby 'crowds of well meaning counsellors descended on survivors and carers alike ...(lurked) around staff rooms trying to spot people in distress'. Staff felt very angry at being forced into sessions that they did not need or want (Rose and Richards, 1991). Iljon Foreman (1991) reports that, on average, victims of the Kings Cross fire were interviewed by 11 different agencies. This form of communication can be anti-therapeutic. Turner *et al.* (1989) suggest that, for most therapeutic effectiveness, a smaller number of longer sessions should be offered, where unpleasant emotional material can gradually become less painful. There is a risk that many brief interventions, perhaps by multiple agencies, will make the individual more sensitive to the event, and they may experience more emotional distress as a result.

Psychotherapy

Psychotherapy places a great focus on the way in which the present trauma revives memories of past experiences. Spragg (1992) argues that various primary treatment methods can be adopted, be they drugs, cognitive behaviour therapy or psychotherapy. However, he stresses that none is likely to succeed, unless the clinician is alert to looking for the unconscious element that underlies the manifest statement. He suggests that throughout the treatment, whatever its length, one cardinal principle prevails. The therapist must remain objective and exercise patience, and resist any temptation to innovate or introduce manoeuvres when progress seems to have halted. If an impasse has been reached, the therapist should consult a colleague, who may be able to perceive elements of transference or counter-transference that have been missed (see Chapter 4). The overriding principle is: 'Do not assume or dictate. Listen and try to understand what is being said.'

Miller *et al.* (1992) add that often the symptomatology associated with traumatic stress generates an avoidant type of personality disturbance – a self-imposed isolation from other people. This becomes a critical factor in the treatment process, and requires the therapist to work towards decreasing the trauma survivor's isolation and to providing a therapeutic component which can address the dissociative aspects of the traumatizing experience. (It is recognized, however, that at times the survivor will have the need for privacy and solitude, and this must be respected, and is therapeutic.)

Niles (1991) refers to the moment of trauma precipitating an instant regression to an infantile state, in which fundamental trust in self and others is disrupted, along with basic assumptions about existence. Therapy requires facilitating the process of reintegration. He adds that medication does not affect such symptoms as mistrust, self-doubt, guilt, isolation, moral pain, and problems with intimacy.

It is stressed by Sturgeon *et al.* (1991) that people who have experienced a disaster often use a variety of psychological defence mechanisms to protect themselves against the psychic pain of the disaster. It is proposed that a psychotherapeutic approach in such cases is vital in assisting recovery.

Allinson (1991) hypothesizes that in delayed PTSD the trauma is internalized to avoid immediate pain.

Five important treatment interventions in working with PTSD have been outlined by Scurfield (1985):

- *Therapeutic trust within the treatment relationship.* It can take longer than a year of therapy before survivors build up enough trust to expose the trauma of sexual abuse, for example.
- *Educating the client regarding the recovery process.*
- *Stress management* or reduction of. It is suggested that this be achieved through a combination of therapeutic endeavours such as behavioural techniques, relaxation exercises, physical exercises and general coping strategies.
- *Helping the patient regress back or re-experience the trauma.* This needs to be done with care and sensitivity, and to consider the client's ability to tolerate this experience. Some clients may feel abused if they are asked to speak about the details of their experiences, or feel totally overwhelmed. If the clinician is too directive, the client may experience the clinician as the torturer. (Allinson, 1991, adds that hypnosis may be used as a technique to facilitate the experience of reliving the event.)
- *An integration of the trauma experience.* This encourages a greater understanding of both the positive and negative aspects.

Timing of the intervention has been considered by several authors. Mejo (1990) suggests that 1–3 months post-trauma is considered optimal, as after that patients begin the process of sealing off the trauma. The rate of drop-out from treatment was 81.6% in a study when treatment began 40 weeks after the trauma (Burstein, 1986).

While the above differs in many ways from the next treatment intervention described, cognitive behaviour therapy, both approaches stress the need to address avoidance behaviour, despite giving different theoretical rationales for the causes of the behaviour.

Cognitive behaviour therapy

Cognitive behaviour therapy emphasizes the understanding of the person's current means of dealing with the stress. Avoidances are examined and decisions reached as to whether these are of a phobic nature, or are based on a new, more accurate perception of the likelihood of danger. Two case studies give an example of the way in which these methods can be applied.

Case 1

A railway worker was told to carry out a certain task, despite inadequate safety precautions. An accident occurred, resulting in him falling onto the electrified line, and suffering a massive electric shock. He survived, despite severe injuries, but presented for psychological help 18 months later, suffering the classic symptoms of PTSD. Treatment focused on explaining the normal responses to trauma, with reassurance that he was not going mad, and that the experience of reliving the electrocution, particularly during nightmares, would not cause heart damage. Withdrawal from sleep medication was achieved, and a return to full working activities was achieved, abolishing the avoidances he had established. Safe working practices were discussed, and it was agreed that if demands were made for unsafe tasks in the future, these would be refused, despite pressure from superiors and colleagues. Within five sessions over a 2-month period, a return to premorbid functioning was established, with reduction in nightmares, improvement in mood, concentration and self-confidence.

A second trauma was then experienced, in which the patient was witness to a roadworker suffering a similar electric shock, and was involved in providing first aid. This experience cause a recurrence of the original flashbacks concerning his own accident, as well as adding extra material to these relating to the horrific sight of the second incident. Two additional sessions of therapeutic support were required to work through this, and once again return to normal functioning was achieved.

Case 2

A woman suffered an unprovoked attack in a pub. She described a complete cessation of social activities and symptoms of panic when she went out of the house. She would only go out if accompanied, and avoided social events wherever possible. Treatment focused on discriminating between safe and dangerous environments, and then testing out the prediction that it was extremely unlikely for such an attack to happen again. She had also stopped dressing attractively and wearing make-up, as a way of presenting a lower profile. The fact that the attack had happened when she was wearing casual clothes, and therefore was unrelated to smart appearance, was discussed, and she agreed to start dressing smartly for occasions for which she would have done so in the past. Over a period of 2 months she reported an increase in self-confidence and was able to return to college and complete her studies. The nightmares gradually ceased, and she also reported that when they did happen, she was able to dismiss then as a normal stress reaction and did not fear that they would last for ever.

Considering overall management of PTSD, in the short term post-disaster period when resources are often scarce, services should be directed at those with greatest risk of developing PTSD. Research quoted by North and Smith (1990) suggests that these are people who have had the greatest exposure or proximity to the disaster event, and those with a past history of psychological problems. If PTSD occurs, the given individual is then at greater risk of developing other psychiatric disorders as well. Systematic screening with these factors in mind may yield a potentially high-risk group for intensive intervention.

Yule and Udwin (1991) point to the paucity of studies of 'psychological triage' with adults, and add that there are no such studies at all on children. Despite the dangers of therapist 'overkill' previously referred to, it is suggested that in the immediate aftermath of a disaster there is a need to provide psychological first aid, and then to consider which survivors are at highest risk of developing further symptoms. Particularly where disasters involve large numbers of survivors, it is crucial to have a means of screening them in order to identify those at high risk for psychological difficulties, so that they can be given immediate access to psychological help and then be monitored over time.

This theme is expanded in a recent article (Joseph *et al.*, 1993) in which crisis support was assessed over an 18-month period following a disaster. Higher crisis support in the immediate aftermath was found to predict less post-traumatic symptomatology at a later period. Joseph and colleagues refer to findings by Cook and Bickman (1990) in which post-traumatic symptoms decline with time elapsed since a disaster. The hypothesis that support received from other people also declines over time was tested by Joseph *et al.* (1993) and found to be the case.

Yule (1992) reports on a study carried out with child survivors of a shipping disaster. The therapy employed a problem-solving approach, based on cognitive behavioural methods to target anxiety, avoidance and intrusive thoughts. Comparing results to a contrasting school where no outside support was accepted until a year after the disaster, he found that pupils in the school that organized early intervention showed significantly lower scores on the Impact of Events scale (Horowitz *et al.*, 1979), especially for intrusive memories.

The implications for treatment identified by Yule (1992) are that the first need is to help children make sense of what has happened to them and to gain mastery over their feelings. They should therefore be treated in small groups, where they are asked to write a detailed account of their experience, and are helped to cope with the emotions that that brings up. In addition, they should be given specific treatment for fears, phobias and any other avoidant behaviours. They should get practical help with sleeping disorders. As intrusive thoughts are often worse at night just before falling asleep, the use of tape-recorded music to distract the children and blot out the thoughts is suggested. With better sleep, the thoughts are more easily dealt with in daylight.

Deblinger *et al.* (1990) report a clinical trial of cognitive behaviour therapy for children suffering from PTSD as a result of sexual abuse, in which the treatment programme includes training of the non-offending adult. The study concludes that treatment appears to result in significant improvement, compared to baseline measures. It is stressed that PTSD can severely disrupt a child's emotional, cognitive and behavioural development, and that the formulation and imple-mentation of an effective treatment programme is imperative.

Another variant of treatment has considered the 'flashback' symptoms of PTSD as aversively conditioned stimuli. The therapy involves 'image habituation training', i.e. the repeated presentation of the aversive event, in imagination, until gradually habituation takes place, and the image no longer triggers avoidance or anxiety. The treatment was reported as especially effective for patients experiencing repeated intrusive images and thoughts, and high levels of arousal (Vaughan and Tarrier, 1992). Richards and Rose (1991) used an audiotaped imaginal exposure as part of a treatment programme incorporating *in vivo* exposure. These authors conclude that when *in vivo* exposure is ineffective with PTSD, imaginal exposure to trauma memories should be employed before abandoning behavioural approaches. They add that controlled research is now indicated to assess the relative importance of *in vivo* and imaginal exposure in PTSD, so that the optimum combination of treatments can be determined.

Thompson (1992) concludes that therapies which are based on habituation and extinction of a conditioned response have a firm theoretical base and appear to be producing powerful results. In the light of present knowledge, he therefore states that this is the treatment of choice for post-trauma reactions.

Drugs

Several case studies and large clinical trials have been reported that antidepressants may alleviate flashbacks, nightmares and panic attacks (APA, 1989; Turchin *et al.*, 1992). The latter study gives two case examples of trimodal therapy for PTSD, including supportive therapy, behavioural interventions and pharmacotherapy. It is suggested that the introduction of antidepressants appears to have been crucial in recovery. However, a detailed description of the other two therapies is not provided, thus leaving open the question of how their effectiveness can be evaluated.

Pharmacological intervention has been documented employing tricyclic antidepressants, monoamine oxidase inhibitors, antipsychotic agents, lithium, beta-blockers, clonidine and benzodiazepines. ECT has also been used in cases presenting with severe depression (Davidson, 1992). Ramsay (1990) reports the hypothesis that there is an underlying organic basis to the response to extreme stress. There can be a generalized suppression of affective arousal or exhaustion of adrenal cortical function following chronic stimulation. The suppression of affective arousal could lead to a numbing of responsiveness. Summarizing the literature on the use of pharmacotherapy in PTSD, Davidson (1992) concludes that the efficacy is certainly less than that seen for depression and panic disorder. However, the conclusion given is that the efficacy of pharmacotherapy has been demonstrated in PTSD. A minimum of 2 months' treatment is likely to be required to achieve a benefit which exceeds that of placebo (Davidson, 1992). Ramsay (1990) adds that drug treatment showed a 70% improvement in patients' motivation to psychotherapy.

Six goals for pharmacotherapy in PTSD are identified by Davidson (1992):

* reduction of phasic intrusive symptoms
* improvement of avoidance symptoms
* reduction of tonic hyperarousal
* relief of depression, anhedonia
* improvement of impulse regulation
* control of acute dissociative and psychotic features.

The use of pharmacotherapy as an adjunct to other forms of treatment is suggested by Friedman (1988), who comments that pharmacotherapy alone is rarely sufficient to provide complete remission of PTSD. Symptom relief provided by medication can enable the patient to participate more thoroughly in individual, behavioural or group psychotherapy. The potential additive effect of both psychotherapy and pharmacological treatment is referred to by several authors (Miller, 1989; Mejo, 1990). However, it is suggested that it is important to wait for specific indications, rather than giving medication immediately after a trauma, in order to see if the person can work through the event without the use of medication (Roth, 1988).

Davidson (1992) emphasizes the need to distinguish between acute and chronic PTSD, as he suggests that there are indications to use different medication for the two conditions. With regard to efficacy, he cites the almost total lack of response to placebo in chronic PTSD.

A warning is sounded when considering using medication for those people with PTSD who are feeling hopeless or out of control, as there is a potential danger of suicide by overdose (Mejo, 1990).

Reference is made to patients with PTSD being at risk for comorbid psychiatric disorders which decrease treatment response (Davidson *et al.*, 1990). Thus the opposite view is also stated – that immediate antidepressant therapy may be protective against the anxious and depressive complications of PTSD, and allow earlier intervention and better response to traditional behavioural and supportive therapies in an individual who has significant signs and symptoms of PTSD, even before meeting the criteria of DSM-III-R.

While it has been mentioned earlier that there is a risk of misdiagnosing PTSD as an organic disorder, the danger of the reverse is mentioned by Roth (1988).

The overall conclusion is thus that controlled research needs to be carried out on the timing of pharmacological intervention in the treatment of PTSD, with respect to both chronology and to the use of multiple therapies.

Nursing management

Several authors describe ways in which the nurse can act as co-therapist in the treatment of PTSD. It may be the nurse to whom the patient speaks about the trauma, thereby having the opportunity to reduce the emotional impact of the experience. Clearly when patients are attending physiotherapy for injuries sustained during trauma, the role of the physiotherapist can parallel that of the nurse with respect to treatment for PTSD. The involvement of physiotherapists in this manner was not referred to in any of the literature which was identified in the research for this chapter. It would seem from conversations with physiotherapists that they clearly have a clinical involvement in the treatment of PTSD, but that published studies describing this are probably few and not well known.

It is also suggested that the nurse can teach such cognitive techniques as thought-stopping, and participate in a graded desensitization programme, such that the patient is gradually reintroduced to the things that they have avoided, for example uniforms, in the case of traumatized soldiers, or other cues associated with the event (Petit, 1991).

The need to have a shared understanding of the proposed underlying causes and maintaining factors of PTSD would seem to be crucial, if more than one therapist is involved. Studies reviewed did not appear to address this issue, nor that of deciding which role is to be taken by each particular therapist, in the case of input from multiple professions such as medicine, nursing, physiotherapy and psychology.

Physiotherapy

Issues within physiotherapy training

Conversations with physiotherapists who have worked with patients suffering from PTSD have highlighted the following needs:

1. The disorder should be addressed during training, thus allowing appropriate recognition and understanding by the physiotherapist. An example was given of a patient, a guitarist, who had suffered severe burns to his hands in the King's Cross fire. He made no eye contact and was almost mute. This was rare in the physiotherapist's experience. Treatment necessitated the provision of analgesics, and a warm, sympathetic but firmly directive approach. The patient was informed that he would receive physiotherapy, whether or not he participated. Once trust was established, and in conjunction with other therapeutic inputs, the social withdrawal gradually lessened and progress was made.
2. The ability to differentiate between people who appear to have 'compensation neurosis' versus genuine PTSD sufferers. This was considered vital to prevent the experience of repeated clinical failure, which could give rise to a self-image of poor competence in the therapist, when the more likely explanation was that the patient needed to maintain the symptoms.
3. To work within a multidisciplinary context, in particular with a psychologist and a doctor. This would enable specific psychological help to be provided, and could enable a joint decision of when to stop offering treatment, in cases where no progress is achieved.

Physiotherapy for survivors of torture and PTSD sufferers

There,
where the light of the sun
lost itself
more than a century ago,
where all gaiety
is impossible
and any smile
is a grimace of irony,
where the stone stench of darkness
inhabits those corners
even the spiders
have abandoned as inhospitable,
and where human pain eludes
that which can be called human
and enters the category
of the unprintable ...
There, I am writing.

[From a Chilean jail, quoted by Sheila Cassidy (1974)]

Background to torture

Torture makes you dead without killing you.*

Torture breaks some fundamental human contract. But over 110 countries are now reported to torture their own citizens (Amnesty International Report, 1993).

* Unattributed quotes are from clients.

Because it is the antithesis of humanity, the concept of torture is difficult to grasp or even accept. But it is more than just the aberrant expression of sadism by individuals in a few wayward banana republics; it is part of the process of government in many countries. The wretchedness of the experience follows survivors and continues to isolate them even in the midst of family life.

It's there 24 hours a day, even when I'm laughing. I'm crying inside.

Effects of torture
Something in you dies when you bear the unbearable (Levine, 1988).

The reactions to these abnormal events can be extreme and are experienced by most survivors. Thus survivors show normal reactions to abnormal events. They need reassurance that these reactions are not signs that they are mentally sick.

Symptoms include chronic hyperventilation, nightmares, phobias, intractable pain, social withdrawal, intense vigilance, an increasingly restricted lifestyle as survivors avoid situations that trigger fear, and a sense of meaningless (Turner and Gorst-Unsworth, 1990). Feelings of guilt, powerlessness and weakness become their new prison (Jacobsen and Vesti, 1990). They may freeze in the street when they see a friendly British policeman.

It is so unusual an experience. You are facing something out of mind, out of biology, out of nature.

Anger at their torturers has had to be suppressed, so it may be turned inward to become depression. This is compounded by a deep sense of loss. Many have lost family, friends, health, culture, self-esteem, sense of self, familiar mechanisms for expressing grief, and belief in the good within themselves and others (Garland, 1993). 'We are men without shadows', one survivor commented. 'I have become a zero', said another. It is as if both internal and external worlds have disintegrated (Bustos, 1990). This destruction of the identity of the victim is one of the main aims of the torturer (Skylv *et al.*, 1990).

The mere act of survival may bring guilt (Turner and Gorst-Unsworth, 1990). This is intensified if survivors' families or friends have been punished for helping them escape, or if they themselves have given away their friends' names under torture. Guilt is compounded by a sense of shame and humiliation, which adds to the difficulty of speaking about the experience. There may also be the fear that putting feelings into words will make the feelings worse.

Survivors diagnosed with PTSD sometimes find that this identification helps to validate their experience. They may have been disbelieved if they attempted to speak about what has happened; they may have come to disbelieve themselves, such is the loss of their sense of self.

When I am with people who were not tortured I cannot speak because there are no words.

Physiotherapy treatment
Working with people who have been tortured requires an acute sensitivity to their responses, an extra awareness of the importance of autonomy, and an understanding of issues of power and helplessness.

The aim of physiotherapy is to act as a bridge between mind and body. It is to facilitate clients in their own physical, mental and spiritual rehabilitation, so that they find strength to recover from their broken expectations of life. It is to enable, not to disable by succumbing to our rescuer instincts.

The pain is not like ordinary pain. With this, something happens in your heart.

Physiotherapy forms a vital link in rebuilding the personality of survivors of torture because trust can be fostered in the context of physical contact. A physical therapist who subsequently trained as a psychotherapist said: 'I often lament how laborious a task it can be to cultivate a relationship with a client when it was so much more accessible in my experience as a physical therapist' (Cimini, 1991).

Verbal expression may be frustrated by a tendency to 'forget' painful experiences. If the mind cannot encompass the task of making sense of what has happened, the body remembers. Physiotherapists are privileged in being authorized to touch. Touch can communicate acceptance and allow clients to connect with a body from which they have become dissociated.

Some clients feel safe to see a physiotherapist because they expect us to work on the physical level without expectation of disclosure. If they are not ready to talk about their experiences, this should be respected. If we follow rather than lead, it is easier to maintain a balance between allowing denial but preventing a form of collusion in which both client and physiotherapist avoid traumatic material by focusing solely on physical symptoms and maintaining a 'conspiracy of silence'.

When survivors are able to speak about their experiences, we need to bear witness. They need to know that their pain can be acknowledged, even if it is beyond the range of our experience. Our job is to both listen and hear, and it is not always easy to hear what they tell us. We must create an environment in which they feel able to talk, be silent, cry, be angry or even laugh. When survivors know that they are given full attention and are believed and responded to, they begin to develop trust.

I realized that pain can increase without end. That feeling is devastating to the mind. The desperation is hard to describe. Suddenly an entire culture collapses. Nothing is possible in such a universe. It is hard to be a survivor.

Precautions. During assessment and treatment, we must maintain vigilance in order to avoid triggering fear. The first session may involve no physical contact, because although touch is particularly healing for survivors, we must be wary of where and how we touch. The intimacy of our relationship with survivors is matched by the perverted intimacy of their previous relationship with their torturer. We always obtain permission before touching, and extra care is taken to respect culture and modesty. All procedures are explained in advance, in detail.

Some discussion is needed to explain what physiotherapy is, to clarify expectations, and identify methods of communication and practice that are culturally appropriate. Questions which mimic interrogation are avoided. Questions such as 'Was the damage here?' are more acceptable than 'What happened here?'

When working with interpreters, it is useful to arrange the chairs in a circle, to talk to the client rather than the interpreter, to avoid jargon, use only a few sentences, and if extra conversation is needed with the interpreter, to explain to the client what is being said. Debriefing sessions with the interpreter are helpful after the session.

During examination, we avoid coming up from behind the client, we avoid bright lights, and we allow them to stay fully clothed if preferred. Techniques to avoid include electrical treatment if they have suffered electric shocks, and water if they have been subjected to near-drowning. Grade five manipulation is seldom used because of the force and noise, and acupuncture rarely because it cannot be guaranteed to be painless. Mirrors should not be visible because many survivors find them disturbing, and traction couches are not used because most survivors have been tied down. Indeed, some find it difficult simply to lie down.

If there is doubt about a treatment technique, it is discussed in detail with the client, and sometimes demonstrated on a volunteer such as the ever-willing interpreter. Most women have been sexually tortured, and may tense up, sometimes barely perceptibly, if there is physical touch near the pelvis.

It is sometimes necessary to resist the need to 'do something' at all costs, when it might be more beneficial to listen, discuss, or simply allow the creative use of silence. 'Being' is often more important than 'doing'.

Once the impossible, the unspeakable, has happened, *nothing* is ever impossible again. Every creak upon the stair is an enemy (Sheila Cassidy, 1988).

Pain. Pain is often closely linked to PTSD. Pain can result from physical injury and/or somatic re-enactment and/or from an attempt to block out the experience of intense emotional pain by a form of 'holding on' to physical pain.

This last form of seemingly intractable pain has similarities to pathological grief reactions (Parkes and Weiss, 1983), which include the unresolved grief of some bereaved people, who fear that letting go of the grief would mean experiencing the loss. In torture survivors there may also be an element of expiation of guilt.

One way of working with this form of pain is to support clients in focusing on the pain rather than avoiding it, to 'breathe into the pain', identify the form it takes and explore what it means. Visualization can be used, clients being asked in imagination to touch, warm, nurture and massage the painful part, to describe its form, colour, texture, weight, taste and smell.

Clients can be asked to tune into their body, to find out what they are feeling: 'What do you think this pain is about? What form does your pain take? Speak as your pain, give it a voice.'Accompanying clients on this journey may assist them to find some meaning to their pain.

Talking about pain often changes it. Sometimes clients also feel able to express emotional pain, which may relieve their physical pain.

Hyperventilation syndrome. The association between breathing and emotion is recognized by the gasp of surprise, the sigh of relief, the disrupted breathing of laughing or crying, and the acute hyperventilation of stress. Chronic hyperventilation is less frequently recognized because sufferers are rarely breathless in an obvious way, and most symptoms are unrelated to breathing.

The hyperventilation syndrome (HVS) is a common response to stress in a society which has little appropriate outlet for the 'fight-or-flight' reaction, but it is notoriously underdiagnosed (Grossman and DeSwart, 1984). The diagnosis is also often missed in survivors of trauma, who have developed it as a useful adaptive response to help dissociation from pain. It is particularly common in survivors who have suffered suffocation or struggled at length to avoid screaming or speaking their friends' names. If HVS becomes established, instead of serving its original purpose it produces an array of alarming and sometimes disabling symptoms (Hough, 1991).

The pattern of HVS is illustrated by a vicious cycle in which hyperventilation, symptoms and anxiety reinforce each other (Figure 20.1). The pattern is maintained by the additional stresses of life for survivors, including loss of family, flight to an unknown country, coping with immigration and state agencies, loneliness, uncertainty, lack of the thread of continuity of life or a context for living. The pattern can be triggered by seemingly insignificant events such as being in an enclosed space or hearing an electrical gadget.

If HVS is identified, it is eminently treatable, with symptoms being abolished in 75% of cases (Lum, 1981). Clients can break out of the cycle by regaining control of their breathing. Physiotherapy can support them in this, but with sensitivity so that panic is not caused by the client feeling that something as personal as their breathing is being interfered with.

Treatment starts with preliminary discussion and explanation, then the client settles comfortably into half-lying or lying, with a pillow under the knees. Awareness of breathing is encouraged by suggesting that he or she visualize air passing down a tube from throat to abdomen.

Breathing cannot usually be re-educated in a stressed person, and a session of relaxation follows. A relaxed state should then be maintained throughout breathing re-education by bringing the client's attention to any areas of tension. Physiotherapists should ensure that they themselves are relaxed because a quiet breathing style is contagious. Relaxation occasionally exacerbates symptoms if letting down the wall of tension releases disturbing feelings. Beware the interpreter falling asleep during relaxation sessions!

Abdominal/diaphragmatic breathing is then taught, taking care to maintain small gentle breaths. Clients are guided towards reducing the rate and, if relevant, the depth, of breathing (Hough, 1991).

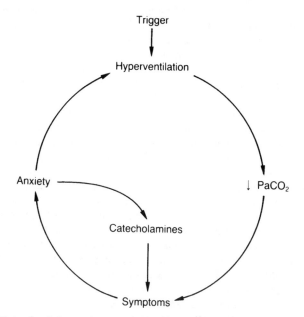

Figure 20.1 Vicious cycle into which people with hyperventilation syndrome become locked

If clients tense up, the emphasis should be on smooth, gentle rhythmic breathing, rather than focusing solely on low, slow breathing. They may need a reminder that slow breathing does not mean deep breathing.

The concept of control is important for people who hyperventilate, because it reduces anxiety and the sense of helplessness that is often a legacy of their experience of torture.

An hour is needed for each session, with regular appointments at the same time each week. This reliability helps to counteract the unpredictability that was fostered by their torturer to engender fear. After discharge, telephone contact is maintained for as long as necessary.

Conclusion. Physiotherapy may be needed for months, healing takes years, and the wound never closes completely. But, with support, the memory gradually becomes less intrusive by day, and nightmares take over less of the night. Survivors learn to trust, to form relationships and to pick up their lives again.

There is no formula for working with the tortured. We continue to refine our understanding of their needs, and we gain much from working with them as they seek to find a sense of creative endeavour in their lives.

My personal revenge will be your children's right to schooling and to flowers.
My personal revenge will be this song bursting for you with no more fears.
My personal revenge will be to offer these hands you once ill treated with all their tenderness intact.

[Thomas Borge, Nicaraguan Minister of the Interior, written in prison to his torturers]

Conclusion

Indicators of good prognosis are summarized by Choy and De Bosset (1992). These include healthy premorbid functioning, trauma of lesser magnitude and brief duration, adequate post-traumatic social support, absence of individual or family history of psychiatric disorder and the absence of medical and psychiatric co-morbidity. Other studies have mentioned early intervention (Sturgeon *et al.*, 1991; Yule, 1992). McFarlane (1989) reiterates the need for further research to target the most appropriate timing for a particular intervention, and also mentions the need for highly experienced therapists.

Although the DSM-III-R does not include the categories of acute and chronic PTSD, such differentiation has clinical utility. Acute disorders, in which symptoms either develop within up to 6 months, and last no longer than a further 6 months, usually have a better prognosis. With severe and prolonged stressors, more victims tend to develop chronic or delayed PTSD. In addition, depression, alcoholism, drug abuse and dependence frequently complicate or are associated with chronic course PTSD.

Despite the number of different forms of treatment available, and the lack of consensus as to which to employ in which particular case, the need for psychological help is overwhelmingly apparent. Gersons and Carlier (1992) state that emergency help in large-scale calamities, accidents at work and violence in the home should be available on request, with opportunity for a subsequent diagnosis of PTSD. They add that PTSD does not only stand for 'crisis' or something like it, but it is also an illness in the sense that it seriously hampers an individual's ability to function socially. As the studies quoted in this chapter indicate, this impairment of functioning ability can be apparent in all aspects of the person's life.

To conclude on a note of optimism, the following aims for the treatment of PTSD are suggested by Mejo (1990) and, if achieved, can go some way toward answering the agonized question, *'Why?'*:

Both client and clinician need to be able to think in terms of helping the client integrate the traumatic episode in such a way that the individual is able to see himself or herself as stronger, wiser and with a new value to his or her life.

References

Allinson, A.J. (1991) Post-traumatic stress disorder: a British perspective. *Medical Science and Law*, **31**, 264–270

Amnesty International Report (1993) AI Publications, London

APA (1952) *Diagnostic and Statistical Manual*, Vol. I, American Psychiatric Association, Washington DC

APA (1968) *Diagnostic and Statistical Manual*, Vol. II, American Psychiatric Association, Washington DC

APA (1980) *Diagnostic and Statistical Manual*, Vol. III, American Psychiatric Association, Washington DC

APA (1987) *Diagnostic and Statistical Manual*, Vol. III (Revised), American Psychiatric Association, Washington DC

Baggaley, M.R. and Rose, J. (1990) Post traumatic stress disorder. *British Journal of Psychiatry*, **156**, 910–911

Baum, A., Fleming, R. and Davidson, L.M. (1983) Natural disaster and technological catastrophe. *Environment and Behaviour*, **15**, 333–354

Beigel, A. and Berren, M.R. (1985) Human-induced disasters. *Psychiatric Annuals*, **15**, 143–150

Breslau, N., Davis, G.C. and Andreski, P. (1990) PTSD: risks for event exposure and syndrome, American Psychiatric Association, *New Research Program and Abstracts*, Abs NR 275, 151

British Library Medical Information Service (1991) Bibliography on treatment of psychological aspects of war 1986–1990. British Library Document Supply Centre, Boston Spa, West Yorkshire, UK

Burgess Watson, P. (1990) Post traumatic stress disorder. *British Journal of Psychiatry*, **156**, 1910–911

Burgess Watson, I.P., Hoffman, L. and Wilson, G.B. (1988) The neuropsychiatry of post-traumatic stress disorder. *British Journal of Psychiatry*, **152**, 164–173

Burstein, A. (1986) Treatment non-compliance in patients with post-traumatic stress disorder. *Psychosomatics*, **27**, 37–40.

Bustos, E. (1990) Dealing with the unbearable. In *Psychology and Torture* (ed. Suedfiedl, P.), Hemisphere, London

Cassidy, S. (1974) *Audacity to Believe*, Darton

Cassidy, S. (1988) *Sharing the Darkness*, Darton

Choy, T. and De Bosset, F. (1992) Post-traumatic stress disorder: an overview. *Canadian Journal of Psychiatry*, **37**, 578–583

Cook, J.D. and Bickman, L. (1990) Social support and psychological symptomatology following a natural disaster. Cited by Joseph, S., Yule, W., Williams, R. and Andrews, B. (1993) Crisis support in the aftermath of disaster: a longitudinal perspective. *British Journal of Clinical Psychology*, **32**, 177–185

Curran, P.S., Bell, P., Murray, A. *et al.* (1990) Psychological consequences of the Enniskillen bombing. *British Journal of Psychiatry*, **156**, 479–482

Daly, R.J. (1983) Samuel Pepys and post traumatic disorder. *British Journal of Psychiatry*, **143**, 64–68

Davidson, J. (1992) Drug therapy of post-traumatic stress disorder. *British Journal of Psychiatry*, **160**, 309–314

Davidson, J.R., Hughes, D., Blazer, D.G. and George, L.K. (1991) Post-traumatic stress disorder in the community: an epidemiological study. *Psychological Medicine*, **21**, 713–721

Davidson, J., Kudler, H. and Smith, R. (1990) Treatment of post-traumatic stress disorder with amitryptaline and placebo. *Archives of General Psychiatry*, **47**, 259–266

Davidson, J.R.T. and Smith, R.D. (1990) Traumatic experience in psychiatric outpatients. *Journal of Traumatic Stress*, **3**, 459–474

Deblinger, E., McLeer, S. and Henry, D. (1990) *Journal of the American Academy of Child and Adolscent Psychiatry*, **29**, 747–752

Donaldson, M.A. and Gardner, R. (1985) Diagnosis and treatment of traumatic stress among women after childhood incest. *Trauma and its Wake* (ed. Figley, C.R.), Brunner/Mazel, New York

Duckworth, D.H. (1991) Managing psychological trauma in the police service: from the Bradford Fire to the Hillsborough Crush. *Journal of Social and Occupational Medicine*, **41**, 171–173

Dyregrov, A. (1988) Critical incident stress debriefings. Unpublished manuscript. Research Center for Occupational Health and Safety, University of Bergen, Norway

Famularo, R., Kinscherff, R. and Fenton, T. (1990) Symptom differences in acute and chronic presentation of childhood post-traumatic stress disorder. *Child Abuse and Neglect*, **14**, 439–444

Famularo, R., Kinscherff, R. and Fenton, T. (1992) Psychiatric diagnoses of maltreated children: preliminary findings. *Journal of the American Academy of Child and Adolscent Psychiatry*, **31**, 863–867

Feinstein, A. and Dolan, R. (1991) Predictors of post-traumatic stress disorder following physical trauma: an examination of the stressor criterion. *Psychological Medicine*, **21**, 85–91

Fisher, S. and Reason, J. (1988) *Handbook of Life, Stress, Cognition and Health*, Wiley

Foa, E. (1992) Treatment of PTSD in civilian contexts. *British Journal of Clinical Psychology*, **31**, 505–506

Friedman, M.J. (1988) Toward rational pharmacotherapy for post-traumatic stress disorder: an interim report. *American Journal of Psychiatry*, **145**, 281–285

Garland, C. (1993) The lasting trauma of the concentration camps. *British Medical Journal*, **307**, 97–104

Gersons, B.P.R. and Carlier, V.E. (1992) Post-traumatic stress disorder: the history of the recent concept. *British Journal of Psychiatry*, **161**, 742–748

Graziano, R. (1992) Treating women incest survivors: a bridge between 'cumulative trauma' and 'post-traumatic stress'. *Social Work in Health Care*, **17**, 69–85

Green, B.L., Grace, M.C., Lindy, J.D. *et al.* (1990) Risk factors for PTSD and other diagnosis in a general sample of Vietnamese veterans. *American Journal of Psychiatry*, **146**, 729–733

Grossman, P. and DeSwart, J.C.G. (1984) Diagnosis of hyperventilation syndrome on the basis of reported complaints. *Journal of Psychosomatic Research*, **28**, 97–104

Helzer, J.E., Robins, L.N. and McEvoy, L. (1987) Post traumatic stress disorder in the general population. *New England Journal of Medicine*, **317**, 1630–1634

Hickling, E.J., Blanchard, E.B., Silverman, D.J. and Schwarz, S.P. (1992) Motor vehicle accidents, headaches and post-traumatic stress disorder: Assessment findings in a consecutive series. *Headache*, 147–151

Hinks, M. (1991) Post-traumatic stress: you'll never walk alone. *Nursing Times*, **87**, 34–35

Horowitz, M.J., Weiss, D.S. and Marmer, C. (1987) Diagnosis of post-traumatic stress disorder. *Journal of Nervous and Mental Disease*, **175**, 267–268

Horowitz, M.J., Wilner, N. and Alvarez, W. (1979) Impact of event scale: a measure of subjective stress. *Psychosomatic Medicine*, **41**, 209–218

Hough, A. (1991) *Physiotherapy in Respiratory Care – a Problem-Solving Approach*, Chapman and Hall, London

Iljon Foreman, E. (1991) Planning disaster response services: the role of a multi-agency steering group. *British Journal of Guidance and Counselling*, **19**, 23–30

Jacobsen, L. and Vesti, P. (1990) *Torture Survivors – A New Group of Patients*, Danish Nurses Organisation, Copenhagen

Joseph, S., Yule, W., Williams, R. and Andrews, B. (1993) Crisis support in the aftermath of disaster: a longitudinal perspective. *British Journal of Clinical Psychology*, **32**, 177–185

Kaplan, P.M. (1989) Post-traumatic stress syndrome and sexual dysfunction. *Journal of Sex and Marital Therapy*, **15**

Kaplan, Z., Singer, Y., Lichtenberg, M.D., Solomon, Z. and Bleich, A. (1992) Post-traumatic stress disorders in Israel during the Gulf War. *Israeli Journal of Psychiatry and Related Science*, **29**, 14–21

Kinchin, D. (1993) High risk PTSD candidates. *Counselling Psychology Review*, **8**, 24–26

Kinzie, J.D. (1989) Post-traumatic stress disorder. In *Comprehensive Textbook of Psychiatry*, 5th edn (eds Kaplan, H.I. and Sadock, B.J.), Williams and Wilkins, Baltimore

Kinzie, D.J., Boehnein, J.K. and Leung, P.K. (1990) The prevalence of post-traumatic stress disorder and its clinical significance among South East Asian refugees. *American Journal of Psychiatry*, **147**, 913–917

Kolb, L. (1989) Editorial in *Psychological Medicine*, **19**, 821–824

Levine, S. (1988) *Who Dies?* Gateway, Bath, UK

Lim, L.C.C. (1991) Delayed emergence of post-traumatic stress disorder. *Singapore Medical Journal*, **32**, 92–93

Lindemann, E. (1944) Symptomatology and management of acute grief. *American Journal of Psychiatry*, **101**, 141–148

Lindy, J.D., Green, B.L. and Grace, M. (1992) Somatic reenactment in the treatment of post-traumatic stress disorder. *Psychotherapy and Psychomatics*, **57**, 180–186

Loughrey, G.C., Bell, P., Kee, M., Roddy, R.J. and Curran, P.S. (1988) Post-traumatic stress disorder and civil violence in Northern Ireland. *British Journal of Psychiatry*, **153**, 554–560

Lovell, K. (1991) Post-traumatic stress management. *Nursing Standard*, **6**, 30–31

Lum, L.C. (1981) Hyperventilation and anxiety state. *Journal of the Royal Society of Medicine*, **74**, 1–4

McFarlane, A.C. (1988) Relationship between psychiatric impairment and a natural disaster: the role of distress. *Psychological Medicine*, **18**, 129–139

McFarlane, A.C. (1989) The treatment of post-traumatic stress disorder. *British Journal of Medical Psychology*, **62**, 81–90

McLeer, S.V., Deblinger, E., Atkins, M., Foa, E. and Ralphe, D. (1988) Post-traumatic stress disorder in sexually abused children: a prospective study. *Journal of the American Academy of Child and Adolescent Psychiatry*, **27**, 650–654

McMillan, M. (1991) Post-traumatic stress disorder and severe head injury. *British Journal of Psychiatry*, **159**, 431–433

March, J.S. (1990) The nosology of post-traumatic stress disorder. *Journal of Anxiety Disorders*, **4**, 61–82

Mejo, S.L. (1990) Post-traumatic stress disorder: an overview of three etiological variables, and psychopharmacologic treatment. *Nurse Practitioner*, **15**, 41–45

Miller, T.W., Kamenchenko, P. and Krasniasnki, A. (1992) Assessment of life stress events: the etiology and measurement of traumatic stress disorder. *International Journal of Social Psychiatry*, **38**, 215–227

Miller, T.W. (1989) *Stressful Life Events*, International Universities Press, Madison, Connecticut

Murray, R. and Huelskotter, M. (1987) *Psychiatric/Mental Health Nursing: Giving Emotional Support*, 2nd edn, Appleton and Lange, Norwalk, Connecticut

Niles, D.P. (1991) War trauma and post-traumatic stress disorder. *American Family Physician*, **44**, 1663–1669

North, D. and Smith, E.M. (1990) Post-traumatic stress disorder in disaster survivors. *Comprehensive Therapy*, **16**, 3–9

O'Brien, L.S. and Hughes, S.J. (1991) Symptoms of post-traumatic stress disorder in Falklands veterans five years after the conflict. *British Journal of Psychiatry*, **159**, 135–141

Parkes, C.M. (1972) *Bereavement: Studies of Grief in Adult Life*, Tavistock, London

Parkes, C.M. and Weiss, R. (1983) *Recovery from Bereavement*, Basic Books

Patterson, D.R., Carrigan, L., Kent, A., Questad, K.A. and Robinson, R.S. (1990) Post-traumatic stress disorder in hospitalised patients with burn injuries. *Journal of Burn Care and Rehabilitation*, **11**, 181–184

Perry, S.W., Cella, D.F. and Falkenburg, J. (1987) Cited by Patterson, D.R., Carrigan, L., Kent, A., Questad, K.A. and Robinson, R.S. Post-traumatic stress disorder in hospitalised patients with burn injuries. *Journal of Burn Care and Rehabilitation*, **11**, 181–184

Petit, M. (1991) Nursing the mind: recognising post-traumatic stress. RN 56–58

Ramsay, R. (1990) Invited review: post-traumatic stress disorders; a new clinical entity? *Journal of Psychosomatic Research*, **34**, 355–365

Richards, D.A. and Rose, J.S. (1991) Exposure therapy for post-traumatic stress disorder. *British Journal of Psychiatry*, **158**, 836–840

Rose, J. and Richards, D. (1991) Post-traumatic stress: healing the mind. *Nursing Times*, **87**, 40–42

Roth, W.T. (1988) The role of medication in post-traumatic stress therapy. In *Post-Traumatic Therapy and Victims of Violence*, Brunner/Mazel, New York

Scurfield, R.M. (1985) Post-trauma stress assessment and treatment: overview and formulations. In *Trauma and its Wake* (ed. Figley, C.R.), Brunner/Mazel, New York

Skylv, G., Block, I., Hohne, L. *et al.* (1990) Muscle tension and articular dysfunction in torture victims. *Journal of Manual Medicine*, **5**, 158–161

Solomon, Z., Bleich, A., Koslowsky, M., Kron, S., Lerer, B and Waysman, M. (1991) Post-traumatic stress disorder: issues of co-morbidity. *Journal of Psychiatric Research*, **25**, 89–94

Solomon, Z. and Flum, H. (1988) Life events, combat stress reaction and post-traumatic stress disorder. *Social Science and Medicine*, **26**, 319–325

Solomon, Z., Mikulincer, M. and Flum, H. (1989) The implications of life events and social integration in the course of combat related post-traumatic stress disorder. *Social Psychiatry and Psychiatric Epidemiology*, **24**, 41–48

Solursh, L.P. (1989) Combat addiction: overview of implications in symptom maintenance and treatment planning. *Journal of Traumatic Stress*, **2**, 451–462

Spragg, G.S. (1992) Post-traumatic stress disorder. *Medical Journal of Australia*, **156**, 731–733

Sturgeon, D., Rosser, R. and Shoenberg, P. (1991) The King's Cross Fire. Part 2: the psychological injuries. *Burns*, **17**, 10–13

Task Force of the American Psychiatric Association (1989) *Treatments of Psychiatric Disorders*, Vol. 3, American Psychiatric Association, Washington DC

Terr, L.C. (1981). Psychic trauma in children: observations following the Chowchilla school-bus kidnapping. *American Journal of Psychiatry*, **138**, 14–19

Thompson, C. (1989) PTSD. *Psychiatry in Practice*, Summer, 17–21

Thompson, J. (1992) Stress theory and therapeutic practice. *Stress Medicine*, **8**, 147–150

Thompson, J. and Solomon, M. Police body recovery teams at disasters: trauma or challenge? *Anxiety Research* (in press)

Toomey, T.C., Hernandez, J.H., Gittelman, D.F. *et al.* (1993) Relationship of sexual and physical abuse to pain and psychological assessment variables in chronic pelvic pain patients. *Pain*, **53**, 105–109

Treishman, R.B. (1980) *Spinal Cord Injuries: Psychological, Social and Vocational Adjustment*. Pergamon Press, New York

Turchin, S.J., Holmes, V. and Wasserman, C.S. (1992) Do tricyclic antidepressants have a protective effect.in post-traumatic stress disorder? *New York State Journal of Medicine*, **92**, 400–402

Turner, S. and Gorst-Unsworth, C. (1990) Psychological sequelae of torture. *British Journal of Psychiatry*, **157**, 476–480

Turner, S.W., Thompson, J.A. and Rosser, R.A. (1989) The King's Cross fire: planning a phase two psychological response. *Disaster Management*, **1**, 31–37

Vaughan, K. and Tarrier, N. (1992) The use of image habituation training with post-traumatic stress disorders. *British Journal of Psychiatry*, **161**, 658–664

Watson, C., Kucala, J., Manifold, V. and Vasser, P. (1991) Childhood stress disorder behaviour in veterans who do not develop PTSD. *Journal of Nervous and Mental Diseases*, **177**, 92–95

Yule, W. (1992) Post-traumatic stress disorder in child survivors of shipping disasters: the sinking of the 'Jupiter'. *Psychotherapy and Psychosomatic Medicine*, **57**, 200–205

Yule, W. and Udwin, O. (1991) Screening childhood survivors for post-traumatic stress disorders: experiences from the 'Jupiter' sinking. *British Journal of Clinical Psychology*, **30**, 131–138

21

Forensic psychiatry

A. Behavioural science in forensic psychiatry

Geoff Barry

Introduction

One of the more recent innovations in the field of forensic psychiatry is the application of behavioural analysis and cognitive problem-solving strategies for interventions with aggressive behaviour. At the present time, on a national level there appear to be no readily available statistics relating to the prevalence of in-patient violence in psychiatric institutions. Although a number of organizations and individuals have expressed concern regarding what they perceive to be a rising tide of assaults on mental health workers, the statistical evidence pointing to this phenomenon being a widespread problem is somewhat lacking (Drinkwater and Gudjonsson, 1989). This is not to say that such a situation does not exist, but for whatever reason, no national information system seems to have been established to monitor the problem.

Most professionals working in the speciality of forensic psychiatry will, at some time in their working lives, either be confronted by, or witness, the consequences of aggression and violence. With this in mind, it has become increasingly important in recent years to develop techniques for helping clients who have problems with violent behaviour. The most promising models have evolved from the fields of social learning theory and cognitive-behavioural therapy and have come to be known as 'anger management'.

When discussing anger, the terms 'aggression' and 'violence' are invariably used to express the social consequences of that emotion. Aggression itself may be seen to take two distinct forms: 'instrumental' aggression is carried out in order to achieve a particular aim, such as using violence in a robbery; 'hostile' aggression differs in that the consequence is not goal-orientated, and the intent is simply to inflict injury to the victim (Buss, 1961).

In this chapter, a model will be proposed for assessment and psychological interventions that are currently under development in order to deal with this problem. The main aim of such a treatment is to help an individual with a propensity for violent responses to develop their behavioural repertoire, so that other non-violent, socially acceptable strategies may be used. Within the confines of this chapter, an exhaustive overview of the concepts and methods relating to dealing with aggression and violence will not be possible.

The emphasis will be on providing background information and practical steps that the reader may take to help clients displaying violent behaviours develop a degree of control over their problem.

Brief overview

The theories that underpin anger and aggression may be seen to reflect the beliefs of three different psychological schools – the psychoanalytic view, the drive theory and the social learning theory.

The psychoanalytic view
Freud proposed that the human psyche consists of two opposing forces, the life force and the death instinct. The life force attempts to displace any excessive psychic energy by directing it outside the body, whilst the death instinct turned such forces inward on the individual themselves (Kutash, 1978). In this analysis, aggression is seen to reside within the individual, i.e. each person has a potential for harm, either to themselves or others. Therefore, it followed that there existed the *aggressive personality*.

The drive theory
Here the concept is slightly different, as internal 'drives' or motivators were believed to be mediated to some degree by learned experience. This particular model became highly developed, reaching its theoretical peak with the work of Berkowitz (1974). However, over time the explanations advanced by this paradigm began to be called into question.

Social learning theory
More recently, it has become accepted that the model of aggression put forward by Bandura (1973) possibly holds the key not only to an empirical analysis of aggressive behaviour, but also practical solutions to deal with these problems.

The social learning model does not deny the fact that people may be born with specific genetic traits. For example, we may inherit our blue eyes from our mother, but we may also inherit particular behavioural predispositions, as pointed out by Skinner (1974) when he discusses 'behavioural imprinting'.

Most importantly, however, Bandura looks at how aggression is a behaviour that can be acquired through learning; this then forms part of the behavioural repertoire of the individual which may be evoked within appropriate situations. This may then be maintained by the consequences of the action, i.e. did the person get what she/he wanted by using this strategy?

An integrated approach

In this field of 'anger management', the work of Novaco (1976) has been out-standing in providing an integrated approach to assessment and intervention. Due to the extremely comprehensive nature of his work, the model is rather complex, taking into account, as it does, a multiplicity of factors which serve as triggers and possible responses which may have an effect on the client and their environment.

Anger and aggression within a social context

If anger is assumed to be a dispositional trait, it is highly unlikely that any therapeutic intervention will be able to help an individual control their violent actions. But over recent years, questions have been asked about what actually constitutes anger: When are we most likely to *feel* angry? Can you remember the last time you became angry? Did the feeling occur totally out of the blue, with no precipitating factors?

The chances are that the anger was provoked in some way, perhaps being caught in a traffic jam when you are in a rush, or somebody insulting you or a member of your family. If we can accept this scenario, then in effect what we are saying is that anger is an emotional response; we are reacting to situations that affect us or our loved ones. If we receive good news, our emotional response is happiness, but bad news may elicit sadness. This may seem simplistic, but it is vital to place anger into the realm of emotional responses. As such, it is then like any other response, amenable to modification.

Over recent years, a great deal of work has been done using psychological treatments for one of the most debilitating of emotional responses – depression. The most promising of these psychotherapeutic approaches is termed cognitive–behavioural therapy. In this field, the work of Beck (1976), particularly, has shown that depression can be alleviated through the use of specific therapeutic techniques.

Anger management is a subject under rapid development, with strong empirically based clinical techniques. What follows consitutes a practical approach, albeit somewhat 'stripped down', that is eminently suitable for use in clinical practice.

Engagement of the client

When initially interviewing the client, the need to establish a collaborative approach cannot be overemphasized. The therapist must show the client that he is not there to 'take away the anger'. Rather it should be acknowledged that anger is a normal human emotion and as such the client is his/her own expert on their own anger.

It may be helpful at this stage to review with the client how exactly aggression has been helpful to them in the past and also how it may have been detrimental. For example: Have they ever been arrested for assault? Have relationships they may have valued broken down because of their violent behaviour?

Possibly violence may be an integral part of the client's livelihood (they may work as a doorman or 'bouncer'), but is the aggression spilling over into their personal lives?

Try to set the scene that this is quite simply a specific problem the client has, and just like any problem, solutions can be found.

Assessment of the problem

A number of psychometric tests are available for the measurement of hostility and aggression. It is not within the scope of this text to enter into a critical account of these tests. For a detailed handbook containing such assessment tools, see Brodsky and Smitherman (1983).

However, if we examine the problem as it directly relates to the client, it may be more appropriate to use a behavioural analysis, as its simplicity and immediacy encourage the client to adopt this technique as a way of evaluating situations for themselves.

Here, the details of the behaviour, along with the accompanying thoughts and feelings, are detailed and broken down into their components. For example, a client may say that he 'felt angry and clobbered the "jerk"'. Although this is descriptive, it gives us no information. Ask the client if they would mind if you broke down this statement into specific points:

(a) Felt angry?
What were the physical feelings?
Did their heart rate increase?
Was their mouth dry?
Were their muscles tense, if so which ones?

What were the thoughts going through their mind?
Did the thoughts say 'She/he's winding me up. ...'
Did the thoughts say 'She/he deserves this. ...'
Did the thoughts say 'I'm going to kill them. ...'

How were they feeling emotionally?
Did they feel happy at the prospect of hitting someone?
Did they feel sad at the prospect of hitting someone?

Ask the client to be as specific as possible, in particular when examining the physical sensations and the thoughts going through their mind.

(b) Clobbered?
Did they use their fists?
Did they head-butt the person?
Did they use their feet?
How many blows were struck?
Did they know that person?
Had that person been insulting them or their loved ones?
What had that person specifically said which had upset them?
Did they believe that person was staring at them?
What harm did they feel that person could seriously inflict on them?

At this point, it may be useful to either note down yourself or ask the client to complete an A:B:C form. This will form the basis of a behavioural analysis which is essential if we are to help the client come to some sort of understanding of the problem. It stands for *A*ntecedents, which are the conditions that precede the violent response, the *B*ehaviour and underlying beliefs, and the *C*onsequences of that behaviour.

The information relating to where and when the violence occurred is written in the first column, including whether or not the client was under the influence of drugs and/or alcohol. What the client actually did, along with what they were thinking and how they were feeling at that time, should be entered in column 'B'. The direct consequences of the violence should be written in column 'C'. Figure 21.1 shows a completed form.

Along with the antecedents, the consequences of the violence must be reviewed with the client. If, because of a violent response, the client were to be arrested, it may be useful to ask outright, 'Was that what you wanted?'. It would be unusual for the client to reply that they did indeed want to be arrested, but

DATE. TIME AND PLACE	WHAT HAPPENED IMMEDIATELY BEFORE THE BEHAVIOUR OCCURRED? 'A'	WHAT ACTUALLY HAPPENED? 'B'	WHAT HAPPENED IMMEDIATELY AFTER THE BEHAVIOUR OCCURRED? 'C'
21/7/92 10-30 p.m. Pub.	Talking to a bloke, saw him looking at my girlfriend I'd drunk about six pints by then.	Felt my heart rate go up. Butterflies in my stomach. Thought — "You can't trust anyone" Felt stupid 'cos I'd been friendly to him.	Police came, I was arrested. That was the last time I saw my girlfriend — she jilted me.

Figure 21.1 An ABC behavioural analysis form

the possibility of such a reply should be borne in mind. More likely would be that they had simply wanted to respond to a situation that they perceived to be threatening or demeaning.

Other ways of reacting to that situation should now be examined. Clients may be asked to think of situations where they had achieved their goals by the use of different strategies, for example negotiating with someone, or walking away from a conflict. Again, this can be written down within an ABC format. Figure 21.2 shows a breakdown of a positive strategy.

Feedback to the client should be couched in positive terms, e.g.: 'You did really well because you must have felt really wound up and angry?' or 'How on earth were you able to control your temper like that, and at the same time get your point across?' The client's answers to these questions can form the basis for developing and enhancing the strategies they may already be using to control the aggressive outbursts.

It may be that the client has already identified that their beliefs and thoughts about the situation are misleading, e.g.: 'I thought at first that he was trying to wind me up, but then I said to myself "Whoa a minute, he's just a little cog in a big machine, he's only trying to do his job".' By giving social praise when the client relates this type of positive response, one not only makes the person more confident about using such a behaviour again, but it may also help the person to

DATE. TIME AND PLACE	WHAT HAPPENED IMMEDIATELY BEFORE THE BEHAVIOUR OCCURRED? 'A'	WHAT ACTUALLY HAPPENED? 'B'	WHAT HAPPENED IMMEDIATELY AFTER THE BEHAVIOUR OCCURRED? 'C'
13/8/92 2 pm. Post Office	Feeling a bit nervous and shaky as I hadn't had a drink. Tried to cash my giro. Postmistress kept saying I had to produce proof of identity.	I didn't have any I. D. on me, and I couldn't get a bus home 'cos I didn't have any money. I started to feel angry, but I explained the problem to her.	She gave me my money !

Figure 21.2 An ABC positive strategy form

realize that they are not 'bad', that they are capable of 'good' as well as 'bad' behaviour.

This technique is termed coping strategy enhancement, and is a powerful tool as it enhances behaviours that the client already possesses. It is also extremely personal to the individual, so that person has a greater sense of 'owning' the solution to the problem, which should serve to further increase the likelihood of that strategy being used in the future.

Relaxation

The vast majority of clients with aggression problems report feelings of anxiety and agitation, particularly in the stages building up to aggressive responses. In these cases it may be helpful to train the client in relaxation techniques such as Jacobsen's progressive muscular relaxation. Unfortunately, this type of exercise requires a good deal of practice as well as motiviation on the part of the client.

Another problem is one of 'temporal contiguity', i.e. the antecedents and the behaviour itself may occur within a very short space of time. The client may literally have only seconds in which to recognize the danger signals and formulate a more appropriate response. In this situation, the relaxation technique is of paramount importance, as the ability of the client to react quickly and effectively will decide upon the outcome of events.

One of the more interesting innovations in the field of stress management, is the application of the Valsalva manoeuvre to panic attacks (Sartory and Olajide, 1988). This technique consists of exerting pressure on the sternum which is believed to stimulate baroreceptors which lower the heart rate. As the authors point out, similar results to Valsalva and progressive muscular relaxation can be achieved by simply applying pressure to the closed eyelid during expiration.

A simple training package, therefore, of deep breathing and self-massage of the closed eyelid appears to be one of the quickest and simplest techniques that may be taught to people who are by definition impulsive and quick to arouse. Although as yet there have been no empirical studies carried out with this intervention, the author's clinical reports from clients seem to indicate that it is a worthwhile strategy in need of further investigation.

Development of subsequent sessions

Once the antecedents and consequences have been identified with the client, subsequent sessions may take the form of homework tasks which the individual can undertake with a reasonable chance of success. For example, it would be unrealistic to ask someone to go back to the pub where they had been involved in a fight and apologise to all concerned (although it has happened!).

Realistically, they should be asked to use the positive strategies that they themselves have identified as being of benefit in controlled situations, such as in a shop when returning faulty goods, or in a benefit office when inquiring about allowances. This involves the client in setting their own achievable goals which have a proven track record of working for them *as an individual.*

Each homework assignment may then be evaluated at the next session, and problems identified and possible solutions generated in a collaborative relationship between therapist and client. Sessions will be seen to build on previous work, almost in the way of a 'stepping stones' approach.

Clients should be told quite explicitly that progress may not always be rapid or smooth, and there may be occasional 'hiccups'. But even the smallest of changes or improvement should be seized upon and discussed with the client. In this way it can be demonstrated that change is possible, and non-violent behaviours can be equally or more effective than violent solutions to problems.

Conclusion

In many circles, individuals who display aggressive behaviours are perhaps not seen as the most rewarding client group with which to work. But the problems they face in their everyday lives are equal to the problems faced by other clients with affective disorders such as mania and depression. In terms of social debilitation, they are certainly on a par with a major mental illness such as schizophrenia.

Helping this client group in controlling their potential to violence should be seen not only as a way of intervening therapeutically for the sake of one individual, but also as a way of helping the client's family and friends understand why that person behaves in that particular way. This can only be achieved by getting rid of the idea of the 'aggressive personality', which assigns the aggression to the person; rather, we should come to terms with how we may help a client control 'violent behaviours', which simply make up one facet of that person's individuality.

References

Bandura, A. (1973) *Aggression: A Social Learning Analysis*, Prentice-Hall, Englewood Cliffs, New Jersey

Beck, A.T. (1976) *Cognitive Therapy and the Emotional Disorders*, International Universities Press, New York

Berkowitz, L. (1974) Some determinants of impulsive aggression: role of mediated associations with reinforcement for aggression. Psychological Review, **81**

Brodsky, S.L. and Smitherman, H.O. (1983) *Handbook of Scales for Research in Crime and Delinquency*, Plenum, New York

Buss, A. (1961) *The Psychology of Aggression,* Wiley, New York

Drinkwater, J. and Gudjonsson, G.H. (1989) The nature of violence in psychiatric hospitals. In *Clinical Approaches to Violence* (eds Howells, K. and Hollin, C.R.) Wiley, Chichester, UK

Kutash, S.B. (1978) Psychoanalytic theories of aggression. In *Violence: Perspectives on Murder and Aggression* (eds Kutash, I.L., Kutash, S.B. and Schlesinger, L.B.), Jossey-Bass, San Francisco

Novaco, R.W. (1976) The functions and regulation of the arousal of anger. *American Journal of Psychiatry, 133,,* 1124–1128

Sartory, G. and Olajide, D. (1988) Vagal innervation techniques in the treatment of panic disorder. *Behavior Research and Therapy, 26*(5), 431–434

Skinner, B.F. (1974) *About Behaviourism,* Jonathan Cape, London

B. Physiotherapy in forensic psychiatry

Jan Fletcher

Forensic psychiatry is concerned with the assessment, diagnosis and treatment of patients whose behaviour, due to mental illness, has brought them, or is likely to bring them, into conflict with the law.

The forensic psychiatry multidisciplinary team

The greater part of this work takes place in a 'forensic' setting, principally a regional secure unit or a secure ward, where the physiotherapist will work within a forensic psychiatry team.

Approaches vary, as each team evolves its own philosophy of care. It is important that the philosophy is shared by all the team members and that the individual member has a clear idea of his role within the team.

Patient assessment

Assessment is ongoing throughout the patient's stay under the team's care. All members of the team have a share in the process. Assessment is primarily of the patient's mental illness, their potential to harm and of their appropriate placement, i.e. the level of security required for their treatment and rehabilitation.

Dangerousness
The Butler Committee (1975) defined dangerousness as 'a propensity to cause serious physical injury or lasting psychological harm'. 'Dangerousness' can refer to dangerousness in a particular situation or a particular state of mind.

The team is therefore continuously observing the patient's behaviour, responses, attitudes and mental state, noting where these are inappropriate or giving cause for concern.

The team, principally the consultant responsible for the patient's care, social worker and psychologist, may be required to write assessment reports for the courts, Home Office and other psychiatry teams. Ideally, they will do this after a team discussion, where all members of the team have the opportunity to report behaviours observed, both on the ward and during therapy time.

Rehabilitation
Patients are placed with the team after an appearance in court, and when transferred from a special hospital. The team's ultimate aim is the rehabilitation of the patients back into the community.

Physiotherapy

The role of the physiotherapist in forensic psychiatry is developing. The physio-therapist is able to contribute to the assessment, treatment and rehabilitation of the patient through physical means in the following ways:

- traditional physiotherapy treatments, e.g. for pain relief, trauma, rehabilitation, etc.
- exercise and sport therapy
- community activities
- anxiety management.

Traditional physiotherapy

As in any other population, psychiatric patients can injure themselves. In addition, some injuries may arise through acting out behaviour or as a result of exercise or sport activity on the unit. Other injuries may predate admission. Treatment in the physiotherapy department may be appropriate, but it must be carried out by a physiotherapist aware of the 'difficulties' of this patient group. In many cases where there is a restriction upon the patient's movements, treatment in the ward environment is the only option.

Exercise and sport therapy

The Butler Committee (1974), in their Interim Report, stated that 'It is our intention that the secure units should be therapeutically orientated, and have the use of workshops and adequate recreational areas'.

The physiotherapist, with knowledge of exercise physiology and injury avoidance, is able to ensure a safe choice of recreational activities that serve a therapeutic purpose as well as being of an exercise or sporting nature. The physiotherapist will also be able to deal with any injuries which may occur.

These exercise and sport activities will form part of a larger patient programme where much of the physiotherapist's time will be spent. The need for safety determines that there should be high staffing levels. Because of this, group work is a more economical use of staff resources. It has many advantages, as it allows several patients and an appropriate number of staff to participate at the same time. This can allow for the assessment, and promotion, of appropriate interactions with other patients and members of staff. Communication, social skills and behaviour can be observed. If necessary, one or two members of the group may be given one-on-one attention, either for observational purposes or to facilitate their participation in the activity.

Resource/facilities
Just what can be offered to this patient group will largely depend on the resources available. The following have been found useful:

- a gym area large enough to play five-a-side games as well as incorporating a full-size badminton court
- an additional area for multi-gym and fitness equipment
- an outdoor recreational area with an appropriate level of security.

The siting of facilities requires forethought regarding the level of security needed. Greater use can be made of facilities if they are open to patients who have no parole.

Patients living within a locked environment, whose movement is subject to restriction, will benefit from the opportunity to exercise and maintain fitness levels. This patient group tend to be heavy smokers and often do not have acceptable levels of fitness.

Activities often work best away from the ward, especially in the outdoors, allowing the patients to break from possible ward tensions. Volleyball or rounders in the ward garden can prove to be very popular. Conversely, activities on the ward can draw in patients who have resisted or declined group attendance.

Equipment can be used as a potential weapon or to inflict self-harm and should therefore be checked back in at the end of a session and kept locked away when not in use. The physiotherapist is advised to have a written policy and guidelines on the use of the equipment to ensure that safety and security are not compromised at any time.

Many units have chosen to use multi-gyms rather than free weights, in an attempt to minimize the potential for harm to individuals or property. Where a multi-gym is in use, it is essential to adopt the system of introductory training sessions, used by many sports centres, before allowing the use of the equipment without the supervision of the physiotherapist. During these introductory sessions, the patient's programme of exercises can be drawn up and recorded. At each subsequent attendance the record sheet should be completed, allowing for monitoring of the patient's progress and any inappropriate use of the equipment.

Staff should be made aware of the safety aspects of using the equipment, and a policy should be devised to ensure all possible prevention of injury and equipment misuse in the physiotherapist's absence.

Exercise and sport activities
These divide into activities which are either more individualistic or which require interaction with others. The majority of forensic patients are male and are aged between 20 and 35. The activity has to interest them. Therefore, identifiable sports may be more acceptable than exercise groups. The small number of female patients will possibly prefer an exercise group. It may be appropriate, where numbers are very small and parole allows, for the women to join a women's group in a general psychiatry setting. They may, however, choose to join in with the men's exercise groups.

Assessment and early rehabilitation stage

On admission. Experience has shown that it is important to allow a patient time to settle into the new environment before beginning to engage in programme activities For some, the gym may be one of the first activities in which they become involved in. This is often on an individual basis, because it can offer an activity which places for mental demands on the patient. The gym may be used in order to begin to engage the patient in exercise and sport activities, paving the way for group participation later.

Aggression and anxiety. A patient may have difficulty in controlling feelings of aggression, anxiety and frustration with the new restricted environment. These may lead to some form of acting-out behaviour. In these circumstances, exercise can be used constructively to channel release of those feelings in an acceptable and positive way. Nursing staff may find it helpful to move a patient to the gym area where they can use a punchball, the multi-gym or do free exercises to ventilate such feelings.

It is important that all staff who make use of the physiotherapy resources in this way are instructed in the safe use of the equipment and of exercise with the patients. Wherever possible, the physiotherapist should be involved in the prior assessment and development of a programme of exercises that can be adhered to in her absence.

Research has demonstrated a relationship between exercise and a reduction in anxiety levels, particularly in the reduction of situational, transitory anxiety which is generally a response to an event or stimulus, (Disham, 1985) and in the somatic symptoms of anxiety in psychotic subjects (Hannaford et al., 1988). Exercise, therefore, offers a practical coping strategy in the treatment of anxiety and some patients will find this approach more acceptable to other forms of treatment, especially in the early stage of admission. Aggression, frustration and anxiety are often interlinked in this patient group, so it could be hypothesized that an activity which has anti-anxiety effects will also influence aggression levels.

Assessment/rehabilitation aims
The following aims are associated both with assessment and with rehabilitation. This is not a definitive list.

1. The provision of a structure and set of rules within which to participate. It may be appropriate to modify the rules of a game to ensure that the game has some structure, but not to have so many that the game is constantly interrupted and hence the patients lose interest. Team games are useful for observing an individual's ability to cope with boundary setting. An inability to grasp the rules may indicate a learning difficulty or area of brain damage.
2. To provide a means of assessing and improving fitness in a confined environment. Lack of fitness is particularly noticeable following transfer from prison where prisoners may spend 23 out of every 24 hours in a cell.
3. To assess and encourage social interaction through team work, developing communication skills.
4. To assess and develop a rapport between patients and staff. This works well where staff join in, acting as role models, and where they are working with the patients towards a common aim i.e. to win! Competitive reactions can also be a very useful assessment tool. Staff who appear disinterested or expect a greater level of participation and behaviour than they themselves are demonstrating, can be disruptive to the group.
5. To assess and promote cohesion and integration of group members. Taking part for the first time can noticeably lead to the patient's acceptance by the others.
6. To facilitate the breaking down of barriers through acceptable physical contact. Physical contact is inevitable when participating in some sports, and

this form of touch is often less threatening and more acceptable to this patient group.

7. To assess and enhance self-esteem through achievement, the learning of new skills and the improvement of skills and fitness. Self-esteem may also be influenced by a positive change in body image and the sense of well-being that accompanies improvement in physical fitness.

8. To assess and encourage the development of appropriate assertion skills. Patients can be allowed a degree of choice regarding the activity or sport undertaken, while the physiotherapist facilitates negotiation between group members.

9. To assess a patient's mental state during the activity, noting, for example, preoccupation, odd behaviours and aggression levels.

10. To improve mental health through participation in regular aerobic exercise. Research suggests that exercise, particularly aerobic exercise, has positive effects on anxiety, depression and level of self-esteem (Glesser and Mendelberg, 1990). It should be noted that the exercise would have to be undertaken on a regular basis to obtain the desired effects.

11. To assess and encourage individual motivation. The programme provides a clearly defined routine and structure which is often an absent feature in the patients' lives.

Individual activities, such as weight training, fitness work and circuit training, can be used to assess and encourage individual motivation. This can be in the form of just a few minutes on various pieces of equipment for example the bicycle or multi-gym, or the use of a planned progressive programme of exercises. It is useful to devise a programme and encourage patients to take responsibility for recording their own activities and progression. Simple forms of fitness testing may act as an added incentive.

Late stage rehabilitation
Groups tend to be smaller, as patients spend more time away from the unit, pursuing activities in preparation for life beyond the unit. However, groups are still important. Sports requiring lower numbers, such as tennis, badminton and bowls, can be more practical with smaller numbers of patients. By this stage, more autonomy can be allowed and patients should be encouraged to make constructive use of their leisure time. Security issues may limit this, but where possible be flexible. For example, patients can be given access to a facility that does not need direct supervision, where they just need to ask for the equipment.

Community activities

Some suggestions for community activities, where possible making use of local leisure centre facilities, include:

- swimming
- badminton
- weight training
- squash
- cycling
- walks
- horse riding

- ten-pin bowling
- ice skating
- roller skating

Find out what is available and what is affordable and be inventive. Encourage walking to the cinema or theatre, or cycling when on parole – it is cheaper than using public transport! Encourage patients to make use of special rates for the unemployed, obtaining passes, etc., as they may then go on to use them on discharge.

Assessment

Activities, with minimal supervision, can be a useful way of assessing a patient's ability to cope in the community. Areas of difficulty may be highlighted, such as dealing with money, people in authority, frustration and strangers. These trips out can be very revealing, as they expand the patient's experience. Removal from the ward environment can result in the disclosure of fears and in exposure to previously tempting situations.

Rehabilitation

Community activities provide an opportunity to develop social skills further by introducing the patient to new people and situations. The therapist's aim should be to normalize these activities.

Choice of activity must take into account the possible difficulties which may arise. It is preferable, where possible, to involve staff in the activity, but it may be appropriate for someone to stand back and observe. Assessing the patient's suitability for the activity is important, as it is unfair to the other group members to include someone who draws attention to the group.

Often patients go on to use the community activities to give a purpose to any parole, a strategy which has proved popular with the Home Office. Longer overnight or weekend trips away are possible. Ideas include a walking weekend in the hills, or a visit to an activity centre to canoe or sail. Good planning is essential. Cost can be prohibitive, as can the large numbers of staff required, and in some cases it is necessary to obtain Home Office permission.

These obstacles can be overcome and the benefit of a real sense of enjoyment, freedom and achievement can be experienced by the patients. This may act as an incentive to maintaining their freedom in the future. These benefits can also be experienced on less ambitious day trips, for example to the seaside or to an amusement park. A regular programme of afternoon trips to a variety of local destinations and activities can prove popular. An air of 'mystery' about each week's destination can be particularly motivating!

Preparation for discharge

Not all patients will pursue these activities on discharge, but a number will develop an interest in a particular activity. This can be supported and provides the patients with an opportunity to use their time constructively and to meet people and make friends. However, the patient needs to be prepared to be asked: "Where have you been living?', 'What have you been doing over the past year?'

Anxiety management

It may be argued that relaxation techniques are not appropriate for this client group. However, patients suffer from anxiety for all sorts of reasons and at varying stages of their rehabilitation.

Physically based, muscle relaxation techniques can prove useful in this patient group. Other techniques which involve guided imagery should be avoided where fantasy can be part of the patient's problem. This will place the physiotherapist as the ideal professional to teach relaxation.

Group or individual sessions and the use of a tape can be considered for the patient who can identify the early signs of his anxiety. However, be prepared for the tape to be damaged on those occasions where it did not prove useful!

A closed anxiety management group, run with a psychology colleague, is another option. They can help patients to understand and identify their anxiety feelings/symptoms and to recognize the behaviours that can ensue.

Coping strategies

This is an interesting, challenging and demanding area of work. Overriding all other factors will be the security of the ward and the safety of staff, patients and the general public. Therapy time can take second place to these factors.

It is essential that good working relationships exist between all team members, and that there are support and supervision mechanisms in place. The high numbers of staff involved may make for areas of role conflict which need to be resolved.

The physiotherapist who works in this field will therefore need to be open to develop a number of interpersonal skills, as well as those of handling aggressive and acting-out behaviour.

Appendix: the Reed Report

The Reed Report is 'a review of the current level, pattern and operation of health and social services for mentally disordered offenders'. The committee was established on 30 November 1990 and is chaired by Dr John L. Reed, Senior Principal Medical Officer at the Department of Health.

The report outlines the urgent need for changes in the way mentally disordered offenders are treated in prison, special hospitals, secure units and the community. It stresses the need for more funding, increased staffing levels and more specialized staff training.

At the time of writing, the report is still in its draft stages but paragraph 4.48 now reads:

We draw attention here to the work of physiotherapists as members of mental health care teams. They have a key role in assessing patients' physical disorders, maintaining and improving their mobility and physical fitness and relieving musculoskeletal pain (e.g. following self-injury). Using various physical methods they can also contribute to the psychological treatment of patients, including programmes to promote their general well-being and self-esteem. Physiotherapy skills are often shared with other staff to ensure safe and effective methods of lifting and handling.

References

Butler Committee (1974) Home Office and DHSS Interim Report of the Committee on Mentally Abnormal Offenders, Chairman Lord Butler of Saffron Walden, Cmnd 5698, HMSO, London

Butler Committee (1975) Home Office and DHSS Report of the Committee on Mentally Abnormal Offenders, Chairman Lord Butler of Saffron Walden, Cmnd 6244, HMSO, London

Dishman, R.K. (1985) Medical psychology in exercise and sport. *Medical Clinics of North America,* **69**(1), 124–143

Glesler, J. and Mendelbeg, H. (1990) Exercise and sport in mental health: a review of the literature. *Israel Journal of Psychiatry and Related Sciences,* **27**(2), 99–112

Hannaford, C.P., Harel, E.H. and Cox, K. (1988) Psychophysiological effects of a running programme on depression and anxiety in a psychiatric population. *The Psychological Record,* **38**, 37–48

22

Dementia

Valerie Pomeroy

Introduction

Dragons are mythical creatures, or are they? Stories often tell of dragons that grow in power until their basis for existence is challenged. The dragon of therapeutic negativity towards elderly people with dementia is now being challenged. One aspect of this challenge is the recognition of how the rehabilitation potential of elderly people with mobility problems may be limited by the ageist attitudes of clinicians (Niewboeur, 1992). Another aspect is the recognition of the need to examine the association between the pathology of dementia and the physical disability experienced by the individual. This chapter will examine information about dementia to explore how much 'clinical knowledge' is mythical and how much has a sound basis. This should aid physiotherapists to design effective intervention programmes.

At present there are two theoretical frameworks for dementia. The biomedical model of dementia implies that a person's functional status is directly a result of neurological impairment arising from the neuropathology. This has been extended by the psychosocial model of the dementing process which implies that functional state is the result of complex interaction between neuropathology, individual brain structure (established through both genetic factors and learning experience) and the psychosocial environment surrounding the individual (Kitwood, 1990; Gilleard, 1992). These two models and the inferences by which they explain observed mobility status are summarized in Table 22.1.

The mobility problems in dementia

Mobility problems associated with dementing illness can be broadly divided into two clinical categories (Sjogren, 1950; Hope and Fairburn, 1990; Jarvick and Wiseman, 1991): (a) people who wander, and (b) people who have increasing difficulty moving and eventually become chair-based.

These problems exist not just in those with severe dementia but also in those with mild and moderate dementia. Consideration of the neuropathology of the two major forms of dementia affecting the elderly would lead to the expectation that those who wander have dementia of the Alzheimer type (DAT) and those who eventually become chair-based suffer from multi-infarct dementia (MID) (Table 22.1).

Table 22.1 Comparison of models of dementia with reference to interpretation of mobility status (From Pomeroy, 1994, by permission of Lawrence Erlbaum Associates Ltd)

	Biomedical model	Psychosocial model
Factors involved in the functional state of the brain	1. Neuropathology – differential diagnosis of DAT, MID, mixed and disease staging (mild, moderate, severe)	Interaction between 1. Neuropathology and 2. Individual brain structure and 3. Psychosocial environment
Inferences by which mobility status is explained	1. A loss of mobility as the disease progresses. Variation exists between those with DAT and MID and also within those with MID because of the differing pathology	1. Variation exists between all people with dementia not just in those with MID
	2. Mobility problems are a direct consequence of the neuropathology and are therefore irremediable	2. Mobility problems are due to a complex interaction between all factors identified in the model
	3. A change in mobility prompts a change in the environment	3. A change in the environment prompts a change in mobility

DAT, dementia of the Alzheimer type; MID, multi-infarct dementia.

A review of the literature suggests that this may not be correct, as variation in mobility appears to be greater than is expected from consideration of neuropathology alone. Not only are there differences as predicted by the biomedical model (Table 22.1) but also between those individuals with a diagnosis of DAT. In addition, there are similarities in the motor impairments of MID and DAT, with Parkinsonian features recorded for both disease processes (Molsa et al., 1982; Chui et al. 1985; Mayeux et al., 1985; Huff and Growdon, 1986; reviewed by Huppert and Tym, 1986; Molsa et al., 1987; Bakchine et al., 1989; Risse et al., 1990; Burns et al., 1991). Most of these studies recognized that neuroleptic drugs used in both DAT and MID can result in motor impairments and due consideration was given to selection of participants.

Precise details of associated mobility problems are scarce, as the majority of research interest has been given to motor impairment rather than functional mobility status. These neurological impairments would be expected to affect several aspects of general function including posture, balance, movement patterns and co-ordination. The following balance and gait parameters have been weakly associated with severity of DAT, being observed in 13% of those with mild dementia and 41% of those with severe dementia (Visser, 1983; Huff and Growdon, 1986):

- decreased arm swing
- postural instability
- shorter step length
- lower gait speed
- lower stepping frequency
- greater step-to-step variability
- greater double support ratio
- greater sway path.

It is important to note that some subjects were excluded from gait analysis because their dementia was too severe for them to understand the instructions. The percentage of those with severe DAT and gait impairment may therefore be higher than 41%. Even so, the implication is that approximately 50% of those with severe DAT may not have gait impairment. Clinical observation of people resident in long-term psychiatric care suggests that individual differences continue until the terminal stages of the disease process. Some people continue to wander, while others are chair-based before admission. It remains unclear whether all wanderers eventually become chair-based and whether functional mobility status is related to differential diagnosis. Other factors may be contributing to the level of disability seen.

Possible influential factors include:

- *Difficulties with differential diagnosis.* Reliability ranges from 64% in clinical practice to 85% in a research series (Wade *et al.*, 1987; Joachin *et al.*, 1988; Galasko *et al.* 1991).
- *Subtypes of DAT.* Subtypes have been proposed based on differences found in motor impairments among those people with a diagnosis of DAT. It remains unclear from experimental studies whether there are distinct neuropathological differences (Chui *et al.*, 1985; Mayeux *et al.*, 1985; Friedland *et al.*, 1988; Risse *et al.*, 1990).
- *Individual differences in brain microstructure.* This hypothesis has been proposed by the psychosocial model and requires testing.
- *Multipathology.* This is a complex area which consequently needs to be fully considered in any assessment or investigation.
- *Environmental stimulation.* Environmental stimulation is thought to affect various aspects of functional status of people with dementia.

Of these, it is environmental stimulation which has received the most therapeutic interest.

Influence of environmental stimulation

Psychosocial theory holds that any individual exists and draws meaning from the complexity of their relationships with other people. Different relationships and experiences engender different emotions, experiences and reactions within an individual and outwards again to other relationships. Elderly people with dementing illness are also exposed to these same influences, but the relationships they experience can produce negative results (Bartol, 1979). Such negative interactions have been called malignant social psychology because of the effects on the person who is neurologically impaired, not because other people have any malevolent intentions.

Kitwood (1990) identifies 10 ways in which this can occur. Those with especial relevance to a physiotherapeutic approach are:

- *Disempowerment.* The person with dementia is able to do the tasks but is not allowed to because it is easier, quicker or less messy for other people to do these themselves.
- *Infantilization.* Treated like a young child.
- *Intimidation.* One example is a professional assessment which is carried out without due consideration given as to how the patient will interpret what is happening. At worst, this can be classified as assault.

- *Labelling*. It is suggested that the label of dementia raises a set of expectations in the affected person, their social and professional contacts. Expectations are known to affect consequent behaviour which in turn reinforces the expectation. In effect, a self-fulfilling prophecy may exist.
- *Outpacing*. The elderly person can get left behind by others, not because they cannot do the task but because they need to function at a slower pace. This need is not recognized by others.
- *Objectification*. The person with dementia is not treated as a person but as an object or as a source of tasks to be completed.

Most physiotherapists would recognize some if not all of the interactions outlined above. However, the extent to which such behaviour influences the mobility of the affected person has not been subjected to systematic enquiry. It is thought that over a period of time these types of interactions compound the effects of neuropathology.

It is known that if opportunities and encouragement to move are not provided, then problems of inactivity – contractures, muscle wasting, osteoporosis and pressure sores – occur in elderly people. Such secondary disability could compound the physical disability resulting from the pathology of dementia, but this is not fully recognized in the current biomedical model of dementia. The complexity of the relationship between environments and functional status ensures that clear research evidence remains difficult to obtain.

Rehabilitative framework for physiotherapy management

Knowledge of functional state in dementia suggests that the environment is important for functional ability. This is not to say that environmental stimulation affects neuropathology or impairments, but it does imply that associated disability and/or handicap may be influenced. Physiotherapists therefore require a biomedical diagnosis which provides information about the underlying pathology and also a functional evaluation which provides information about the disability and handicap.

Already examined in this chapter is the way in which individual differences exist between pathology and disability. Clinical practice requires that these are fully explored. For example, several people presenting with the same clinical differential diagnosis and an inability to walk independently could have different 'functional diagnoses'. These could include muscle weakness, decreased exercise tolerance, poor balance, inappropriate walking aids and care-giver behaviour. The range of possible functional diagnoses taken in conjunction with both the biomedical and psychosocial influences on functional ability suggest that neither the biomedical nor the psychosocial model alone is sufficient framework for physiotherapy practice. Physiotherapists need to integrate approaches to dementia. Use of this conceptual framework allows all levels of the disease process, from pathology to handicap, to be considered. It also provides the opportunity for research findings from several disciplines to be incorporated into clinical practice more easily. The integrated framework also promotes effective interdisciplinary teamwork which must be acknowledged, even though this chapter concentrates on physiotherapy. A physiotherapist works across the biomedical and psychosocial models of dementia, moving from the molecular level of pathology to the holistic level of environment. In effect, physiotherapists adopt a biopsychosocial framework for practice (Engel, 1980).

Each of the 'functional diagnoses' given as examples above indicates a specific course for physiotherapy intervention which, while not effecting a cure, should improve or maintain functional mobility. Rehabilitation is now recognized as being much more than a return to premorbid function. The maintenance of optimal functional ability throughout the course of a progressive disease should be the aim of physiotherapy intervention (Eisdorfer, 1986; Pope, 1988; Condie, 1992).

Knowledge of all aspects of the disease process, from pathology to handicap, combined with active management provides a dynamic framework for clinical physiotherapy with elderly people with dementia.

Are reservations to the adoption of a rehabilitative approach justified?

Acceptance of the above framework is often hindered by reservations about a rehabilitative approach to elderly people with dementia. Implicit in rehabilitation of mobility is change in motor behaviour, which in turn implies that some learning has taken place. Essentially, the neurological impairment associated with dementia is loss of cognitive skill. Consequently, what is expected is that the affected person will not be able to communicate effectively, integrate stimuli at a central level, or remember what happened during a treatment session, and thus will be unable to learn or relearn motor skills. This section will examine whether this expectation can be justified.

Appropriate motor behaviour depends on:

- sensory input
- sensory nerve efficiency
- central nervous system (CNS) structures involved in information processing (CNS integration of all sensory input with the current CNS programme of body image to execute appropriate motor action)
- motor nerve efficiency.

In relation to dementia, a decrease in sensory nerve efficiency is unlikely to affect motor response adversely, as sensory nerve conduction velocity is probably unaffected by dementing illness (Levy *et al.*, 1970). Decreased motor response could result from a decrease in motor nerve conduction and power. This is unlikely in dementia, as handgrip strength (which is used as a measure of these factors) has not been related to dementia (Milne and Maule, 1984). This leaves sensory input and neural integration.

Diffuse cerebral pathology, such as that resulting from a dementing illness, would be expected to hinder information processing and therefore motor performance. But observed variation in activities in daily living (ADL), like motor impairment, is not fully explained by severity of dementia as measured by mental status tests (Galasko *et al.*, 1991). In addition, experimental evidence suggests that appropriate environmental input (e.g. encouraging physical and social activity) improve functional state (Rovner *et al.*, 1990; Pomeroy, 1993). So, although neurological pathology reduces the capacity for appropriate motor behaviour, the provision of sensory stimulation may result in a higher level of functional status.

Clinicians report success in teaching motor skills to elderly people with dementing illness. Activities such as learning to walk with an aid which is new to the individual can be accomplished with continual practice and reinforcement (Davis, 1986). These activities can mainly be classified as stimulating the expression of retained continuous motor skills, but also include an element of new learning which would not be expected from cognitive learning theory.

People with moderate dementia have been shown to have the ability to learn a motor skill, although they were unable to learn a list of 10 related items or recognize eight unfamiliar faces (Eslinger and Damasio, 1986). The implication is that the learning of motor skills may involve different neural structures than the hippocampus (a major site of neuropathology in DAT) which is involved in other forms of learning. Physiotherapeutic interventions aimed at improving mobility status may therefore be successful.

An example of the use of appropriate stimulation is given by reference to an observational study of communication. Tanner and Daniels (1990) identified carer behaviour which decreases and that which increases communication with the affected individual. Identified strategies which emerged as important for effective communication were those such as ensuring the listener's attention is gained by eye contact and touch and emphasizing the informer's body language and facial expression. This work suggests that what is required for optimal function is the accentuated use of existing environmental stimulation. Carers who accentuated the normal body and facial language involved in communication were more effective than those who did not. Demonstration and repetition of the message has also been advised as an effective strategy (Knopman and Sawyer De-Maris, 1990). These communication techniques could be employed during therapeutic interaction. Often a verbal request to 'stand up' is insufficient. It may be better to precede the request with physical prompts and performing the activity with the affected person. Oddy (1987) provides several good clinical examples of this.

Physiotherapy assessment

Physiotherapy assessment for the person with severe dementia is essentially to provide a functional evaluation to establish measurable goals. To achieve this, assessment needs to identify what the person can do, where movement becomes difficult and why. The major part of the 'why' is to differentiate between what is directly as a result of the neuropathology, what arises from other pathology and what may result from environmental influences. This is not an easy task because of the complexities of the interactions between pathology and environment on functional status. Additionally, some standard clinical tests such as those used for joint range, muscle power and balance may not be appropriate to use with all people referred. These are likely to be classified as intimidation (discussed earlier in this chapter). Strategies which are based ADL tend to be most useful.

Assessment needs to take time to examine the range of normal variability in mobility skills. Elderly people with a dementing illness have a clinical reputation for being able to walk one day and not the next. Often medication patterns or time of day explain this variability.

As with any physiotherapy assessment, it is very important to collect information from other professionals, the patient and appropriate carers, in addition to performing both a neuromuscular (as able) and functional examination. In particular, carers' knowledge about how they manage the patient should not be ignored. Often they have gained specific expertise which can be of enormous help to professionals. The assessment process should also take full account of carers' coping mechanisms and whether they could continue to manage if mobility state altered.

Specific guidelines to help physiotherapists new to this field decide whether a physiotherapy programme is likely to be of benefit have not yet emerged from the small amount of published research. The only help which can be offered at present is a suggestion that those patients with very severe dementia who are unable to maintain unsupported sitting may be unlikely to benefit from physiotherapy treatment (Pomeroy, 1994). But this finding should be approached cautiously until further testing has been completed.

Goals derived from the assessment findings must be achievable and measurable. Suggestions of specific methods are given later in this chapter, though not all goals set will be encompassed by these. Common broad objectives which are set include (Hare, 1986; Oddy, 1987):

- restore/maintain optimal functional mobility
- ease the physical handling problems of carers
- provision of adequate seating for comfort, pressure care, maintenance of joint range and enablement of functional ability
- maintain the comfort of the affected person through terminal care.

Physiotherapy intervention

From the assessment and goal-setting process, a plan of intervention is derived. Essentially, physiotherapy techniques do not differ markedly for people with dementia than for other elderly people, although the approach is adapted. Time has to be allowed for repetition of cues and delayed responses. The physiotherapist has to be prepared to change direction during treatment sessions according to the inclinations of the patient. As cognitive impairment increases, non-verbal cues become more important and flexible and creative approaches have to be employed. The differing degrees of cognitive impairment require an intervention programme to comprise differing combinations of the following:

- body awareness training
- music and movement
- functional mobility training
- seating and positioning for activity and comfort
- advice and training for carers.

Details of all of these are provided in the following text and include the rationale and schedules used in a recent studies (Pomeroy, 1993; Pomeroy, 1994). This preliminary work has suggested that $1\frac{1}{2}$ hours of physiotherapy treatment a week for approximately 10 weeks may be required to obtain optimal functional mobility in people with a severe dementia. Whether these improvements are maintained once physiotherapy ceases, remains equivocal.

Body awareness

Identification of the possible importance of the level and type of environmental stimulation for functional status has encouraged the development of sensory integration therapy. Price (1977) defined sensory integration as 'the neurophysiology of somatosensory functions and integration phenomena, mediated in the brain stem, which control posture, motor activity, perception and attention, powerfully influence the other senses and cognition, and are essential for motivation, self concept and self control'. The sensory integration concept proposes that by increasing the level of sensory stimulation, responses become more appropriate. Input is divided into the following sections (Richman, 1969; Price, 1977; Ross and Burdick, 1981):

* kinaesthetic and proprioceptive
* tactile
* auditory
* visual
* social and cognitive.

Examination of concepts of information processing and sensory integration therapy suggest that physiotherapeutic techniques based on tactile stimuli may facilitate motor response in elderly people with dementing illness. All physiotherapists use physical prompts to stimulate functional skills. Two simple examples are moving a walking frame forwards to elicit stepping and pelvic resistance of rolling to facilitate reaching. Such techniques cause difficulties if used with people who have a severe dementia. Their application can be classified as intimidation, part of the malignant social psychology discussed earlier in this chapter. Misinterpretation of therapeutic intervention can result in aggression or withdrawal. Either way the end result is of no use to the patient, carer or physiotherapist. The pure application of most neurologically based physiotherapeutic techniques for elderly people with dementia is inappropriate. Adaptation and innovation which is based on both neurological and biomechanical principles is necessary.

Physiotherapists working in this area of health care have developed approaches which emphasize tactile, proprioceptive and kinaesthetic input. It is thought these help develop a subcortical body image which facilitates appropriate motor behaviour. The physical aspects of this therapeutic activity need to be accompanied by a sensitivity to the reactions of the patient. This must be appreciated in the clinical application of the following treatment schedule.

Physiotherapy schedule – body awareness
The aim is to enhance information processing and thus improve motor reactions:

* participants to be seated in chairs which allow a symmetrical upright posture with hips, knees and ankles at 90°
* six participants in each group
* one leader and one or two helpers
* group session to last approximately 30 minutes.

1. Circle formed with subjects in wheelchairs, feet flat on the floor, sitting with hips well back in the chair so that the spine is as vertical as possible.

2. 'Hello' to each participant in turn, using their name and shaking hands. Smile and seek to establish eye contact.
3. Head and cervical spine:
   (a) Therapist standing behind participant. Light circular fingertip massage to the scalp area.
   (b) Therapist standing behind participant. Hold participant's head, thumbs under occiput and palms along parietal region, fingers spreading upwards. Gentle pressure in and up – passive or assisted movements of cervical spine, flexion, extension, side flexion left, and right and rotation left and right – three times each pair of movements.
4. Trunk:
   (a) Therapist at side of participant with hands around the lateral costal region. Light pressure inwards and upwards following the natural breathing pattern of participant. Maintain for 2 minutes and then repeat on the other side.
   (b) Therapist at the side of participant inward and opposite pressure with hands placed on the sternum and thoracolumbar spine to encourage extension. Maintain pressure for 15–30 seconds and repeat 4–5 times.
5. Upper limbs:
   (a) Therapist at side of participant with hands along the line of the clavicle and encompassing scapula. Sustain pressure inwards and repeat 3 times each side.
   (b) Therapist in front of participant, stroking from scapulae down to fingertips on the extensor surface bilaterally, encouraging protraction of scapulae, flexion/external rotation of the glenohumeral joint, extension of elbow, wrist and fingers until hands are resting comfortably on knees.
   (c) Therapist in front of participant with hands around participant's scapulae using arm on arm support – encourage forward/backward movement of the trunk, gradually withdrawing support as appropriate until hand on hand support is achieved.
6. Lower limbs:
   (a) Therapist in front of the participant with hands on top of participant's knees exerting pressure down through feet which are directly under knees. Maintain pressure while rocking knees from side to side twice. Repeat 5 times.
   (b) Therapist in front of participant with one hand under lower third of participant's thigh and the other hand under instep. Facilitate stamping of feet on the ground 5 times each leg, with impact being taken mostly by the heel. Remove support as appropriate.
7. Integration activity:
   (a) Large (95 cm dia.) gym ball in centre of circle, participant's hands on ball with knees also in contact. Leader to bang ball, helpers to assist participants to maintain vibratory contact.
   (b) Encourage participants to bang on the ball, hand-on-hand facilitation if necessary.
   (c) Leader lifts ball up and down, helpers encourage/assist participants to keep hands on the ball.
   (d) Enlarge the circle. Each subject called by their preferred name and encourage to push or kick the ball back.
8. Individual 'goodbye' to each participant, using their name, shaking hands and encouraging eye contact.

Music and movement

Physiotherapists working with individuals with a dementing illness frequently use music to encourage movement, often as part of a sensory training programme (Wolfe, 1983). Music is used to arouse attention, maintain attention, aid memory (both recall and expectation) and assist the temporal organization of activity (Knill, 1983). Music is also proposed as a medium for communication with people with very severe dementia who appear to be unaware of their environment and may use self-stimulating behaviour (Norberg *et al.*, 1986). Clinical reports of music and movement groups have noted increases in verbalization, spontaneous expression of feelings, interaction, assertiveness and mobility skills (Needler and Baer, 1982; Wolfe, 1983; Dunachie and Budd, 1985).

Henson (1977), in a review of electromyographical studies, provides some justification for music and movement therapy. These indicate an increase in muscular activity during the process of listening to music while no muscular activity was observed. Lullabies were found to decrease and march songs to increase muscular reaction. Predominantly, motor responses were produced by march rhythms, while other rhythms were more likely to produce respiratory or cardiovascular responses. These autonomic reactions (changes in blood pressure, pulse rate and respiration) may also result when musical sounds are not consciously perceived. As well as these physiological responses, links between rhythm and simple emotion have been shown. The theory suggests that the rhythmical component of the auditory input has an impact on the whole cerebral cortex and also on large subcortical areas via the extensive connections of the reticular formation.

Physiotherapy schedule – music and movement
The aim is to arouse attention, increase muscular activity and increase temporal organization of activity:

• participants seated in chairs which allow a symmetrical erect posture with hips, knees and ankles at 90°
• six participants in each group
• one leader and one or two helpers
• group session to last approximately 30 minutes.
• all verbal instructions to be rhythmical and reinforced by gesture if necessary; physical prompts to be given as appropriate.

1. Circle formed with subjects in wheelchairs – feet flat on the floor. Sitting with hips well back in the chair so that the spine is as vertical as possible.
2. Individual greeting and welcome, then general 'hello'.
3. Cheerful familiar music to catch attention:
   (a) body sway side to side
   (b) body sway forward and backward
   (c) trunk rotation.
   Helper facilitating or assisting movement as appropriate, with support to participant's arms.
4. Vigorous music. Shaking hands with helper – bilaterally and rhythmically.
5. Slow grand music. Participant clasps hands (helper facilitate if necessary – hands on hands) and moves arms up and down, side to side and circle.

6. March music:
   (a) banging and/or shaking tambourine (only if this is not resulting in infantilization – see above)
   (b) stamping feet on the floor.
7. Slow waltz:
   (a) reaching for feet – forward and back with trunk
   (b) standing – weight transference side to side.
8. Dance music:
   (a) stamping feet on floor
   (b) encourage and/or facilitate dancing.
9. Hokey-cokey (only if this is not resulting in infantilization – see above). In sitting or standing, helpers to assist participants as necessary.
10. Individual 'goodbye' to each participant, shaking hands and encouraging eye contact.

Functional mobility training

Standard physiotherapeutic techniques to improve muscle strength, an important factor in gait performance, involve a degree of new learning (Bohannon, 1989). New tasks, such as the use of an unfamiliar walking aid, requesting the repetition of a small part of the gait cycle or any use of resistance to movement, are unlikely to succeed with people who have a severe dementia.

To facilitate and then reinforce functional mobility the therapist needs an understanding of how movement patterns vary throughout the life span and the effects of individual variability. Movement patterns are influenced in the individual by premorbid activity level, body dimensions and the effects of any disease process (VanSant, 1990). Observation of any group of elderly people performing an everyday task such as getting out of bed will reveal the many different movement patterns which can be considered normal. Any attempt therefore to produce total conformity in physiotherapeutic techniques will neglect this variability. Remembering individual differences, movement can be facilitated by using non-verbal cues, especially tactile ones (see the body awareness and music and movement schedules above).

Physiotherapy schedule – functional mobility training
The aim is to maintain/improve movement in joints, flexibility of soft tissues and functional movement:

• One therapist and one assistant as necessary.

1. Passive movement – aim for full range of movement in each joint. The same procedure to be used in side lying left and right.
   (a) rotation of trunk – shoulder on pelvic girdle
   (b) scapular movement
   (c) glenohumeral joint
   (d) elbow joint
   (e) wrist and hand
   (f) hip joint
   (g) knee joint
   (h) ankle and foot.
2. Prone lying – 10–15 minutes if participant will tolerate this.

3. Practice of areas of functional mobility which the mobility scale indicates as difficult.
4. Practice of walking in parallel bars.
5. Introduction of and practice with walking aids as appropriate.

Seating and positioning

The problem of inappropriate seating is one that most physiotherapists will have experienced some frustration about. The affected person spends the majority of their time sitting in a chair and therefore comfort, posture, hygiene, safety and optimal functional ability all need to be considered. It is not often, however, that physiotherapists working with elderly people with a dementia have access to the resources needed to provide adequate seating. Adaptations can be made to wheelchairs, but it is not socially desirable for people to sit in these all day. After all, which of us can sit in the same chair in the same position for up to 4 hours at a time without becoming stiff and sore? So even if adequate seating is provided, attention to positional changes still has to be given.

Advice and training for carers

Advice and training for carers form a large and important part of the role of a physiotherapist working in this aspect of health care. Before outlining the areas that physiotherapists may need to contribute to, it will be helpful to give some attention to carers themselves.

Carers, whether formal or informal, need to incorporate advice and instructions for specific aspects of care into the total care which they provide for the elderly person. Informal carers provide this care 'at home', often alone, with professional support being available. This includes home care, community psychiatric nurse (CPN) visits and respite care admissions. But most of the time they are providing care alone. Formal carers, in contrast, normally have a working structure within which they are supported. They also do not have the emotional aspects of caring which arise from family relationships. The approach of a physiotherapist who has some advice and training to offer therefore needs to differ between these two broad groups. For both, however, it is important to remember that what is offered needs to be relevant to the carer, fully considers their capabilities and recognizes the specific expertise gained from working intensively with the affected person. These considerations are of especial importance for informal carers.

Although it is clear that precise details of advice and training cannot be given, it is possible to outline the major issues which physiotherapists become involved in:

• Highlighting the movement abilities of the affected person and discussing with the carer how these can be utilized even if the tasks take a long time (disempowerment, discussed earlier in this chapter). An example might be walking to the dining room rather than being pushed in a wheelchair.
• Training of moving and handling techniques which facilitate the affected person to be as active as possible whilst minimizing physical stress on the carer.
• Advice and training which relates to speed of response (outpacing, discussed earlier in this chapter). For example, frequently the affected person will not

stand and walk when asked by a carer but will when asked by a physio-therapist. Often some simple explanation about the need for repetition of verbal commands, reinforcement by gesture and demonstration and time for response is enough. If not, the advice needs to be accompanied by training in gaining attention and then facilitating activity by physical prompts.

- Providing information and explanation about the affected person's disabilities and planning with the carer how compensations can be made. Simple adjustments to the environment, such as correct footwear, the height of a chair or the side of the bed which the patient gets in and out of, often solves the problem. Even if the problem is irremediable the resultant tension can be alleviated if the carer knows the cause.

Physiotherapy evaluation

Formal evaluation of intervention provided is an essential area of practice but one which many physiotherapists tend to neglect. In general, evaluation happens on an informal level as part of clinical decision-making. These clinical evaluations are important, but without the information provided by reliable and valid outcome measures cannot be used to evaluate the effectiveness of physiotherapy intervention. One reason given for not using formal evaluation is that physiotherapists work as part of a team. But if physiotherapists are being effective as experts in mobility, they should be involved in much more than the 'hands on' treatment. The advice and training they provide is designed to be beneficial. This requires to be evaluated as much as specific therapy. Another reason which is commonly given for not using formal outcome measures is that those available do not cover all the areas that physiotherapists consider important. However, it is very unlikely that a perfect measure will ever exist and without any outcome measures at all it is impossible to justify use of physiotherapy resources, compare different types of interventions and collate information from more than one department. Physiotherapists need to become more familiar with the outcome measures which do exist. They also need to gain an understanding of the basic properties of a 'good' outcome measure. Specific details can be obtained by consulting relevant textbooks (Streiner and Norman, 1989; Wade, 1992), but briefly these properties are:

- sensitivity – a measure needs to have the ability to detect clinically significant change
- reliability – the measure used for the same patient by different therapists has to produce essentially the same result
- validity – a measure has to measure what it claims to measure.

Outcome measures which can be used to evaluate change in functional mobility skills of elderly people with dementing illness are:

- two-minute walking test (Stewart *et al.*, 1990)
- Rivermead Mobility Index (Collen *et al.*, 1991)
- Southampton Assessment of Mobility (Pomeroy, 1990).

These will be outlined in turn.

The two-minute walking test is very simple, requiring only a stopwatch and a measured length of corridor. It requires the participant to walk in their normal manner for 2 minutes. Verbal encouragement is provided and a turn is allowed if the end of the corridor is reached before the 2 minutes have passed. This has been shown to be a sensitive measure of change in mobility in elderly people, but it must be remembered that individual variability of approximately 20% can occur with timed walking tests (Collen *et al.*, 1990).

The Rivermead Mobility Index is a hierarchical assessment of functional ability (a person failing on three consecutive items is unlikely to pass any further items). Scoring is either 'yes' or 'no' and covers abilities from turning over in bed (score 1) to running 10 metres in 4 seconds (score 15). Although not validated on an elderly population with a dementia, clinical use has found it to be a useful indicator of functional ability.

The Southampton Assessment of Mobility was specifically designed for use with elderly people with a dementing illness (Pomeroy, 1990); see also the Appendix to this chapter. The scale is based on a biomechanical analysis of sitting to standing and walking a few steps. Abilities covered range from immobile (score 0) to walk four steps (score 18). Inter-rater reliability, construct validity and content validity have been established.

All of these measures are completed easily and quickly and can be used in conjunction with existing informal clinical evaluation. Although not perfect, they represent a step forward in evaluating the effects of physiotherapy intervention. Physiotherapists must, however, ensure that those to whom this information is given appreciate both the progressive nature of dementia and the limitations of the measures being used.

Conclusion

Therapeutic optimism towards elderly people with a dementia and a mobility problem is recommended. Rehabilitation is a more comprehensive concept than just a return to premorbid function. It entails maintenance of optimal function throughout the course of a progressive neurological disease such as dementia. This requires a physiotherapist to:

- have a full understanding of the biomedical and psychosocial components of the dementing process
- have a full understanding of motor learning
- be highly trained in biomechanical and neurological therapeutic techniques
- have the ability to be innovative in effective application of principles of these techniques
- have communication skills which facilitate a relationship with elderly people whose dementia can be so severe that they do not even know their own name
- be an effective teacher for carers and other professional staff
- be able fully to evaluate interventions provided.

These are not simple requirements, but expert physiotherapists make them look easy!

Acknowledgements

I gratefully acknowledge the grant provided by Research Into Ageing. I also thank Professor R.S.J. Briggs for his support and advice. Thanks are also due to my colleagues Mrs E. Sandford and Dr C. Fulton for their helpful comments on an earlier draft of this chapter.

Appendix:

Southampton ADL Orientated Assessment of Mobility. (From Pomeroy, 1990, by permission of *Physiotherapy*)

General instructions.
- At the beginning of the assessment the subject is to be seated in a chair with armrests, which allows hips and knees to be flexed to 90°.
- All commands are shown in the scale (in italics) and should be both verbal and gestural. Demonstration is permissible if necessary.
- Any additional assistance allowable is indicated in the appropriate section.

Scoring.
Score 1 for does and 0 for does not. Total possible score is 18.

ASSESSMENT

Score

SECTION A. SITTING TO STANDING   *Stand up please*
1. Leans forward with feet flat on the floor   [ ]
2. Takes weight through feet and lifts hips clear of surface, hand
   support allowed   [ ]
3. Hips level with arms of chair   [ ]
4. Weight bears through feet only   [ ]

SECTION B. STANDING BALANCE   *Stand still please*
Use of support object, e.g. table or walking aid allowed.

5. Is steady first 3–5 seconds   [ ]
6. Stands 15 seconds   [ ]
7. Stands 30 seconds   [ ]
8. Stands 45 seconds   [ ]
9. Stands 1 minute or more   [ ]
                                    Stand still please
10. Remains steady – eyes open – when pushed lightly on sternum
    3 times. Normal stepping reactions allowed.   [ ]

SECTION C. GAIT   *Walk forward please*
Assistance of one person or use of aid allowed.

11. Transfers weight side to side   [ ]
12. Brings weight forward   [ ]
13. Walk 4 steps forward   [ ]
                                    Walk backwards please
14. Walks 4 steps backwards

SECTION D. STANDING TO SITTING   *Sit down please*
15. Brings weight forward   [ ]
16. Bends hips and knees   [ ]
17. Lowers smoothly into chair   [ ]
18. Moves hips to back of chair from the front   [ ]
                                    Total score   ____

References

Bakchine, S., Lacomblez, L., Palisson, E. *et al.* (1989) Relationship between primitive reflexes, extra-pyramidal signs, reflective apraxia and severity of cognitive impairment in dementia of the Alzheimer type. *Acta Neurologica Scandinavica,* **79**, 38–46

Bartol, M.A. (1979) Nonverbal communication in patients with Alzheimer's disease. *Journal of Gerontological Nursing,* **5**, 21–31.

Bohannon, R.W. (1989) Relevance of muscle strength to gait performance in patients with neurologic disability. *Journal of Neurological Rehabilitation,* **3**, 97–100

Burns, A., Jacoby, R. and Levy, R. (1991) Neurological signs in Alzheimer's disease. *Age and Ageing,* **20**, 45–51

Chui, H.C., Teng, E.L., Henderson, V.W. *et al.* (1985) Clinical subtypes of dementia of the Alzheimer type. *Neurology,* **35**, 1544–1550

Collen, F.M., Wade, D.T. and Bradshaw, C.M. (1990) Mobility after stroke: reliability of measures of impairment and disability. *International Journal of Disability Studies,* **12**, 6–9

Collen, F.M., Wade, D.T., Robb, G.F. *et al.* (1991) The Rivermead Mobility Index: a further development of the Rivermead Motor Assessment. *International Journal of Disability Studies,* **13**, 50–54

Condie, E. (1992) A therapeutic approach to physical disability. *Physiotherapy Canada,* **44**, 7–12

Davis, C.M. (1986) The role of the physical and occupational therapist in caring for the victim of Alzheimer's disease. In *Therapeutic Interventions for the Person with Dementia* (ed Taira, E.D.), The Haworth Press, New York, pp. 15–27

Dunachie, S. and Budd, B. (1985) Music and physiotherapy: A combined approach. *Physiotherapy Practice,* **1**, 27–30

Eisdorfer, C. (1986) Ageing and rehabilitation: summary of meeting. In *Ageing and Rehabilitation* (eds Brody, S.J. and Ruff, G.E.), Springer, New York, pp. 357–364

Engel, G.L. (1980) The clinical application of the biopsychosocial model. *American Journal of Psychiatry,* **137**, 535–544

Eslinger, P.J. and Damasio, A.R. (1986) Preserved motor learning in Alzheimer's disease: implications for anatomy and behaviour. *Journal of Neurosciences,* **6**, 3006–3009

Friedland, R.P., Koss, E., Haxby, J.V. *et al.* (1988) Alzheimer disease: clinical and biological heterogeneity. *Annals of Internal Medicine,* **109**, 298–311

Galasko, D., Corey-Bloom, J. and Thal, L.J. (1991) Monitoring progression in Alzheimer's disease. *Journal of the American Geriatrics Society,* **39**, 932–941

Gilleard, C. (1992) Losing one's mind and losing one's place. A psychosocial model of dementia. In *Gerontology. Responding to an Ageing Society* (ed. Morgan, K) Biddles, Guildford, UK, pp. 149–156

Hare, M. 1986 Mental illness in the elderly. In *Physiotherapy in Psychiatry,* Heinemann, London, pp. 66–93

Henson, R.A. (1977) Neurological aspects of musical experience. In *Music and the Brain. Studies in the Neurology of Music* (eds Critchley, M. and Henson, R.A.), Heinemann, London, pp. 233–254

Hope, R.A. and Fairburn, C.G. (1990) The nature of wandering in dementia: a community based study. *International Journal of Geriatric Psychiatry,* **5**, 239–245

Huff, F.J. and Growdon, J.H. (1986) Neurological abnormalities associated with severity of dementia in Alzheimer's disease. *Canadian Journal Neurological Sciences,* **13**, 403–405

Huppert, F.A. and Tym, E. (1986) Clinical and neuropsychological assessment of dementia. *British Medical Bulletin,* **42**, 11–18

Jarvik, L.F. and Wiseman, E.J. (1991) A checklist for managing the dementia patient. *Geriatrics,* **46**, 31–40

Joachin, C.L., Morris, J.H. and Selkoe, D.J. (1988) Clinically diagnosed Alzheimer's disease: autopsy results in 150 cases. *Annals of Neurology,* **24**, 50–56

Kitwood, T. (1990) The dialectics of dementia: with particular reference to Alzheimer's Disease. *Ageing and Society,* **10**, 177–196

Knill, C. (1983) Body awareness communication and development: a programme employing music with the profoundly handicapped. *International Journal of Rehabilitation Research,* **6**, 489–492

Knopman, D.S. and Sawyer-DeMaris, S. (1990) Practical approach to managing behavioural problems in dementia patients. *Geriatrics,* **45**, 27–35

Levy, R., Issacs, A. and Hawks, F. (1970) Neurophysiological correlates of senile dementia. 1 Motor and sensory nerve conduction velocity. *Psychological Medicine,* **1**, 40–47

Mayeux, R., Stern, Y. and Spanton, S. (1985) Heterogeneity in dementia of the Alzheimer type: evidence of subgroups. *Neurology,* **35**, 453–461

Milne, J.S and Maule, M.M. (1984) A longitudinal study of handgrip and dementia in older people. *Age and Ageing,* **13**, 42–48

Molsa, P.K., Marttila, R.J. and Rinne, U.K. (1982) Extrapyramidal symptoms in dementia. *Acta Neurologica Scandinavica,* **90**, (Supl.), 298–299

Molsa, P.K., Sako, E., Paljarvi, L. *et al.* (1987) Alzheimer's disease: neuropathological correlates of cognitive and motor disorders. *Acta Neurologica Scandinavica,* **75**, 376–384

Needler, W. and Baer, M.A. (1982) Movement, music, and remotivation with the regressed elderly. *Journal of Gerontological Nursing,* **8**, 497–503

Nieuwboer, A.M. (1992) Attitudes towards working with older patients: physiotherapist's responses to video presentations of post-amputation gait training for an older and a younger patient. *Physiotherapy Theory and Practice,* **8**, 27–37

Norberg, A., Melin, E. and Asplund, K. (1986) Reactions to music, touch and object presentation in the final stage of dementia. An exploratory study. *International Journal of Nursing Studies,* **3**, 315–323

Oddy, R. (1987) Promoting mobility in patients with dementia: some suggested strategies for physiotherapists. *Physiotherapy Practice,* **3**, 18–27

Pomeroy, V. (1990) Development of an ADL orientated assessment of mobility scale suitable for use with elderly people with dementia. *Physiotherapy,* **76**, 446–448

Pomeroy, V.M. (1993) The effect of physiotherapy input on mobility skills of elderly people with severe dementing illness. *Clinical Rehabilitation,* **7**, 163–170

Pomeroy, V.M. (1994) Mobility, dementia and rehabilitation. *Physiotherapy Theory and Practice,* **10**, 35–43

Pomeroy, V.M. (1994) Immobility and severe dementia. When is physiotherapy treatment appropriate? *Clinical Rehabilitation,* **8**, 226–232

Pope, P.M. (1988) A model for evaluation of input in relation to outcome in severely brain damaged patients. *Physiotherapy,* **74**, 647–650

Price, A. (1977) Sensory integration in occupational therapy. *American Journal of Occupational Therapy,* **31**, 287–289

Richman, L. (1969) Sensory training for geriatric patients. *American Journal of Occupational Therapy,* **23**, 254–257

Risse, S.C., Lampe, T.H., Bird, T.D. *et al.* (1990) Myoclonus, seizures and paratonia in Alzheimer's disease. *Alzheimer Disease and Related Disorders,* **4**, 217–225

Ross, M. and Burdick, D. (1981) *A Training Manual for Therapists and Teachers for Regressed Psychiatric and Geriatric Patient Groups,* Slack, Thorofare, New Jersey

Rovner, B.W., Lucas-Blaustein, J., Folstein, M.F. *et al.* (1990) Stability over one year in patients admitted to a nursing home dementia unit. *International Journal of Geriatric Psychiatry,* **5**, 77–82

Sjogren, H. (1950) Twenty four cases of Alzheimer's disease. A clinical analysis. *Acta Medica Scandinavica,* **246** (suppl. 1), 225–233

Stewart, D.A., Burns, J.M.A., Dunn, S.G. *et al.* (1990) The two-minute walking test: a sensitive index of mobility in the rehabilitation of elderly patients. *Clinical Rehabilitation,* **4**, 273–276

Streiner, D.L. and Norman, G.R. (1989) *Health Measurement Scales. A Practical Guide to their Development and Use,* Oxford University Press, Oxford

Tanner, B.B. and Daniels, K.A. (1990) An observation study of communication between carers and their relatives in dementia. *Care of the Elderly,* **2**, 247–250

VanSant, A.F. (1990) Lifespan development in functional tasks. *Physical Therapy,* **70**, 788–798

Visser, H. (1983) Gait and balance in senile dementia of Alzheimer's type. *Age and Ageing,* **12**, 296–301

Wade, D.T. (1992) *Measurement in Neurological Rehabilitation,* Oxford Medical Publications, Oxford

Wade, J.P.H., Mirsen, T.R., Hachinski, V.C. *et al,* (1987) The clinical diagnosis of Alzheimer's disease. *Archives of Neurology,* **44**, 24–29

Wolfe, J.R. (1983) The use of music in a group sensory training programme for regressed geriatric patients. *Activities, Adaptations and Ageing,* **4**, 49–62

23

Mental illness in old age

Lynne Kendall

Introduction

This chapter inevitably overlaps with other chapters. For example, Chapter 22 is devoted to dementia which is often the first psychiatric condition thought of when considering elderly people's mental health. Other psychiatric disorders and their treatment are also dealt with elsewhere in this book. So what is the purpose of devoting a separate chapter to 'Mental illness in old age'? What difference does age make when considering mental illness?

There are very many significant circumstantial changes associated with the onset of old age, e.g. changes in financial and social status, and in physical health. While these changes by no means occur automatically with increasing age, they do tend to occur more commonly and have a very significant effect on life within an older age group. Of course, all elderly people will react differently to these changes. How they react depends on many factors, but principally on the way that they have learnt to deal with problems in their younger years. All elderly people will have spent a lifetime dealing with a variety of problems and difficulties, and the way they face old age will depend crucially on what they have learnt from those experiences. This means that each aging person will bring a characteristic response to the process of aging; some will bring wisdom, openness, flexibility, gentleness and kindness; others will bring prejudice, dissatisfaction, rigidity, frustration and aggression.

For most people, however they come to terms with the aging process, all these changes will not result in any form of mental illness. But there are those for whom the changes may trigger a temporary or even long-term mental illness. There are also those people who were already suffering some form of mental illness and for whom old age brings added complications which are hard to deal with and may exacerbate their existing condition.

Changing services

Care and treatment of mentally ill patients in large psychiatric institutions is now almost at an end in Britain and the implementation of the Care in the Community Act is aimed at providing care for people in their own homes wherever possible. In most areas this has led to a closing or reduction in care given in these institutions. Much effort is made to enable people to remain in their own homes and a part of this has been the formation of Community Mental Health teams. For those for whom it is not possible to remain in their own home, then ideally care is provided in small units close to their own home. The involvement of the private sector in the provision of this care is variable according to geographical area.

Even more variable is the provision of physiotherapy to this client group. When care was provided in centralized, large institutions, many had a physiotherapy department of some description, and most were staffed by physiotherapists who had some experience of working in psychiatry and were in constant contact with other disciplines from whom they could learn more. This was a two-way process where other staff could learn from the physiotherapist's expertise in the physical field. However, such physiotherapists were relatively small in number, and in many areas the decentralization of services has meant that this expertise and experience has become very thinly spread and may not be available at all. Decentralization has, however, meant the growth of more generic community physiotherapy services. It is important that the physiotherapists providing this service are not reluctant or fearful of becoming professionally involved with mentally ill people. They need to have an understanding of the problems of elderly people with mental illness and realize the potential for effective physiotherapy intervention, provided that a good relationship can be developed between physiotherapist and client.

The psychiatric team and facilities for the elderly

The concept of the multidisciplinary team is, in most areas, well established in the field of mental illness in elderly people. The potential for complicated multipathology within this field, coupled with a possible myriad of social problems, means that there is likely to be a large number of different services and people involved with the client. The core psychiatric team would normally be made up of representatives of the following professions: medical, nursing, occupational therapy, physiotherapy, psychology, social work. While the primary medical input would come from a psychiatrist, there must be close involvement from a physician in geriatric medicine.

The team should function both in the hospital setting and in the community and, if possible, cross the boundaries between hospital and local authority services so that local authority social workers can be as much members of the team as health service workers. The management of the physiotherapy input depends very much on local arrangements, but ideally a physiotherapist experienced in this field should be available in all the settings that the rest of the team service. It is important that the physiotherapist should have an in-depth working knowledge of psychiatry and close, supportive relationships with other members of the team.

Many areas now have Community Mental Health teams, some working in Community Mental Health centres and some in general practices. The remit of some of these teams is to assess, treat and support elderly people with mental illness, dealing both with clients with organic psychiatric problems (dementia, acute confusional states, etc.) and functional psychiatric problems (depression, anxiety, schizophrenia, etc.). Clients are sometimes seen first in their own home or at the general practice. There are then a whole range of possible locations for ongoing assessment/treatment if this is appropriate: client's home, general practice, Community Mental Health centre, day centre, day hospital, hospital ward. If the referral to the team was prompted by a crisis in the client's condition or behaviour, then the initial assessment and treatment may be more appropriately undertaken as a hospital inpatient. The team should also be able to offer advice and treatment in residential and nursing homes.

It may be that treatment as such is either inappropriate or not possible, in which case social/physical support is the main issue, and the team will become involved in a multidisciplinary assessment of the client's needs in order to remain in their own home, or assessment for appropriate placement elsewhere. At the moment, availability of the necessary support varies considerably with geographical area, but the use of services such as night and day sitters, and respite/programmed care are certainly well used where they are available. Admissions for respite care are sometimes useful for reassessment by a physiotherapist and more intensive episodes of physiotherapy treatment if appropriate.

Functional psychiatric problems

Dementia has been dealt with elsewhere in this book, so there is no need to touch on the subject in detail here. Similarly other psychiatric disorders have been described, but there is a need to discuss the implications of these functional disorders occurring in old age.

Depression

Seligman (1975) describes depression as the common cold of psychiatry, and it is the most common psychiatric disorder in old age (Gurland and Toner, 1982). Changes in lifestyle, loss of role, changes in social circumstances, loss of relatives or old friends, and physical illness or disability, are all possible occurrences in old age, and may be expected to lead to a natural sadness or sense of bereavement. However, there is always a danger than an elderly person's family, friends and even their GP may take this negative emotional state as inevitable and not register the transition to a clinical and treatable depression. If this delay in diagnosis persists, it can become life-threatening.

There is a particularly close association between physical illness and depressive reactions in old age (Pfeiffer and Busse, 1973). Older persons seem to tolerate the loss of close relatives and prestige better than a decline in physical health (Busse, 1965). Professor Elaine Murphy states that physical illness of a severe, chronic kind likely to shorten life and affect adversely the quality of life of the older person is found in up to 60% of elderly patients suffering from depression (Murphy, 1984). She goes on to suggest that prevention of physical illness and the alleviation of accompanying handicaps might have substantial impact on the occurrence of depression in the elderly.

Of course, once clinical depression is present, the associated reduction in activity and loss of motivation can exacerbate the original physical problem, thus leading to a deteriorating downward spiral.

CASE STUDY 1. Until the age of 72, Mr Jones had enjoyed very good health, and being an enthusiastic golfer he was very fit for his age. He then developed osteoarthritis of the right knee and was soon unable to pursue his golf which was his only hobby and motivation to exercise. After 6 months of being relatively inactive and spending most of his time at home, he underwent a total knee replacement and was discharged from hospital with a regimen of exercises to follow at home. It had not been noticed that, during his enforced inactivity before surgery, Mr Jones had become depressed and was therefore insufficiently motivated to carry out his home exercises. As his right leg consequently became more wasted, his knee became more painful and so his depression grew worse. Eventually he was admitted to a psychiatric ward where the physiotherapist worked with the other staff to combine a graduated, supervised exercise regimen with pharmacological treatment of his depression. Within 3 months he was able to resume his golf.

Conversely, it is possible that an elderly person may be diagnosed as being depressed when there is actually an underlying physical condition presenting with similar symptoms to that of depression. For instance, the decreased mobility, weakness and slowness caused by congestive heart failure may resemble the physical signs of depression, or the mask-like face and decreased speech often associated with Parkinson's disease may be mistaken for poverty of thought or negativism. Therefore, physiotherapists working with depressed patients should be alert to the possibilities of other physical causes of these symptoms and if they have any doubts they must have the confidence to discuss these with the relevant medical staff.

Elderly people are particularly likely to be taking drugs as treatment for a medical condition and may display depressive side effects and unwanted toxic effects of the drugs. Drugs used to treat a wide variety of medical conditions are capable of producing central nervous system symptoms or mood depression, and diagnosis of depression in an elderly person should include a careful evaluation of concurrent medication. Elderly people are also likely to be taking several drugs at once and interaction between drugs can sometimes produce depressive states.

While evidence for an increasing suicide rate with increasing age is inconclusive (Stenback, 1980) older people as a group tend to have a higher rate of fatal suicide attempts in relation to non-fatal attempts (Gurland and Cross, 1983). Therefore, should an elderly client express suicidal thoughts to a physiotherapist, it is essential that this is taken seriously and advice sought from the relevant medical officer.

In some areas, severe, life-threatening depression may be treated with electroconvulsive therapy carried out under general anaesthetic. This may have physiotherapeutic implications in helping to prepare the patient for anaesthetic and in dealing with any possible respiratory after-effects.

Anxiety/hypochondriasis

Anxiety reactions in older persons may be a continuation of the pattern of a lifetime or may be the reaction to losses occurring in later life (Gurland and Cross, 1983). Anxiety in old age can arise from the fear of losing control or mastery of one's life. Linked with this is the fear of becoming a burden and the ensuing fear of being abandoned. An elderly person may be filled with anxious depression when realization occurs that time is insufficient to achieve goals set earlier in life.

The physical symptoms of anxiety, e.g. breathlessness, palpitations, headaches, muscular aches and pains, can increase the feeling of fear of physical illness and frailty. It is important that a physiotherapist is able to reassure clients with such symptoms by giving clear simple explanations of those symptoms and teaching effective relaxation techniques to help reduce them. The physiotherapist has an important role to play in assessing and advising on the client's potential to improve their physical abilities and in guiding and assisting the client in maximizing this potential.

Hypochondriacal complaints sometimes seem to be a means of communicating the need for support and attention by older people. It has been frequently found that, while the basic problems of older persons may be social, economic, or related to the external environment, the person communicates the problem as a bodily complaint (Blum and Weiner, 1979). The physiotherapist should remember that, while they may not be able to find a significant physical cause of the reported symptoms, those symptoms, nevertheless remain very real to the client and should be approached with empathy and understanding, while helping the multidisciplinary team investigate the underlying non-physical problem.

Schizophrenia and late life paranoid states

A physiotherapist working in psychiatry is likely to encounter a proportion of elderly patients who have suffered from chronic schizophrenia since early adulthood. While treatment is likely to continue in a similar way to earlier life, persons who were hospitalized for long periods of time may have severe behavioural deficits in addition to their thought disorder. They may need more help in meeting the everyday demands of elderly life, such as physical illness, bereavement and social changes. Many who spent long periods in institutions may have inherited some physical consequences of the lifestyle that institutionalization included. Many long-term patients were very heavy smokers and now suffer consequent respiratory and cardiovascular disorders, which may require physiotherapy interventions. Very few had access to or were motivated to make use of opportunities for regular exercise and may therefore be more prone to heart disease, high blood pressure and joint stiffness. Some may suffer the long-term effects of past episodes of self-harm or even injuries caused by other patients.

It is possible for an elderly person to develop a late onset paranoid state. Indeed, paranoid reactions show an increased incidence in old age (Post, 1980; Butler and Lewis, 1982). This may accompany either acute confusional states, including those brought about by toxic levels of medication, or senile dementia. Some people always tend to blame others if things go wrong. Elderly people with this kind of personality are very likely to accuse other people of stealing from them or interfering with their property if they become forgetful. Two other factors in the aetiology of late life paranoid states are social isolation and sensory losses. The prior social adjustment of many paranoid patients has often been poor, and it appears that deafness and paranoid reactions are particularly related (Post, 1980; Zimbardo *et al.*, 1981). Hallucinations and delusions frequently include the hearing of voices via a hearing aid, or the belief that someone is to influence or harm the patient by directing radio waves or gases at a hearing aid.

Such delusions often result in intense suspicion of attempts at treatment for whatever purpose, even to the extent of refusing food and drink which is believed to be poisoned. This can sometimes severely hamper attempts at physiotherapy treatment and it is vital that the physiotherapist concerned be fully informed of the nature of any such delusions, so that treatment attempts can be tailored to avoid conflict and suspicion. For example, it would be very unwise to attempt a form of electrical treatment with a patient suffering from paranoid delusions.

Substance misuse

Although this area has been covered in Chapter 19, there are implications very specific to elderly persons.

Alcoholism in an elderly person may be of chronic, long-standing duration, or it may be of recent onset. When it occurs as a late onset disorder, it may be due to age-related stresses or the removal of work-related constraints on drinking (Simon, 1980). Based on community surveys, it has been estimated that between 2% and 10% of elderly people are alcoholics, with the figures higher for widowed persons and those having medical problems (Schuckit, 1977). Alcoholism can be complicated by the special physical and psychological problems of old age and is often an unrecognized and therefore untreated problem of older people because of its confusion with other age-related disorders such as dementia (Wood, 1978; Simon, 1980).

Physiotherapists may encounter elderly patients suffering from a variety of neurological symptoms and syndromes caused by alcohol abuse, such as peripheral neuropathy, and cerebellar and cerebral degeneration involving both mobility and cognitive problems. As a member of the multidisciplinary team, the physiotherapist should be aware of alcohol abuse as the potential cause of the physical symptoms referred for treatment and report back to the rest of the team should there be a suspicion that this may be the underlying problem.

The term 'drug abuse' can be synonymous with drug misuse. The adverse effects of drugs on an elderly person can be a result of a deliberate act on that person's part, or the inadvertent, inappropriate use of drugs intended for therapeutic purposes. Recent research has shown elderly persons as over-users of medication and their physicians as over-prescribers (Whittington, 1983). Older people are more vulnerable to the inapproapriate use of drugs, as they are more likely to have concurrent medical problems for which they are taking potentially interacting medication, and may have physiological changes which alter the action of drugs in their body.

Sleep disorders

Many psychiatric conditions include alterations in sleep patterns and, generally speaking, people need less sleep as they age. This is sometimes associated with a reduction in physical activity, and physiotherapy can have a part to play in providing more opportunity for such activity, or in reassuring the client that the change in their sleep pattern is a normal response to their changing lifestyle. However, some form of relaxation may also be useful.

Death and dying

Old age is a time of reduced physiological function, but a proportion of the general population has an exaggerated view of the physical deterioration that should be expected as inevitable with aging. Some elderly people find themselves becoming progressively more anxious about their health and the possibility of death. As death still tends to be a taboo subject, an elderly person may not have the opportunity to express their fears, and therefore may not receive the subsequent reassurance that expression of those fears may bring. A physiotherapist is often in the privileged position of being able to help an elderly patient address those fears by using their professional standing to dispel some of the myths surrounding aging. However, when there is genuine physical deterioration, it is the author's experience that an elderly person usually appreciates and respects a physiotherapist as the major source of realistic and truthful information about their physical health.

Grief and mourning

The loss of a loved one, particularly a spouse, is a highly stressful event that has been found to be associated with an increased incidence of physical and mental symptoms. It is postulated that such loss and the subsequent problems in re-adjustment make the bereaved more vulnerable to a variety of disease processes (Rahe, 1972). Therefore, the physiotherapist may encounter recently bereaved patients, possibly suffering from a severe depressive reaction, coupled with one or more physical complaints, needing treatment. It is likely that the patient may find the physical treatment acts as a catalyst to the release of many previously suppressed emotions such as guilt, resentment and anger which need to be dealt with openly and empathically. Should the physiotherapist not feel able to deal with such a release of emotion adequately, it is vital that another member of the multidisciplinary team be called to help support the patient. As in all areas of psychiatry, a physiotherapist will find a grounding in counselling skills invaluable when working in this area.

The role of physiotherapy

The physiotherapist

The role of physiotherapy in the care of elderly mentally ill people overlaps greatly with that of physiotherapy in general care of the elderly and that in psychiatry with younger patients, as well as that with elderly people suffering from dementia. It is an intricate field, where the potential for physical pathology can be complicated or even masked by psychiatric functional behavioural problems. No one person can be expert in all the problems faced by patients in this area, which is why it is so vital that the physiotherapist works closely as part of the multidisciplinary team, supporting and being supported by the other team members. The ultimate aim has to be to pool the skills of all disciplines to provide the highest standard of diagnosis and care/treatment possible for each individual client.

Many surveys of perceptions of the personality traits of older people, carried out with all age groups under the age of 50 (Aaronson, 1966; McTavish, 1971; Braceland, 1972), have shown that younger people tend to consider older people as stubborn, touchy, bossy, complaining, incompetent, passive, dependent, rigid, extreme in behaviour, bored, indolent, resigned and lacking in trust. Ageism in our society is being increasingly recognized as a powerful influence, developing a stereotype of 'old people' which diminishes and undermines their social status. Elderly people are often represented as physically and mentally frail, rigid in their thinking and immutably set in their ways.

There is no factual evidence to support this. Contrary to the prevailing public, and in some cases, professional stereotypes of the aged personality, there is no universal trend towards change in personality traits in the transition from middle to old age. This has been shown to be true by research based on many studies of healthy, aged persons living outside of institutions (Reichard *et al.*, 1962; Britton and Britton, 1972; Schaie and Parham, 1976). Psychological studies indicate that the incidence of most personality traits is the same in old age as in younger years. Therefore, adjustments to old age is often influenced by patterns established in earlier years.

It is extremely important that any physiotherapist working in any field with older people has examined their own beliefs about elderly people and can say with total honesty that they do not bring any preconceived ideas or prejudices into their work. This is even more important when working with elderly people with mental illness, as so much of the work is concerned with multidisciplinary assessment of a client's problems and pathology, and we must be sure that this is not influenced by unfounded ideas about what is 'normal' in an elderly person.

The role of the physiotherapist within the team is as follows:

- to assess and treat appropriately specific physical pathologies with traditional physiotherapeutic techniques
- to assist in the assessment of the degree of functional limitation resulting from physical pathology and that resulting from a psychiatric condition
- to advise the multidisciplinary team of the functional ability it would be reasonable to expect individual clients to achieve in various circumstances
- to participate in the goal-setting process
- to participate in team treatment programmes, e.g. behavioural therapy, stress management
- to use physiotherapeutic techniques to improve the psychological health of patients
- to use physiotherapy to maintain physical and psychological health
- to educate and advise other team members, patients, other physiotherapists and the general public in the role and value of physiotherapy in the field of mental illness in old age.

Physical assessment

When dealing with elderly patients in psychiatry, the medical assessment is obviously vital in eliminating physical pathology which may be the cause of psychiatric problems. However, in dealing with functional psychiatric disorders, there are many grey areas in which physiotherapy assessment has a major part to play in assisting the multidisciplinary team in formulating a complete picture of the patient's problems. Without the complete picture, it is very difficult to plan a treatment programme with realistic and relevent goals.

The most common area for physiotherapy involvement is in assessment of physical function, especially in relation to pain, musculoskeletal or neurological disorders. First, there is a need to establish whether or not there is a genuine physical reason for a patient's functional limitation and, more importantly, to qualify this limitation. The author's experience has shown that it is not enough, when dealing with elderly people simply to say a patient can or cannot peform a particular activity. Account must be taken of variations in ability according to time of day, other recent activity, interval since last dose of medication, height of furniture available, etc. This is particularly important for the rest of the multidisciplinary team to know, especially psychiatrically trained nurses and therapists who may not have the depth of physical knowledge to appreciate the theories of muscle fatigue, disinhibition of reflexes, overnight stiffening of joints, facilitation of normal movement, etc.

CASE STUDY 2. Mrs Edwards was admitted from a residential home to hospital for psychiatric assessment. She was known to suffer from Parkinson's disease, but was usually able to dress independently and was mobile around the home with minimal assistance. In recent weeks she had 'refused' to get out of bed in the morning and care staff needed to give considerable assistance with dressing. It was only after great 'persuasion' on the part of the staff that Mrs Edwards would begin to 'make an effort'. The day after admission, a physiotherapy assessment concluded that Mrs Edwards was still physically capable of the level of self-care previously reported, and it was suspected that there was an underlying psychological reason for the reduction in function in the home. However, when the hospital staff reported that this lady professed to be very happy with the residential home and made every effort to be independent and co-operative, it was hard to believe that the reported problems really existed. The physiotherapist decided to make further enquiries of the residential home. It transpired that there had been a change of routine at the home. Previously, residents had received a cup of tea and the first dose of any medication before getting out of bed in the morning. The new routine meant that getting out of bed became the first activity of the day and, not having had medication for her Parkinson's disease, Mrs Edwards was less able to do this unaided, whereas on the hospital ward she received her medication first and therefore was able to comply. The delay in the first dose of medication also resulted in reduction in facial expression and communication which the home's staff had interpreted as withdrawal and stubbornness. Mrs Edwards returned to the home which reverted to the original routine and no further investigations were necessary.

It is hardly ever possible to make a full and thorough assessment of a patient with a functional psychiatric disorder in one session, and sometimes several sessions are necessary to be sure that the assessment is accurate. An anxious, depressed or paranoid patient may take quite some time to feel comfortable enough with a new person to be willing to have their abilities tested. It may be that their physical symptoms have been challenged by professionals several times in the past and the patient may be feeling resentful and defensive about yet another assessment, however kindly presented and well motivated that assessment might be.

Time is never wasted in this area, when taken to form a friendly and trusting relationship with the client. Whatever the conclusion drawn from the final assessment, results of future work with the client will depend very much on the relationship built up during the assessment period. Therefore, despite the pressures of our modern working environment, time should always be taken to get to know the client, their family relationships, life history, view of his past and present life and regrets, pleasures and aspirations for the future. An outline of this can be obtained from other members of the team, but there is no substitute for discussing this with the client, if they feel comfortable in doing so.

Even if it is felt that there is no genuine physical cause for the client's functional limitation, or that those limitations are more than would normally be expected, the client should be told this, but in a supportive, non-judgmental way. It should be made clear that, whatever the cause of their problems, the physiotherapist is there to work with them to overcome those problems, or at least to minimize them.

Where there is no underlying physical pathology, it is important to note any secondary effects of a reduction in function and activity, e.g. muscle wasting, soft-tissue shortening, contractures, etc. It is vital that psychiatrically trained staff working with the client have the implications of these secondary effects explained to them, as they can very easily assume that the lack of a primary physical pathology means that any inability on the patient's part is entirely behavioural in origin, when this is not necessarily so.

CASE STUDY 3. While resident in the North of England, Mrs Foster had complained of diverse recurrent joint pains which her GP had suggested may be some form of arthritis, for which he would carry out tests should it occur again. Before these tests could be done, Mrs Foster moved house to a town several hundred miles away, but carried with her the idea that her continually recurring pains were due to arthritis. As these painful episodes became more frequent she naturally reduced her activity to try to reduce the pain. This situation deteriorated very rapidly, to the point where she was not eating adequately and was neglecting her hygiene because moving to do so was too painful. Eventually she was admitted to a psychiatric ward where she was initially, thoroughly medically screened. On admission, the nursing staff were happy to help her with all her physical needs and activities for the short time until it was decided by the medical staff that there was no physical pathology causing her pain. At this time they withdrew all physical assistance and told Mrs Foster that she was perfectly capable of looking after herself. The medical staff referred this lady to the physiotherapist for assessment and this revealed extensive disuse muscle wasting and early contracture of both knees which meant that she had a genuine functional limitation, even though these changes were secondary to her belief in the arthritis, rather than a primary physical pathology.

There then followed a period of intense education of the nursing staff, by the physiotherapist, coupled with detailed documentation of the patient's true functional abilities according to what other activities she had already undertaken which may have caused fatigue. A graduated exercise programme helped restore muscle strength and joint range. It was eventually decided that the joint pain was due to tension-related postural changes, and a team approach by nurses, physiotherapist and psychologist using counselling, relaxation and posture correction gradually reduced the pain to tolerable levels so that Mrs Foster could resume a relatively normal life.

Goal-setting

Obviously, if there is a real physical problem which is likely to respond to physiotherapy, then the first part of the goal-setting process is to explain to the client exactly what the physical problem is and how physiotherapy might help. As in all fields of physiotherapy, it is important to describe the client's part in the process of recovery and the extent of their responsibility for this process. However, it is vital to emphasize that the physiotherapist will be there to guide and support them through that process and will be feeding back reports of their progress to the rest of the team.

If there is no primary physical problem, then there should be a detailed multi-disciplinary discussion about the client's problems and needs, from which should come the aims of physiotherapy involvement in the client's treatment, e.g. to provide a suitable exercise programme to help promote relief from tension, and increase confidence and self-esteem.

It is essential that the whole team have a uniform and consistent approach in their dealings with clients so that they feel secure and not confused, e.g. when a client complains that they find it too difficult to perform a specific activity, should staff give minimal help with lots of encouragement, or should they insist on the client persevering unaided? The policy needs to be recorded in the care plan and adhered to without exception, if changes in behaviour are to be achieved.

A client should feel that they have a part to play in any goal-setting process, and those goals should be relevant to the client in order to ensure ongoing motivation for involvement and co-operation.

CASE STUDY 4. Mr Harper had been admitted to a small assessment unit for elderly patients with functional psychiatric disorders. He was 78 years old and lived with his 75-year-old wife. He had been a very active man all his life and a keen walker, until 4 years previously when he developed low back pain and X-rays showed mild degenerative changes in the lumbar spine. He found it very hard to accept the reduction in activity caused by his back pain and gradually became depressed, morose and withdrawn until his wife had to care for him completely.

Physiotherapy assessment revealed a marked decrease in Mr Harper's lumbar lordosis with other associated postural changes which could be expected to cause diffuse aches and pains, but with great potential for improvement with treatment using exercise, postural correction and education in back care. It seemed that, as often happens, Mr Harper's GP, not realizing the impact it would have on Mr Harper, had told him that he had signs of wear and tear in his lower back which would probably get worse and was not curable. This was the first time Mr Harper had been confronted with the vulnerability of his ailing body. The physiotherapist explained her findings to both the client and the nursing staff, including her theory that it was probably the reduced activity caused by the depression which had worsened the physical symptoms. When seeking realistic goals for future treatment, it was not possible to predict whether return to walking very long distances was likely to be achievable and was therefore dismissed as an unrealistic initial goal.

Mr Harper had also been a keen gardener and had expressed a wish to be able to get out in his garden, but when this was suggested as an initial goal it was dismissed as unrealistic by the client himself. His depression was such that he could not envisage his pain reducing sufficiently for him to be able to do this. Eventually he agreed to set an initial goal of being able to walk comfortably the length of the corridor in the ward. Because he was able to concede that this might just be possible, he was well motivated to persevere with the exercise programme. Once he could see that the first goal had been achieved relatively easily, he became quite enthusiastic about setting further goals.

Treatment

Any elderly person with mental illness may also be suffering from a physical problem sometimes associated with old age, e.g. osteoarthritis, CVA, Parkinson's disease, respiratory disease, or a fall resulting in a fracture or other injury. There may be a physical problem as a side effect of medication or as a result of self-harm or self-neglect. Whatever the physical pathology is, the general principles of physiotherapy intervention remain the same as for any other client group. The method of this intervention, however, may have to be adapted on occasions.

As already mentioned, careful consideration should be given to the effect any sort of electrical treatment may have on the psychological state of a paranoid patient. Indeed, great care should be taken that any form of treatment or activity is not perceived as a threat by the client.

A depressed or anxious patient may be poorly motivated, and they are un-likely to respond to misguided overenthusiasm and unrealistic goal-setting. A low-key, gradual approach is much more likely to suceed. It may even be necessary to let the client just sit quietly and watch other people having physio-therapy before they will agree to participate themselves. This can seem to be inappropriate in today's climate of striving to achieve cost-effective, speedy treatment outcomes. But with this particular client group, a little time taken to win someone's trust can be very effective in achieving long-term gains.

An anxious patient with low self-esteem desperately needs achievable goals to aim for, and consistent reinforcement of any signs of improvement. This requires infinite patience on the part of the physiotherapist and can be quite wearing at times. So it is useful if more than one member of the physiotherapy department can be involved with the client to provide a supportive environment for the staff.

There is also a part for physiotherapy to play in helping to improve the client's psychiatric problems.

Exercise

A prime example is the use of exercise in the alleviation of anxiety and depression (Greist *et al.*, 1979; Ledwidge, 1980). Laboratory research has indicated that improvement in fitness level allows an individual to cope better with emotional stress (Keller, 1980). Jasneski *et al.* (1981) found that some of the important personal changes associated with physical fitness training, such as improvement in self-perceived abilities and confidence, are partly due to group participation. Chastain and Shapiro (1987) found that psychiatric patients having difficulty with self-esteem and body image, who join a physical fitness programme, can achieve a sense of accomplishment that is often elusive in other aspects of psychiatric care.

Therefore, it seems that some form of moderate aerobic exercise, preferably with the socialization effect of a group setting, can be very therapeutic. Yet we must be sensitive to the fact that we may be dealing with some people for whom physical exercise other than work has never played a part in their life, or whose body image would make the idea of exercising in front of other people abhorrent. It is easy to allow an exercise group to deteriorate into a patronizing, childish situation, which should be avoided at all costs.

The author's experience is that elderly people appreciate exercise to music when an effort is made to bring it as close as possible to dance. Games are quite successful in motivating participants as long as they are reasonably adult in nature, e..g. carpet bowls, target bowls, giant dice games involving simple calculations, seated indoor hockey, ball games involving sequences and counting.

It is often beneficial to introduce activities that require some form of group co-ordination and co-operation, but where less able members can be discreetly helped by more able members of the group, e.g. tasks using the Lanmoor activity canopy. This is a large circle of brightly coloured parachute material which has canvas handles around its circumference. The group can be asked to throw a light ball up and down on it, or to co-ordinate its movements to make the ball travel around the circle. There are many imaginative combinations of movement that the group can be asked to do, in both sitting or standing, according to the client group's capabilities.

Exercise circuits are usually associated with young and active people, but such a circuit can be devised for less active patients, from those who can walk independently to those who must remain seated. These circuits are useful in allowing a client to repeat standard tasks on a regular basis and so monitor their own improvement. In this setting, however, it is usually wise to actively discourage comparison and competition between individuals.

Relaxation

Although exercise has been researched as an effective form of relaxation, there are some elderly people who are too physically unwell to exercise sufficiently to produce significant reduction in tension, or some who just do not feel able to cope psychologically with exercise. Therefore, it is often useful to introduce specific relaxation techniques. Mary Hare states that relaxation therapy is important in helping to alleviate the symptoms of anxiety, and the method of relaxation to suit the client should be taught and applied both as a method of resting and for use in problem situations (Hare, 1986). The chapter goes on to say that it is best if the physiotherapist can acquaint herself with several different ways of teaching relaxation. While she may then tend to favour one method and use it predominantly, clients who do not respond can be found an alternative.

A physiotherapist with an in-depth knowledge of the musculoskeletal system is well placed to teach relaxation techniques, although other professionals may teach them just as competently, and this duty is often shared within the multi-disciplinary team. However, a physiotherapist's expertise in the physical field can provide invaluable advice on how to adapt relaxation methods in order to accommodate physical pathologies, e.g. a client with respiratory disease will not be able to lie flat for relaxation sessions.

Traditional methods of relaxation, which are well documented are Jacobsen's Contrast Technique (Jacobsen, 1938), the Laura Mitchell method (Mitchell, 1977), yoga (Silva and Mehta, 1990) and breathing techniques (Lumm, 1977; Cluff, 1984). Other alternatives are the Whitchurch method (Ricketts and Cross, 1985), the Alexander technique (Alexander and Maisel, 1975; Gelb, 1987). Meditation (Fenwick, 1973, 1983; Camp, 1973; Bloomfield *et al.*, 1975; Paterson, 1979; Benson, 1980), autogenic training (Schultz and Luthe, 1969), imagery and t'ai chi (Soo, 1984). A very popular and effective form of relaxation among this elderly client group is massage, particularly for those who have stiff and painful joints or fibromyalgia (Lidell *et al.*, 1984) – see Chapter 12.

It must be remembered that, as in many other areas of mental health, the relationship with the client is all important. There may be times when the physiotherapist, through no personal fault, finds it impossible to form a relationship with a particular client. In these circumstances it might be beneficial to introduce some modified form of therapeutic intervention via a third party, such as a psychiatric nurse or a relative. The closer the working relationships within the multidisciplinary team, the more easily this can be achieved.

Care in the community

It is vital that health care professionals have close working relationships with social services teams, especially in light of the community care legislation which came into operation in April 1993. Social services departments are responsible for the assessment of the need for care, the purchasing of care from a range of service providers and for arranging further specialist assessment and management if it is thought necessary. Effective co-operation between community mental health teams and social services staff is essential to enable elderly people who have both mental health problems and functional impairment to be cared for in the community or, if necessary, have ready access to high-quality, appropriate residential care. This co-operation and liaison is inevitably better in some areas than others.

The geographical distribution of private sector residential and nursing homes can be somewhat uneven, and in areas of over-provision, price cutting may lead to a drop in quality of care, home closures, or a reluctance to accept patients with a history of mental illness as they may present with more complex future management problems and require higher staffing levels.

This volatile, changeable provision by the private sector makes it very difficult for statutory health and social care bodies to plan their own future provision accurately (Murphy and Banerjee, 1993).

Most elderly people with mental health problems present to and are managed by GPs, and 71% of mental health team community psychiatric nurses regularly work in surgeries and health centres (Banerjee *et al.,* 1993). Therefore it is important that GPs and CPNs have easy access to very experienced community physiotherapists, at least, if not to a physiotherapist specializing in mental health, in order to make full assessments of their clients problems and needs. The shift of focus of physiotherapy from hospital to community must continue.

Conclusion

In recent years, not only has there been a shift of care of all mentally ill clients from large psychiatric institutions into smaller units and into the community, but in the case of the elderly mentally ill there has been a major transfer of some remaining beds into district general hospitals (Schulman and Arie, 1991). This move recognizes the great relationship between physical and mental disorders in elderly people, the need for greater liaison between geriatric medicine services and psychiatry of old age services, and the value of a truly holistic approach. Physiotherapy has a significant role to play in building bridges between the general, medical and psychiatric services.

It is hoped that a part of this would be the recognition by physiotherapists that, in caring for elderly mentally ill people, the evaluation of an intervention must take into account the client's subjective view of the improvement or otherwise of their quality of life, and not just conventional objective measurements. In other words, physiotherapists should endeavour to develop services that are patient-led and fully respect and respond to the views of clients and their carers.

References and further reading

Aaronsen, B.S. (1966) Personality stereotypes of ageing. *Journal of Gerontology*, **21**, 458–462

Alexander, F.M. and Maisel, E. (1975) *The Alexander Technique*, Thames and Hudson, London

Banerjee, S., Lindesay, J. and Murphy, E. (1993) Psychogeriatricians and general practitioners – a national survey. *Health Trends* (in press)

Benson, H. (1980) *The Relaxation Response*, Collins, Glasgow

Birren, J.E. and Sloane, R.B. (1980) *Handbook of Mental Health and Ageing*, Prentice-Hall, Englewood Cliffs, New Jersey

Blum, J.E. and Weiner, M.B. (1979) Neurosis in the older adult. *Psychopathlogy of Ageing* (ed. Kaplan, O.J.), Academic Press, New York

Bloomfield, H.H., Cain, M.P., Jaffe, D.T. and Kory, R.B. (1975) *T.M. – Discovering Inner Energy and Overcoming Stress*, Dell, New York

Braceland, F.J. (1972) Senescence: the inside story. *Psychiatric Annals*, **2** (Pt 1), 48–62

Britton, J.H. and Britton, J.O. (1972) *Personality Changes in Ageing*, Springer, New York

Busse, E.W. (1965) Research on ageing: some methods and findings. In *Psychiatry: Grief, Loss, and Emotional Disorders in the Ageing Process* (eds Berezin, M.A. and Cath, S.H.), Ontario University Press, New York

Butler, R.N. and Lewis, M.I. (1982) *Ageing and Mental Health*, 2nd edn, C.J. Mosby, St. Louis

Camp, J. (1973) Think deep, think happy, think healthy. *World Medicine*, 5 Sept.

Chastain, P.B. and Shapiro, G.E. (1987) Physical fitness programme for patients with psychiatric disorders. *Physical Therapy*, **67** (4), 545–548

Cluff, R.A. (1984) Chronic hyperventilation and its treatment by physiotherapy: discussion paper. *Journal of the Royal Society of Medicine*, **77**, 855–862

Fenwick, P. (1973) Meeting life with a mantra. *The Times*, 17 Feb.

Fenwick, P. (1983) Can we still recommend meditation? *British Medical Journal*, **287**, 1401

Gelb, M. (1987) *Body Learning: An Introduction to the Alexander Technique*, Aurum Press, London

Greist, J.H., Klein, M.H., Eischens, R.R. *et al.* (1979) Running as treatment for depression. *Comprehensive Psychiatry*, **20**, 41–54

Gurland, B.J. and Cross, P.S. (1983) Suicide among the elderly. In *The Acting-out Elderly* (eds Aronsen, M.K., Bennett, R. and Gurland, B.J.), Haworth Press, New York

Gurland, B.J. and Toner, J.A. (1982) Depression in the elderly: a review of recently published studies. In *Annual Review of Geriatrics and Gerontology* (ed. Eisadorfe, C), Springer, New York

Hare, M. (1986) *Physiotherapy in Psychiatry*, Heinemann, London

Jacobsen, E. (1938) *Progressive Relaxation*, University of Chicago Press, Chicago

Janoski, M.L., Holmes, D.S., Solomon, S. and Aquar, C. (1981) Exercise, changes in aerobic fitness and changes in self-perception: an experimental investigation. *Journal of Research in Personality*, **15**, 460–466

Keller, S.M. (1980) Physical fitness hastens recovery from psychological stress. *Med. & Sci. Sports and Exercise*, **12**, 118–119

Kermis, M.D. (1986) *Mental Health in Late Life. The Adaptive Process*, Jones and Bartlett, Boston

Kleinman, A. (1988) *The Illness Narratives. Suffering, Healing and the Human Condition*, Basic Books, USA

Ledwidge, B. (1980) Run for your mind: aerobic exercise as a means of alleviating anxiety and depression. *Canadian Journal of Behavioural Science*, **12**, 127–140

Lidell, L., Thomas, S., Beresford-Cooke, C. and Porter, A. (1984) *The Book of Massage*, Gala Books, London

Lumm, L.C. (1977) Breathing exercises in the treatment of hyperventilation and chronic anxiety states. *Chest, Heart and Stroke Journal*, **2**, 9

McTavish, D.G. (1971) Perceptions of old people. A review of research methodologies and findings. *Gerontologist*, **11**(4), Pt II, 90–102

Mitchell, L. (1977) *Simple Relaxation*, Murray, London

Murphy, E. and Banerjee, S. (1993) *Reviews in Clinical Gerontology*, **3**, 367–378

Paterson, W.P. (1979) *Medication Made Easy*, Franklin Watts, New York

Pfeiffer, E. and Busse, E.W. (1973) Affective disorders. In *Mental Illness in Later Life*, American Psychiatric Association, Washington, DC

Pitt, B. (1982) *Psychogeriatrics. An Introduction to the Psychiatry of Old Age*, Churchill Livingstone, London

Post, F. (1980) Paranoid, schizophrenia-like and schizophrenic states in the aged. In *Handbook of Mental Health and Ageing* (eds Birren, J.E. and Sloane, R.B.), Prentice-Hall, Englewood Cliffs, New Jersey

Rahe, R.H. (1972) Subjects' recent life changes and their near-future illness reports. *Annals of Clinical Research*, **4**, 250–265

Raskin, A. and Jarvik, L.F. (1979) *Psychiatric Symptoms and Cognitive Loss in the Elderly*, Hemisphere, Washington, DC

Reichard, S., Livson, F. and Peterson, P.G. (1962) *Ageing and Personality. A Study of 87 Older Men*, Wiley, New York

Ricketts, E. and Cross, E. (1985) The Whitchurch method of stress management by relaxation exercises. *Physiotherapy*, June, 262–264

Schaie, K.W. and Parham, I.A. (1976) Stability of adult personality traits. Fact or fable? *Journal of Personality and Social Psychology*, **34**, 146–154

Schuckit, M.A. (1977) Geriatric alcoholism and drug abuse. *Gerontologist*, **17**, 168–174

Schulman, K. and Arie, T. (1991) U.K. survey of psychiatric services for the elderly: direction for developing services. *Canadian Journal of Psychiatry*, **36**, 169–175

Schultz, J. and Luthe, W. (1969) *Autogenic Therapy, Autogenic Methods*, Grune and Stratton, New York

Seligman, M.E.P. (1975) *Helplesness: On depression, Development and Death*, W.H. Freeman, San Francisco

Silva, M. and Mehta, S. (1990) *Yoga the Iyengar Way*, Dorling Kindersley, London

Simon, A. (1980) The neuroses, personality disorders, alcoholism, drug use and misuse and crime in the aged. In *Handbook of Mental Health and Ageing* (eds Birren, J.E. and Sloane, R.B.), Prentice-Hall, Englewood Cliffs, New Jersey

Soo, Chee (1984) *Tai Chi Chuan: The Taoist Way to Mental and Physical Health*, The Aquarian Press, Wellingborough

Stenback, A. (1980) Depression and suicidal behaviour. In *Handbook of Mental Health and Ageing* (eds Birren, J.E. and Sloane, R.B.), Prentice-Hall, London

Whitehead, T. (1979) *Psychiatric Disorders of Old Age. A Handbook for the Clinical Team*, 2nd edn, H.M. & M. Publishers, Aylesbury, UK

Whittington, F.J. (1983) Misuse of legal drugs and compliance with prescription directions. In *Drugs and the Elderly Adult* (eds Glantz, M.D., Peterson, D.M. and Whittington, F.J.), Department of Health and Human Services, Washington, DC

Wood, W.G. (1978) The elderly alcoholis: some diagnostic problems and considerations. In *The Clinical Psychology of Ageing* (eds Storandt, M., Siegler, I.C. and Elias, M.F.), Plenum, New York

Zarit, S.H. (1980) *Ageing and Mental Disorders. Psychological Approaches to Assessment and Treatment*, Free Press, New York

Zimbardo, P.G., Anderson, S.M. and Kobat, L.G. (1981) Induced hearing deficit generates experimental paranoia. *Science*, **212**, 1529–1531

Coventry University

Index

ABC form, 370–1, 372 (fig.)
Acetylcholine, 21
Acupressure, 141, 322
Acupuncture, 253, 331–3
  auricular, 333
Acute (organic) confusion, 7 (table)
Adrenal cortical insufficiency, 130
Adrenal corticosteroids, 121–2
Adrenaline, 162–3
Adrenergic fibres, 113–14
Adrenocorticotrophin (ACTH), 116, 121
Aggression, 143–52, 368–9
  breakaway technique, 150
  coping strategies, 151–2
  dealing with, 148–51
  factors increasing likelihood of, 145–6
  legal aspects, 150–1
  theories, 144–6
    frustration hypothesis, 144–5
    instinct hypothesis, 144
    learned response, 145
  types, 144 (fig.)
  warning signs, 146–8
Agoraphobia, 226–32
Air pollution, 146
Alcoholic dementia (Korsakoff's
  syndrome), 21, 313–14, 314
Alcoholism, 214, 313, 314
  in elderly person, 405
  exercise for, 214
  genetics, 22
Aldosteronism, 130
Alexander technique, 69, 70, 179
Allodynia, 105
Alzheimer's disease, 21, 23, *see also*
  Dementia
Amitriptyline, 14
Amputation, 7
Amyotrophic lateral sclerosis, 130
Anaemia, 130
Anger, 368–9
  management, 368
Anorexia nervosa, 5 (table), 296–311

complications of low weight, 302–4
epidemiology, 297
medical symptoms, 305 (table)
nature of illness, 299–300
pattern of illness/movement through it,
  300–2
social/cultural context, 297–9
therapy, 304–11
  group work, 307–8
  physiotherapy techniques, 308–11
Antidepressants, 14–15, 211
Antinociceptive response, 103
Antipsychotics, 15, 355
Antisocial behaviour, 12
Anxiety, 5 (table), 11
  exercise for, 212–13
Anxiety spiral, 323, 324 (fig.)
Apricot kernel oil, 260–1
Aromatherapy, 253–63, 322–3
  carrier oil, 260
  essences, 257–8
  essential oils, 260–2
    hazards, 261–2
    uses in practice, 262
  hand massage, 258–9
  qualification, 256–7
  self-massage, 259
Aromatherapy for the Family, 257
Assertiveness training, 175–6
Association of Chartered Physiotherapists
  in Reflex Therapy, 266
Association for Dance Movement Therapy
  UK, 249
Asymmetrical tonic neck reflex, 227
Atlanto-axial joint, 139 (fig.), 140 (fig.)
Autogenic training, 201
Autonomic nervous system, 104
Avocado, 261

BASICID chart (modality profile), 172,
  173 (table)